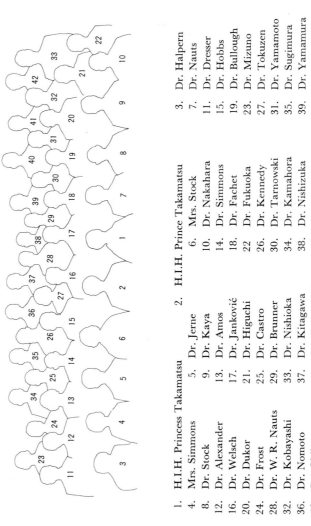

1. H.I.H. Princess Takamatsu
2. H.I.H. Prince Takamatsu
3. Dr. Halpern
4. Mrs. Simmons
5. Dr. Jerne
6. Mrs. Stock
7. Dr. Nauts
8. Dr. Stock
9. Dr. Kaya
10. Dr. Nakahara
11. Dr. Dresser
12. Dr. Alexander
13. Dr. Amos
14. Dr. Simmons
15. Dr. Hobbs
16. Dr. Welsch
17. Dr. Janković
18. Dr. Fachet
19. Dr. Bullough
20. Dr. Dukor
21. Dr. Higuchi
22 Dr. Fukuoka
23. Dr. Mizuno
24. Dr. Frost
25. Dr. Castro
26. Dr. Kennedy
27. Dr. Tokuzen
28. Dr. W. R. Nauts
29. Dr. Brunner
30. Dr. Tarnowski
31. Dr. Yamamoto
32. Dr. Kobayashi
33. Dr. Nishioka
34. Dr. Kamahora
35. Dr. Sugimura
36. Dr. Nomoto
37. Dr. Kitagawa
38. Dr. Nishizuka
39. Dr. Yamamura
40. Dr. Chihara
41. Dr. Tsukagoshi
42. Dr. Sugano

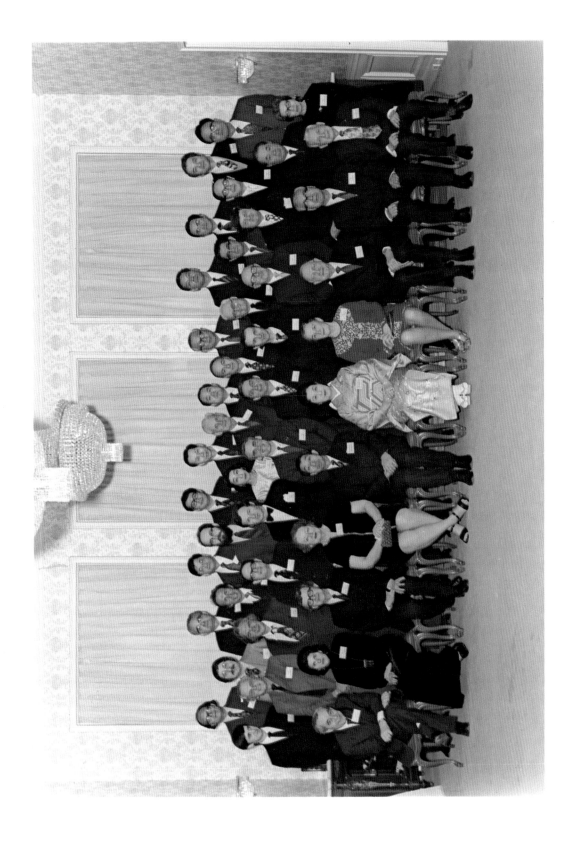

HOST DEFENSE AGAINST CANCER
AND ITS POTENTIATION

Proceedings of the 5th International Symposium of
The Princess Takamatsu Cancer Research Fund, Tokyo, 1975

HOST DEFENSE
AGAINST CANCER AND
ITS POTENTIATION

Edited by
DEN'ICHI MIZUNO, GORO CHIHARA, FUMIKO FUKUOKA,
TADASHI YAMAMOTO, and YUICHI YAMAMURA

UNIVERSITY PARK PRESS
Baltimore · London · Tokyo

UNIVERSITY PARK PRESS
Baltimore · London · Tokyo

Library of Congress Cataloging in Publication Data
Main entry under title:

Host defense against cancer and its potentiation.

   Includes bibliographies.
   1. Cancer—Immunological aspects—Congresses.
2. Immunotherapy—Congresses. I. Mizuno, Den'ichi.
II. Takamatsu no Miya Hi Gan Kenkyū kikin.
[DNLM: 1. Neoplasms—Immunology—Congresses.
QZ200 H831 1975]
RC271.I45H67   616.9′94′079   75-44226
ISBN 0-8391-0854-0

© UNIVERSITY OF TOKYO PRESS, 1975
UTP No. 3047-68343-5149
Printed in Japan.

Originally published by
UNIVERSITY OF TOKYO PRESS

Princess Takamatsu Cancer Research Fund

Organizing Committee of the 5th International Symposium

Den'ichi MIZUNO
   Faculty of Pharmaceutical Sciences, University of Tokyo, Tokyo, Japan
Goro CHIHARA
   National Cancer Center Research Institute, Tokyo, Japan
Fumiko FUKUOKA
   National Cancer Center Research Institute, Tokyo, Japan
Tadashi YAMAMOTO
   Institute of Medical Science, University of Tokyo, Tokyo, Japan
Yuichi YAMAMURA
   Osaka University Medical School, Osaka, Japan

Participants

ALEXANDER, P.
Chester Beatty Research Institute, Institute of Cancer Research, Royal Cancer Hospital, Clifton Avenue, Belmont, Sutton, Surrey, SM2 5PX, England

AMOS, B.
Division of Immunology, Department of Microbiology and Immunology, Duke University Medical Center, Durham, North Carolina 27710, U.S.A.

BRUNNER, K. T.
Institut Suisse de Recherches Expèrimentales sur le Cancer, Bugnon 21, 1011 Lausanne, Switzerland

BULLOUGH, W. S.
Mitosis Research Laboratory, Department of Zoology, Birkbeck College, University of London, Malet St., London, WC1E 7HX, England

CASTRO, J. E.
Department of Surgery, Royal Postgraduate Medical School, University of London, Hammersmith Hospital, DuCane Rd., London, W12 OHS, England

CHIHARA, G.
National Cancer Center Research Institute, Tsukiji 5-1-1, Chuo-ku, Tokyo 104, Japan

DRESSER, D. W.
MRC, National Institute for Medical Research, The Ridgeway, Mill Hill, London, NW7 1AA, England

DUKOR, P.
Research Laboratories of the Pharmaceuticals Division, Ciba-Geigy Ltd., CH-4002 Basel,

Switzerland

FACHET, J.
Institute of Genetics, Biological Research Center, Hungarian Academy of Sciences, Szeged, P.O.B. 521, Hungary

FROST, P.
Department of Immunology and Microbiology, Wayne State University School of Medicine, Scott Hall, 540 East Canfield Avenue, Detroit, Michigan 48201, U.S.A.

HALPERN, B.
Chaire de Médecine expérimentale, College de France, 11 Place Marcelin-Berthelot, 75 Paris 5ᵉ, France

HOBBS, J. R.
Department of Chemical Pathology, Westminster Medical School, University of London, 17 Page St., London, SW1P 2AR, England

JANKOVIĆ, B. D.
Immunology Research Center, Vojvode Stepe 458, P.O. Box 979, 11000 Belgrade, Yugoslavia

JERNE, N. K.
Basel Institute for Immunology, 487 Grenzacherstrasse, CH 4058 Basel, Switzerland

KENNEDY, J. C.
Cancer Research Division, Department of Pathology, Queen's University, Kingston, Ontario, K7L 3N6, Canada

KITAGAWA, M.
Institute for Cancer Research, Osaka University Medical School, Dojimahamadori 3, Osaka 553, Japan

KOBAYASHI, H.
Laboratory of Pathology, Cancer Institute, Hokkaido University School of Medicine, Nishi 7-chome, Kita 15-jo, Kita-ku, Sapporo 060, Japan

MIZUNO, D.
Faculty of Pharmaceutical Sciences, University of Tokyo, Hongo 7-3-1, Bunkyo-ku, Tokyo 113, Japan

NAKAHARA, W.
National Cancer Center, Tsukiji 5-1-1, Chuo-ku, Tokyo 104, Japan

NAUTS, H. C.
Cancer Research Institute Inc., 1225 Park Avenue, New York, New York 10028, U.S.A.

NISHIOKA, K.
National Cancer Center Research Institute, Tsukiji 5-1-1, Chuo-ku, Tokyo 104, Japan

NISHIZUKA, Y.
Laboratory of Experimental Pathology, Aichi Cancer Center Research Institute, Tashiro-cho, Chikusa-ku, Nagoya 464, Japan

NOMOTO, K.
Department of Microbiology, Kyushu University School of Medicine, Maidashi 3-1-1, Higashi-ku, Fukuoka 812, Japan

SIMMONS, R. L.
Department of Surgery, University of Minnesota Medical School, Mayo Memorial Building, Minneapolis, Minnesota 55455, U.S.A.

STOCK, C. C.
Walker Laboratory, Sloan-Kettering Institute for Cancer Research, 145 Boston Post Rd., Rye, New York 10580, U.S.A.

TARNOWSKI, G. S.
Walker Laboratory, Sloan-Kettering Institute for Cancer Research, 145 Boston Post Rd., Rye, New York 10580, U.S.A.

TOKUZEN, R.
National Cancer Center Research Institute, Tsukiji 5-1-1, Chuo-ku, Tokyo 104, Japan

TSUKAGOSHI, S.
Cancer Chemotherapy Center, Japanese Foundation for Cancer Research, Kami-Ikebukuro 1-37-1, Toshima-ku, Tokyo 170, Japan

WELSCH, C. W.
Department of Anatomy, Michigan State University, East Lansing, Michigan 48824, U.S.A.

YAMAMOTO, T.
Institute of Medical Science, University of Tokyo, Shirokanedai 4-6-1, Minato-ku, Tokyo 108, Japan

YAMAMURA, Y.
The Third Department of Internal Medicine, Osaka University Medical School, Dojima-hamadori 3, Osaka 553, Japan

Observers

SHICHIRO AKIYA, Showa University School of Pharmacy, Tokyo

TAKEHISA AKIYAMA, Kitasato University School of Medicine, Sagamihara

MINORU AMANO, National Cancer Center Research Institute, Tokyo

MICHIKO AOSHIMA, Cancer Chemotherapy Center, Japanese Foundation for Cancer Research, Tokyo

ICHIRO AZUMA, Osaka University Medical School, Osaka

TSUNEO BABA, Cancer Research Institute, Kyushu University, Fukuoka

KOJI EGAWA, Institute of Medical Science, University of Tokyo, Tokyo

GENSHICHIRO FUJII, Institute of Medical Science, University of Tokyo, Tokyo

HIROSHI FUJITA, Tsurumi University School of Dental Medicine, Yokohama

MICHIRO FUJIWARA, Institute of Medical Science, University of Tokyo, Tokyo

TOSHIYUKI HAMAOKA, Institute for Cancer Research, Osaka University Medical School, Osaka

JUNJI HAMURO, Ajinomoto Central Research Laboratories, Kawasaki

YOSHIYUKI HASHIMOTO, Tokyo Biochemical Research Institute, Tokyo

TOJU HATA, Kitasato University, Tokyo

TAKAO HATTORI, Research Institute for Nuclear Medicine and Biology, Hiroshima University, Hiroshima

SHINJI HAYASHI, National Cancer Center Research Institute, Tokyo

HIDEMATSU HIRAI, Hokkaido University School of Medicine, Sapporo

TAKESHI HIRAYAMA, National Cancer Center Research Institute, Tokyo

YUZURU HOMMA, Institute of Medical Science, University of Tokyo, Tokyo

HIROSHI HOSHINO, National Cancer Center Research Institute, Tokyo

MASUO HOSOKAWA, Cancer Institute, Hokkaido University School of Medicine, Sapporo

MOTOO HOZUMI, National Cancer Center Research Institute, Tokyo

TSUYOSHI IIDA, Central Institute of Sankyo Co., Tokyo

YOJI IKAWA, Cancer Institute, Japanese Foundation for Cancer Research, Tokyo

TETSURO IKEKAWA, National Cancer Center Research Institute, Tokyo

MOTOI ISHIDATE, National Institute of

x

NAGAHIRO SAIJO, National Cancer Center Hospital, Tokyo

KAZUHISA SAITO, Keio University School of Medicine, Tokyo

TERUYO SAKAKURA, Aichi Cancer Center Research Institute, Nagoya

YOSHIO SAKURAI, Cancer Chemotherapy Center, Japanese Foundation for Cancer Research, Tokyo

TAKUMA SASAKI, National Cancer Center Research Institute, Tokyo

HARUO SATO, Research Institute for Tuberculosis, Leprosy and Cancer, Tohoku University, Sendai

MORIMASA SEKIGUCHI, Institute of Medical Science, University of Tokyo, Tokyo

FUJIRO SENDO, Cancer Institute, Hokkaido University School of Medicine, Sapporo

SHOJI SHIBATA, Faculty of Pharmaceutical Sciences, University of Tokyo, Tokyo

TSUYOSHI SHIIO, Research Institute of Life Science, Ajinomoto Co., Yokohama

HARUO SUGANO, Cancer Institute, Japanese Foundation for Cancer Research, Tokyo

MASANOBU SUGIMOTO, National Institute of Health of Japan, Tokyo

TAKASHI SUGIMURA, National Cancer Center Research Institute, Tokyo

MASUKO SUZUKI, Tohoku College of Pharmacy, Sendai

SHIGEO SUZUKI, Tohoku College of Pharmacy, Sendai

TOMIO TADA, Chiba University School of Medicine, Chiba

TETSUO TAGUCHI, Research Institute for Microbial Diseases, Osaka University, Osaka

SHOZO TAKAYAMA, Cancer Institute, Japanese Foundation for Cancer Research, Tokyo

MIEKO TAKEUCHI, Nippon Roche Research Center, Kamakura

SHOSHICHI TAKEUCHI, Niigata University School of Medicine, Niigata

TOMIO TAKEUCHI, Institute of Microbial Chemistry, Tokyo

KENJI TAKEYA, Kyushu University School of Medicine, Fukuoka

TOMIKO TANAKA, National Cancer Center Research Institute, Tokyo

TAKAE TANINO, Institute of Medical Science, University of Tokyo, Tokyo

HIROSHI TERAYAMA, Faculty of Science, University of Tokyo, Tokyo

TOHRU TOKUNAGA, National Institute of Health of Japan, Tokyo

EIRO TSUBURA, Tokushima University School of Medicine, Tokushima

MASAHARU TSUCHIYA, Keio University School of Medicine, Tokyo

KIMIYOSHI TSUJI, Tokai University School of Mecicine, Isehara

TORU TSUMITA, Institute of Medical Science, University of Tokyo, Tokyo

HAMAO UMEZAWA, Institute of Microbial Chemistry, Tokyo

ICHIRO URUSHIZAKI, Cancer Research Institute, Sapporo Medical College, Sapporo

TAKESHI WATANABE, Osaka University Medical School, Osaka

KAZUMASA YAMADA, Nagoya University School of Medicine, Nagoya

IKUO YAMASHINA, Faculty of Pharmaceutical Sciences, Kyoto University, Kyoto

UKI YAMASHITA, Institute for Cancer Research, Osaka University Medical School, Osaka

REIKO YANAI, National Cancer Center Research Institute, Tokyo

YOSHIHITO YAOI, National Cancer Center Research Institute, Tokyo

KENJIRO YOKORO, Research Institute for Nuclear Medicine and Biology, Hiroshima University, Hiroshima

TAKATO YOSHIDA, Hamamatsu University School of Medicine, Hamamatsu

CHIKAO YOSHIKUMI, Tokyo Research Laboratories of Kureha Chemical Industry, Tokyo

YASUMI YUGARI, Research Institute of Life Science, Ajinomoto Co., Kawasaki

Opening Address

H.I.H. Princess Kikuko Takamatsu

It is with great pleasure that I attend this opening meeting of the Fifth International Symposium of our Cancer Research Fund, to personally greet all the participants, and especially to extend my cordial welcome to the invited speakers from overseas.

We are well aware that in the treatment of cancer timely surgical and radiological interventions have proved their merits, and chemotherapy also is being approved to a certain extent as a useful adjunct. In recent years a fourth possible approach to the problem has come to be actively discussed, and this is the so-called immunotherapy.

I am told that there is sufficient evidence to show the existence in our bodies of some sort of resistance against cancer cells. To find out the nature of this cancer resistance and to see how this resistance mechanism can be mobilized so as to attain the destruction of cancer would be a real great challenge, and the present Symposium is intended as a preliminary attempt to meet this challenge. It was organized to afford an opportunity for reviewing and evaluating our present knowledge on the host defence against cancer and the possibility of its potentiation.

It is my earnest hope that the discussion among the world's top scientists in this special field who are gathered together in this Symposium may be fruitful in forming a first step along the long and difficult road to our final objective, which is an epoch for the welfare of the humanity in general.

With these few words, and expression of my appreciation to the Organizing Committee for its efforts, I wish to declare open the Fifth International Symposium of our Cancer Research Fund.

Prof. NIELS KAJ JERNE

Your Imperial Highness. It is a great honour to reply to the kind and gracious words you have spoken to open this Fifth Symposium of the Princess Takamatsu Cancer Research Fund. I am speaking on behalf of all participants, and in particular on behalf of those that have come from overseas, in thanking Your Highness for inviting us and for welcoming us to discuss with our distinguished Japanese colleagues the problems of host defense against cancer and its potentiation.

When considering host defense, our attention is naturally drawn to immunology because this science deals with the defense system in our body that is directed against invading foreign antigens. Accordingly, most contributions to our symposium will deal with many aspects of the immune response.

There are several examples of a successful mobilisation of the immune system against specific diseases. The earliest is vaccination against smallpox which was actually practised in what we called the Far East several centuries before knowledge of this effective procedure penetrated into Europe. Studies toward more general applications of immunization lead to the development of the science of immunology which is often said to have originated in the year 1890 when Shibasaburo Kitasato, together with Emil von Behring, discovered diphtheria antitoxin and thus the existence of antibody molecules.

Immunologists are now faced with the challenge of cancer: Can we devise methods for mobilizing the immune system against cancer cells, or for interfering with the immuno-suppressive mechanisms by which a developing cancer escapes this host defense? The present symposium, so effectively organized by Drs. Waro Nakahara, Den'ichi Mizuno, Goro Chihara, Fumiko Fukuoka, Yuichi Yamamura, and Tadashi Yamamoto, will approach these questions from various perspectives. In all modesty, we share the hope, expressed by Your Imperial Highness, that our discussions will add a fruitful step on the road to our common objective. We are happy to have this opportunity for visiting your beautiful country and for strengthening the friendships and cooperation with our Japanese colleagues.

Opening Remarks

Prof. DEN'ICHI MIZUNO

Our honorable guests from abroad and ladies and gentlemen :

It is with a profound sense of pleasure and privilege that I, on behalf of the Organizing Committee of this Symposium, extend a hearty welcome to you all, especially to a number of distinguished guests from abroad. At the outset, I want all of you to join with me in expressing our sincere gratitude to Her Imperial Highness Princess Takamatsu, under whose generous sponsorship we could arrange the holding of this international meeting.

It seems to be a prevalent idea nowadays that the chemotherapy of cancer has fallen into a state of deadlock. Among many difficulties met in the field of cancer chemotherapy, the most serious one is in finding out the high selective toxicity against cancers. About 10 years ago, Dr. Waro Nakahara of this country found that some polysaccharides of plant origin had a marked effect against transplanted tumor cells. Since then, many other agents of natural origin having similar effects such as lentinan, PSK, GE-2, some terpenoids and *etc.*, were discovered in this country. All these agents seemed to have the effect of stimulation, more or less, on the defense mechanism of the hosts against cancers. Thus, there seemed to appear a new avenue of approach to the utilization of such substances for the experimental as well as clinical cancer chemotherapy which was called "host mediated therapy." Since about 50 years ago, attempts have been made of using live cells of some bacteria or extracts of them for curing cancers. These agents might also have contained some substances having an effect similar to that mentioned above. The mode of action of all these agents may be called "potentiating" of the defense by host against cancers.

On the other hand, immunology of cancer has made a remarkable progress in recent years, and has begun to penetrate the domain of cancer therapy. Interest has been focussed on the cytotoxicity against cancer cells of lymphocytes, macrophage and humoral factors including the complements. The cytotoxicity can be obtained also with tumor cells modified in some way by the treatments which bring about the potentiation of defense by hosts. Studies on the inhibition of the immune mechanism are also of great importance, since the blocking of this inhibition can be converted to a complete immune stage.

Now the extensive studies on the mechanism of potentiation of the defense by host has revealed that the immunology of cancer is intimately related to this problem. The studies along this line have yielded a number of unexpected results which seem to be of great significance from the viewpoint of cancer chemotherapy as well as of pure immunology.

The extensive studies on the mechanism of potentiation of the defense by host has also revealed that the study of hormones in view of carcinogenesis and of carcinocidal effect is also intimately related to this problem. So far, we do not know whether or not the hormonal control is directly connected with the cytotoxic effect on cancer cells. However, hormones should play a role, directly or indirectly, in controlling the defense of host against cancer.

Problems relating to some clinical trials employing various potentiating agents will also be dealt with in this meeting. Although some of the research to be reported might still be in quite rudimentary stages, report and discussion on them will give undoubtedly encouraging effect on further development of studies along relevant lines, especially for workers in fundamental fields.

Needless to say, cancer cells must be killed selectively, and this selection is most elegantly done by the cells or humoral factors of host organisms, themselves. Discussion of the problems from this angle with the view to find out the most effective method of cancer therapy is the object of this Symposium having the title: "Host Defense against Cancer and Its Protentiation."

Thank you for your kind attention.

Contents

HOST DEFENSE AGAINST CANCER AND ITS POTENTIATION, D. MIZUNO ET AL. (EDS.),
UNIV. OF TOKYO PRESS, TOKYO / UNIV. PARK PRESS, BALTIMORE, PP. 1-11, 1975

Regulatory Aspects of the Immune System

Niels Kaj JERNE

Basel Institute for Immunology, Basel, Switzerland

Abstract: The proposition that the immune system plays a defensive role against cancer is an old one and the experimental attempts to demonstrate immune surveillance in cancer have been presented and debated in many recent conferences and symposia. There exist in fact many experiments which demonstrate that the immune system responds to the occurrence in the organism of cancer cells and that it may, in many cases, prevent such cells from establishing themselves and to develop. From that point of view the prevention of cancer may be postulated to be one of the main tasks of the immune system, and as certain experimental evidence shows that partial immunity against certain cancers can be induced by immunization, we might conclude that the actual occurrence of cancer rests on a failure of the immune system to respond adequately, or on a distortion of the immune response that occurs. The question then becomes to study the malfunction of the immune system in certain such situations, but it seems rather obvious, generally, that it is not possible to study the malfunction of a system before you know how it functions normally. This is the reason why basic immunology focusses its attention on the physiology of the normal immune system rather than on the pathology of the malfunctioning immune system. There are two essential problems in basic immunology, one of which is the question how the immune system arose in evolution or arises in ontogeny, the second being how it functions and how it is regulated. The two questions are not strictly separable because the system may partly arise in ontogeny whilst it functions, but in the context of the response of the immune system to antigens, including cancer antigens, the main knowledge we need is how the system is regulated. We can distinguish between two types of heterogeneity among antibody molecules and lymphocytes. Heterogeneity I concerns the occurrence of different classes of antibody molecules and of different stages of differentiation of lymphocytes. Heterogeneity II is a consequence of antibody diversity which is based on the occurrence of a large repertoire of variable regions displayed by antibody molecules and antibody-like cell receptors. These variable regions must be the target of any specific regulatory mechanisms in the immune system.

Two proposals towards describing specific regulation are considered. A minimal model makes use only of interactions of the combining sites of the variable regions with antigen that is external to the system, whereas a network model admits the importance in regulation also of the idiotypic properties of the variable regions, *i.e.*, of internal antigen-antibody interactions within the immune system.

In considering the question of the response of the immune system to cancer, the hope is naturally to discover a procedure of intervening in such a way that the immune system becomes more effective in controlling and eliminating cancer cells. Many laboratories study the immunological phenomena that can actually be observed in cancer patients, and in experimental animals exposed to cancer cells. A search is made for the expression by cancer cells of foreign antigenic determinants, or of factors which may inhibit lymphocytes from developing an immune defense. This type of research suffers from the essential difficulty that we lack, at present, sufficient basic knowledge of the regulatory mechanisms that govern the immune system. Instead of concentrating first on studying the immune system itself, a search is made for a lucky short cut towards a solution of the medical problem. The history of immunology shows a number of successful short cuts, such as prophylactic immunizations and the inhibition of the formation of anti-rhesus antibodies in rhesus-negative women by the injection of inhibitory antibody. On the other hand, it seems reasonable to expect that, in the long run, only a better understanding of the basic properties of the immune system will enable us to manipulate the system in the directions we desire. Basic immunological research therefore remains a task to which many laboratories should direct their efforts, even if their long-term aim is to find immunological solutions to cancer problems.

I intend to outline some recent concepts concerning the properties of the normal immune system and its regulation. I shall define the immune system as consisting of antibody molecules and of cells that synthesize antibody molecules, and I shall start out by describing some of the properties of these elements. Then, in turning to a discussion of specific regulatory mechanisms, I shall assume that clonal selection is essentially correct, or in other words that there is now overwhelming evidence for at least one basic law of immunology, namely that one lymphocyte and its descendant cells produce antibodies of only one specificity. I shall try to demonstrate that the target of any specific regulatory mechanism must be the variable region of the antibody molecule. Two models simulating the regulation of the immune system will be discussed. One makes use only of interactions of the antibody combining site with antigens that are "external" to the immune system. The other admits the regulatory importance of idiotopes, *i.e.*, of "internal" antigenic determinants situated on the variable regions of antibody molecules, implying that the immune system functions as a network (*1, 2*).

Antibody Molecules: Heterogeneities I and II

The existence of antibody molecules was discovered in 1890 by Shibasaburo

Kitasato and Emil von Behring. The general shape and primary structure of these protein molecules have been clarified during the past 15 years. Two identical light polypeptide chains and two identical heavy polypeptide chains (consisting of linear sequences of about 200 and 400 amino acid residues) make up the basic structure of an antibody molecule.

Antibody specificity, *i.e.*, its ability to combine with certain antigens, is a property of two identical combining sites that occur in the two "variable regions" of the molecule. The structure of these regions is determined by the variable sequences of about 100 amino acids at the amino-terminal ends of the polypeptide chains. The remainder of the molecule, its "constant regions," displays properties (such as complement fixation) that antibodies of different specificity have in common.

On this basis, we can distinguish between two types of heterogeneity among antibody molecules. Heterogeneity I results from the occurrence of about 20 different regions. Accordingly, antibody molecules fall into about 20 classes with differing general properties. Heterogeneity II, called antibody diversity, results from the enormous variety of variable regions. The number of different variable regions that occur at a given moment on the antibodies of one individual animal is the antibody repertoire of that animal. Well-founded estimates of repertoire size are not available, but we may assume that it exceeds one million in adult animals of many species.

Lymphocytes: Heterogeneities I and II

Cells producing antibody molecules were identified as plasma cells in the 1940s. It was soon shown that plasma cells are capable of synthesizing and secreting a few thousand antibody molecules per second, and it has since become established that all antibody molecules released by a single cell have the same specificity, *i.e.*, have identical variable regions. Plasma cells were shown to be differentiated descendants of small lymphocytes in the early 1960s. It is now clear that small lymphocytes are precursor cells that can be stimulated to divide into clones of cells that include plasma cells. On the basis of these advances in our knowledge we can now simplify the description of the immune system by boldly stating that it consists, in an adult person, of about 10^{12} lymphocytes and about 10^{20} antibody molecules. It is true, of course, that the system is scattered throughout our body, in bone-marrow, thymus, spleen, lymph-nodes, lymphatics, blood, *etc.* The simplified description seems justified, however, by the experiment of Mishell and Dutton (*3*), who showed that lymphocytes from a normal animal when suspended in tissue culture medium would respond to added antigen with the synthesis of specific antibody. This experiment demonstrated that the finer architecture of lymphatic organs was not a prerequisite for antibody formation, and that the presence of other organs, such as the nervous system, was not needed. One of the main tasks of basic immunology is now to unravel the mechanisms by which this system of 10^{12} lymphocytes, 10^{20} antibody molecules (and other lymphocyte products) is kept intact and functional. We must here distinguish between general and specific regulatory mechanisms. General mechanisms regulate the size of the system. In man, about 2% of all antibody molecules, and probably a similar percentage of lymphocytes, decay every day, and must be replaced by lymphocyte proliferation and antibody synthesis. The immune system thus must produce about 2×10^{18} antibody molecules per day, equivalent to the continuous output of 10^{10} plasma cells. We can interfere with this general homeostatic situation, for example by applying cytostatic drugs, anti-lymphocyte serum, or cortisone. More important is the understanding of the specific regulatory mechanisms. What are the signals that govern a specific immune response or specific paralysis of responsiveness? What mechanisms restrict immune responses, keep the total system functional, and maintain its diversity of responsiveness?

To approach such questions we must study the properties of lymphocytes. The lymphocyte population, like the antibody molecules, presents two types of heterogeneity. Heterogeneity I concerns the distinction of lymphocyte classes and differentiation stages. First, a fundamental distinction is made between bone marrow-derived (B) lymphocytes and thymus-dependent (T) lymphocytes. Morphologically, both these types of cells are small lymphocytes; and the immune system contains about an equal number of each. Only B lymphocytes can develop into antibody secreting plasma cells. The outer membrane of most B lymphocytes presents several thousand antibody-like molecules which can be easily demonstrated. It has been shown that these antibody-like "receptor" molecules are produced by the B cell that carries them, and that all receptor molecules on one B cell have the same specificity, i.e., the same "variable region." Antigen molecules can attach to a B cell if they fit to the combining sites displayed by the variable regions of its receptors. It would seem that a given B cell is committed to the expression of antibody molecules with a given "variable region," and that this commitment is retained by the cells of the clone arising from a proliferating B cell. Thus, the specificity of the antibody molecules produced by a plasma cell is the same as the specificity displayed by the receptor molecules of the B cell from which this plasma cell arose.

T lymphocytes likewise appear to be monospecific, and they can bind antigen, though the demonstration of membrane receptor molecules on T cells has proven so difficult that their antibody-like nature remains controversial. Like B lymphocytes, T lymphocytes can proliferate after an antigenic stimulus. They do not develop into plasma cells, but yield cell types showing a variety of properties, such as the abilities to kill target cells, to suppress B cells, or to cooperate with B cells. Most antigens cannot induce B cells to develop into plasma cells without the presence of cooperating T cells. In spite of these complications we would not anticipate a very extensive heterogeneity I among lymphocytes. If there are, say, ten differentiation stages in both the B-cell and the T-cell series, we might have to distinguish between 20 classes of lymphocytes with different properties.

The Target of Specific Regulation

Heterogeneity II of lymphocytes, as for antibody molecules, reflects the enormous diversity of specificities which these cells represent. Two B lymphocytes of different specificity, i.e., displaying antibody-like receptor molecules that have different variable regions, must express different genes encoding the primary structures of these variable regions. If we consider two such lymphocytes, and imagine that both are in the same stage of differentiation, displaying the same number of receptors of the same antibody class, then we must conclude that any specific regulatory mechanism that discriminates between these two cells must act *via* the variable regions of the receptors.

Having thus identified the variable regions of the antibody-like receptor molecules of lymphocytes as the targets of specific regulation of the immune system, we must focus on the properties of these variable regions. It is clear that a variable region contains the structure known as combining site, to which a fitting antigen can attach. Since the early 1960s another property of these variable regions has become the subject of study, namely the presence on these regions of antigenic determinants ("idiotopes") capable of inducing the formation of specific anti-idiotypic antibodies.

External Regulation by Epitopes

In the present stage of our knowledge, we cannot hope to describe the regulation of the immune system in all its complexities. We can only attempt to retain the dominating features in a simplified model. Before considering the possibility that the idiotypic properties of the variable regions are involved in the specific regulation of the immune system, I shall briefly outline a regulatory model, proposed by Bell (*4*), which does not make use of these properties. This minimal model starts out with a situation in which the immune system is confronted with a certain concentration of an antigen. The system is assumed to contain a very small fraction of lymphocytes that can potentially respond to this antigen. This group of cells consists of subpopulations that differ with respect to the association constant of the cell receptors toward the antigen. Interaction of antigen with cell receptors and with free antibody molecules leads to a chemical equilibrium determining the average number of antigen-bound receptors on a given target cell. A target cell can respond in three ways: a) by paralysis if the fraction of antigen-bound receptors is large, b) by division into two proliferating cells if the fraction of antigen-bound receptors is smaller, or c) by division either into two plasma cells (considered to be end-cells) or into a plasma cell and a memory cell (considered to be a new target cell), if the fraction of antigen-bound receptors is below a certain minimum. Proliferating cells and plasma cells secrete antibody molecules which compete for antigen and speed up its elimination, thus bringing the response to a halt. This model is embodied in a set of differential equations which can be handled by a computer after introducing certain reasonable parameters for cell numbers, receptor numbers, cell proliferation times, and decay rates. The model simulates experimental antibody responses quite well, and it accounts for high-zone tolerance (by cell paralysis) and for low-zone tolerance (by forcing target cells to yield small clones of plasma cells leading to target cell elimination). The target cells to a given antigen, and their offspring, are assumed to respond independently from the remainder of the immune system of which they are only a minor part.

The model thus disregards the occurrence of suppressor cells and suppressing antibody molecules which have been demonstrated to exist and are needed to account for such phenomena as allotype and idiotype suppression, and for the transfer of suppressive and tolerant states to normal animals by the transfer of cells.

Internal Regulation by Idiotopes

I have therefore proposed to include the idiotypic properties of the variable regions into a future model for the specific regulation of the immune system (*1, 2, 5*). It was clear from the early work on idiotypes (*6, 7*) that the number of different idiotypic determinants (idiotopes) which a single animal is capable of synthesizing is enormously large. In fact, there is reason to believe that this number is of the same magnitude as the number of different combining sites. After all, the repertoire of combining sites and the repertoire of idiotopes both reflect the repertoire of variable regions.

Assuming both repertoires to be of the order of 10^7 in the immune system of a given animal, and recalling that a given antigenic determinant can combine (with different association constants) with a large variety of different combining sites, it seems reasonable to conclude that every combining site in the immune system can recognize a number of different idiotopes present in the same system, and *vice versa*. It is difficult to analyse or predict the properties of the resulting network of cellular and molecular interactions, though some partial models have already been proposed (*8, 9*). At present, I shall limit myself to mentioning a few findings that have now been experimentally demonstrated.

1)   A mouse of an inbred strain can produce anti-idiotypic antibodies to antibodies produced by another mouse of that same strain. Of particular interest to our present discussions are the experiments of Eisen *et al.* (*10*), who showed that normal BALB/c mice can produce anti-idiotypic antibodies upon immunization with BALB/c myeloma protein, and that this immunization leads to a degree of protection against the acceptance of transferred myeloma cells producing this protein.

2)   A rabbit can produce anti-idiotypic antibodies to stored antibodies produced by this same rabbit a year earlier (*11*).

3)   Mice and rats producing antibodies to pneumococcal antigens (*12, 13*) or to histocompatibility antigens (*14*) have been shown simultaneously to produce anti-idiotypic antibodies to their own antibodies.

4)   The injection of anti-idiotypic antibodies into normal recipients has repeatedly been shown to suppress the formation of antibodies of the corresponding idiotype (*15–17*). In one case, using anti-idiotypic antibodies of a given heavy chain class, enhancement was observed instead of suppression (*17*). Chronic anti-idiotypic suppression initiated in this way appears to be sustained specifically by T cells, and can be transferred to normal recipient animals with the transfer of such cells (*20*).

5)   Anti-idiotypic antibodies at low concentrations have been shown capable of inducing, in lymphocyte cultures, the formation of antibodies displaying the corresponding idiotype (*18*).

As I have said earlier, the target for specific regulation of the immune system must be the variable region of the receptor molecules of lymphocytes. By taking the idiotypic properties of this region into account, we can now conclude that the target region can be acted upon not only by antigen that is external to the immune system, but also by idiotypic interactions within the system itself. The combining sites of the variable regions of the receptors can also recognize idiotopes on receptors of other cells and on free antibody molecules. These idiotopes would, on the average, resemble the external antigen. Conversely, the idiotopes displayed by the variable regions of the antigen recognizing cell can be recognized by combining sites of receptors of other cells and of free antibody molecules. The latter are anti-idiotypic antibodies, and since many of these have been shown experimentally to compete with antigen for attachment to the idiotypic sites ("ligand inhibition") it seems possible that idiotopes overlap structurally with combining sites. In that case the combining sites of the anti-idiotypic antibodies would also, on the average, bear resemblance to the external antigen, and there would be no clear distinction between the idiotopes recognized by a given variable region, and the anti-idiotypic antibodies recognizing this same variable region. It remains a formidable task to build a realistic though simplified model on these insights. Even if we assume that the idiotype-anti-idiotype network constitutes the major regulatory system, we must know which interactions are suppressive or stimulatory, and demonstrate how the stability and diversity of the system would be maintained. Moreover, the role of T cells needs clarification, also with respect to idiotypic interactions. There are some recent indications that anti-idiotypic antibodies can recognize (19) and recruit (20) T cells. A description of the role of the immune system when faced with a developing cancer still seems beyond our predictive possibilities, at present. In the minimal model of Bell, a developing cancer would present the requirement for obtaining low-zone tolerance. Any network model would likewise have to specify the mechanism by which a developing cancer produces a tolerant or suppressed state of the immune system. The value of a model in this context would mainly lie in its predictive capacity, parti- cularly in its specification of the type of interventions that could abrogate the tolerant or suppressive state. Immunology can be approached in many ways, and I hope to have outlined one of the approaches that may contribute to our concerted efforts towards understanding the immune system and towards marshalling its defensive potentialities against cancer.

REFERENCES

1. Jerne, N. K. The immune system. Sci. Am., *229*: 52–60, 1973.
2. Jerne, N. K. Towards a network theory of the immune system. Ann. Immunol. (Inst. Pasteur), *125 C*: 373–389, 1974.
3. Mishell, R. I. and Dutton, R. W. Immunization of dissociated spleen cell cultures from normal mice. J. Exp. Med., *126*: 423–442, 1967.
4. Bell, G. I. Mathematical model of clonal selection and antibody production. J. Theor. Biol., *29*: 191–232, 1970; *33*: 339–378, 1971.
5. Jerne, N. K. Clonal selection in a lymphocyte network. *In;* G. M. Edelman (ed.),

Cellular Selection and Regulation in the Immune Response, pp. 39–48, Raven Press, New York, 1974.

6. Oudin, J. and Michel, M. Sur les spécificités idiotypiques des anticorps de lapin anti-S. typhi. C. R. Acad. Sci. (Paris) (Sér. D), *268*: 230–233, 1969.

7. Kelus, A. S. and Gell, P. G. H. Immunological analysis of rabbit anti-antibody systems. J. Exp. Med., *127*: 215–234, 1968.

8. Richter, P. H. A network theory of the immune system. Eur. J. Immunol., *5*: 350–354, 1975.

9. Hoffmann, G. W. Regulation and self non-self discrimination in an immune network. Personal communication.

10. Lynch, R. G., Graff, R. J., Sirisinha, S., Simms, E. S., and Eisen, H. N. Myeloma proteins as tumor-specific transplantation antigens. Proc. Natl. Acad. Sci. U.S., *69*: 1540–1544, 1972.

11. Scott Rodkey, L. Studies of idiotypic antibodies. J. Exp. Med., *139*: 712–720, 1974.

12. Kluskens, L. and Köhler, H. Regulation of immune response by autogenous anti-receptor antibody. Proc. Natl. Acad. Sci. U.S., in press.

13. Cosenza, H. Personal communication.

14. Fitch, F. W. Personal communication.

15. Cosenza, H. and Köhler, H. Specific suppression of the antibody response by antibodies to receptors. Proc. Natl. Acad. Sci. U.S., *69*: 2701–2705, 1972.

16. Hart, D. A., Pawlak, L. L., and Nisonoff, A. Nature of anti-hapten antibodies arising after immune suppression of a set of cross-reactive idiotypic specificities. Eur. J. Immunol., *3*: 44–48, 1973.

17. Eichmann, K. Idiotype suppression. Eur. J. Immunol., *4*: 296–302, 1974.

18. Trenkner, E. and Riblet, R. Induction of anti-phosphorylcholine antibody formation by anti-idiotypic antibodies. Personal communication.

19. Coutinho, A. Personal communication.

20. Rajewsky, K. and Eichmann, K. Personal communication.

Discussion of Paper of Dr. Jerne

Dr. Hobbs: Perhaps an additional mode of regulation of the immune system, complementing those which you have here proposed, might involve variability in antibody of type I in your scheme, so that one particular individual produces IgE against a pollen, while another forms mainly IgG. Are the idiotopes on these IgE molecules the same as those of class IgG? Also, why do some individuals produce augmented levels of IgE to certain antigens while others do not?

Dr. Jerne: IgE and IgG share identical idiotopes in one individual, as these antibodies possess the same set of heavy and light chain variable regions. However, an anti-idiotypic antibody of one class may not act in the same manner as an anti-idiotypic antibody of a different class. Dr. Eichmann in Cologne has discovered that if guinea pig IgG_1 and IgG_2 anti-idiotypic antibodies to mouse antibody are isolated, IgG_2 will suppress the immune response of that idiotype in a normal mouse, whereas IgG_1, even when employing only 10^{12} molecules, will instead enhance it. This enhancing antibody appears to act on T lymphocytes, presenting an enigma as it was produced by immunization with immunoglobulin, *i.e.*, a B cell product. I believe the problem of immunoregulation is enormously complex, rendering a complete answer to your questions as yet impossible.

Dr. Kennedy: I wonder about possible pragmatic applications of your regulatory scheme. I realize that if one desires to promote an immune response to a certain antigen, in theory this could be easily accomplished, for one need be concerned with but a single idiotope. However, if one wants rather to suppress the response to a single antigen, wouldn't there exist myriad types of idiotope to that antigen, making such selective abrogation very difficult?

Dr. Jerne: Surely. It has been shown that in response to a given antigen, an animal will produce a great array of antibody molecules differing in many respects, including idiotopes, so that abolishment of this array by idiotype suppression does not seem feasible. However, before we engage in extensive speculation on the possibilities of interfering in the network model I have presented, one must first gain an understanding of how it normally functions, how it retains its diversity and develops a memory, and how certain distortions of this network remain fairly constant.

DR. JANKOVIĆ: I was quite impressed by the repertoires of combining sites (10^7) and idiotipy variations (10^7). By simple pairing between those two repertoires one can obtain such a number of possible expressions that even an astronomer may be astound. I wonder where is the place of the clonal selection theory in the system of your predictions.

DR. JERNE: The diversity in this scheme evolves from the combination of two variable regions so that the number of divergent variable regions need approximate only the square root of your figure, that is, 10^3–10^4, which is not an obstacle.

DR. ALEXANDER: Do you anticipate finding anti-idiotypic antibodies to idiotypes on previously formed anti-idiotypic antibodies?

DR. JERNE: Definitely, and that is the crux of the network model. Two papers attempting to explain the mechanism of high-and low-zone tolerance will soon appear in the Eur. J. Immunol. by Hoffmann and by Richter. The latter employs a new terminology in a network model created to simplify the expression of the concept of antibodies to antibodies, *etc*. Ab1 is used to designate the antibody to the original antigen, Ab2 is the anti-idiotypic antibody of Ab1, Ab3 is the anti-idiotypic antibody to Ab2, and so on.

DR. FROST: How can you account for the phenomenon of immunologic memory in this system? There is usually a dramatic antibody response upon re-introduction of antigen, and one might expect a smaller response in the presence of anti-idiotypic antibodies?

DR. JERNE: The Richter model, which I noted, is soon to appear in the Eur. J. Immunol., attempts to answer your question. He hypothesizes that if one administers a high dose of an antigen to an individual, production of Ab1 is stimulated, which, in turn, will stimulate Ab2, which then leads to formation of Ab3, *etc*. But Ab3 can suppress the production of Ab2. Introduction of too small a dose of antigen results in suppression of Ab1 by Ab2, while a larger initial load results in abrogation of Ab2.

DR. FROST: Aren't anti-idiotype antibodies produced in response to a small amount of antigen as compared with the original antigenic dose? How can an individual continue forming antibodies 3, 4, 5, *etc*., when the amount of antigen evoking each future response is continuously diminishing?

DR. JERNE: If an individual forms, for example, 100 different immunoglobulin molecules all termed Ab1, each of these may stimulate 100 other classes of Ab2, already accounting for 10^4 different molecules. Thus, the successive responses in this direction will soon encompass the entire system.

DR. T. TADA (Chiba University School of Medicine, Chiba):   Dr. Herzenberg has observed that allotype suppression is maintained by T cells. Do you think that idiotype suppression is continued by a similar mechanism?

DR. JERNE: Yes. Herzenberg has shown that allotype suppression is initiated by anti-idiotypic antibody and maintained for long periods by T lymphocytes. Eichmann's group in Cologne recently demonstrated that idiotype suppression is comparable in that it is evoked by anti-idiotypic antibody and prolonged by specific anti-idiotype T cells.

DR. DRESSER: In this network model, you suggest that anti-antibodies continue along an extended chain. Is it not implicit in that scheme that Ab3 could be identical to Ab1, forming a circular system?

DR. JERNE: Yes, and this raises the question of the exact site of the idiotypic determinant. Previously, it was presumed that the idiotope fits somewhere in the variable region, with the combining site situated elsewhere in this area. However, it now seems that these two areas may overlap, so that the idiotope, in being part of the antibody combining site, can compete with it. In various experiments, anti-idiotypic antibody, Ab2, competes with the antigen for the original antibody, Ab1. In this sense, on the average, Ab2 would become an image of the antigen, Ab3 the image of Ab1, *etc.*

DR. DRESSER: Isn't that reminiscent of a very old model, proposed by Abderhalden, which suggested that antibody was in some manner a reflection of antigen?

DR. JERNE: I'm not sure. I must return to that reference.

DR. HOBBS: M. G. Lewis and K. B. Cooke have suggested that one of the inhibitory factors often demonstrated in the sera of patients with malignant melanoma may be an anti-idiotypic antibody directed against an original anti-melanoma immunoglobulin. I was wondering if anyone here has made similar observations that a blocking factor can, at least occasionally, be an anti-idiotypic antibody, for it is important to substantiate this one claim.

DR. JERNE: There appear to be no responses.

HOST DEFENSE AGAINST CANCER AND ITS POTENTIATION, D. MIZUNO ET AL. (EDS.),
UNIV. OF TOKYO PRESS, TOKYO / UNIV. PARK PRESS, BALTIMORE, PP. 13–29, 1975

Selective Immunopotentiation

J. M. Phillips and D. W. Dresser

National Institute for Medical Research, London, U.K.

Abstract: In immunological manipulations selectivity, as distinct from specificity, is an important consideration. Specificity involves an interaction between antigen and antibody, whereas selectivity concerns an ability to affect cellular compartments concerned in the formation of the cells which produce specific antibody. Selectivity may involve a potentiating effect which is activated by a molecular recognition which is distinct from the primary antigen-antibody interaction of a particular (experimental) situation. For example, antilymphocyte serum can selectively suppress a thymus-dependent cell (T cell) response by virtue of an affinity for T cells in general, which is independent of the specific responsiveness of any individual T cell.

We have shown that lipopolysaccharide and *Lentinus edodes* are adjuvants which are selective for bone marrow-derived cells (B cells) and T cells respectively. Since it is known that T cells may be helpers or suppressors of humoral immunity or that an individual T cell may be solely concerned with cell-mediated immunity, it follows that potentiation of the "wrong kind" of T cell could be disastrous in a clinical context. It will therefore be important in the future, both to gain information about the precise nature of such sub-categories of T, B, or macrophage cells (M cells) but also to learn how to manipulate each independently of the other.

It is clear that adjuvants can potentiate immune responses in one or more of several ways, such as depot effects, increased cell interaction or post-induction mitotic stimulation. However, we believe that an important function of an "adjuvant" is to block an innate tendency for an antigen sensitive cell to react to contact with antigen by becoming immunologically tolerant. In this case, the kind of tolerance being referred to is of the long-lasting kind induced by low concentrations of non-immunogenic antigen, and distinct from the forms of short-lived (reversible?) tolerance sometimes included under the headings of receptor blockade and high dose paralysis. We have interpreted our conclusions about adjuvant action in terms of the model for cellular growth and differentiation developed by D. B. Thomas and his colleagues.

The immune response can be manipulated in both a positive and a negative sense, independently of its specificity for antigen. In purely empirical terms therefore, it is possible to look on immunopotentiation and immunosuppression as complementary, although opposite, effects. The complexity of the immune response means that its successful manipulation depends on a sufficient knowledge of its component parts together with a means to potentiate or suppress these components independently.

Evolution, as a result of selective pressures for economy, flexibility, and control has produced an immune response mechanism not only with a great discriminatory capacity (specificity) but also a mechanism of great inherent complexity. As a consequence, despite more than a century of effort, the immune response is not properly understood and efforts to manipulate parts of the mechanism by nonspecific (antigen unrelated) agents often result in effects quite opposite to those expected. In recent years, however, information has accrued, sufficient to form a framework for the design of experiments with putative selective immunopotentiating or suppressing agents.

Whilst not producing humoral antibodies themselves, lymphocytes of thymic origin (T) were shown some years ago to help lymphocytes of bone marrow or bursal origin (B) to produce antibody (1–5). Although many antigens have been shown to be T-dependent and to elicit significant IgG as well as IgM responses, there are some antigens, mostly polysaccharides, such as pneumococcus (SIII), which are T-independent and induce a response which is mostly IgM: it seems that they are capable of stimulating B lymphocytes directly (6). Certain antigens, xenogeneic erythrocytes may be an example, probably require to be processed by macrophages (M cells) if they are to become fully effective (7, 8). The helper effect of T cells depends on an element of specificity for the antigenic molecule (9), whereas the auxiliary role of the M cell most probably depends on the physical nature of the antigen and not its specificity in an immunological sense.

Although T lymphocytes can be physically separated on the basis of such parameters as the amount of θ antigen expressed on the cell membrane (10), it is not at all clear if the different physiological functions which have been ascribed to T lymphocytes can all be assigned to the same cell. It is certainly possible that cell-mediated immunity, help, and suppression are generated by distinct and separately differentiated lines of cells. Furthermore, it is possible that one kind of T lymphocyte can help the development of immunity in another line of T lymphocyte. Control of the specificity of the humoral (11) response can be exercised at the level of general cellular homeostatic mechanisms such as those which operate in liver regeneration (12) or at an immunological level. The effective concentration of antigen binding to an antigen sensitive cell (ASC) can be altered by antibody (13) and by the activity of M cells (8). It is not impossible that suppression and stimulation of a humoral response by antibody may be due to a direct differentiational stimulus on the lymphocytes themselves and not to competition for antigen between membrane receptor and free antibody (14). Suppressor T lymphocytes have been pro-

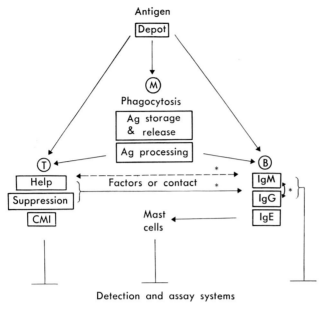

FIG. 1. An outline plan of where an adjuvant might act. An adjuvant can be selective at the level of cell types (circled) or at the level of functional subtypes of cells (boxed). Positive and negative feedback by humoral factors, including antibody, can occur within the B-cell system or also with T cells(*).

posed recently (*15, 16*) and might be considered as "anti-helpers" with specificity for at least part of the antigenic molecule.

A summary of the interactions between antigen, cells, and the various processes in the immune response can be seen in Fig. 1.

Adjuvant Action at a Gross Level

An enormous number of substances have been shown to have adjuvant activity, ranging from the early observations of Ramon (*17*), who used tapioca, and Glenny and colleagues (*18*), using alum-precipitated diphtheria toxoid, to recent studies with chemically well-defined materials (*19*). Three important factors stand out: (1) the slow release of antigen from a depot, such as the site of the injection of incomplete Freund's adjuvant (IFA), results in higher titres of antibody than injection of the same amount of antigen as a solution, (2) polymerized or particulate antigen is a more powerful immunogen than the same antigen in soluble form, and (3) adjuvant substances tend to be toxic in a general sense, causing inflammation at the site of injection (*20*), perhaps mediated by cytotoxicity due to labilization of cell membranes (*21*). The possibility that crosslinking of receptors by polymerized antigen or chemical insults to an immunocyte membrane can give the recipient cell some kind of stimulus activating a differentiational signal will be discussed.

If the immune response is dependent to some degree on the conjunction of two or more of at least four components (Antigen, T, B, and M), then any physiological response which tends to achieve this end is likely to result in a potentiated immune response. It has been shown that several adjuvants could initiate the trapping of circulatory lymphocytes in a lymph node draining an injection site (22, 23). Although Frost and Lance (24) have argued that this mechanism is activated by M cells as the primary target of the adjuvant action, it seems just as likely from earlier work (25, 26) that the litoral cells of the efferent sinuses are the primary targets.

Cellular Targets for Adjuvants

The nature of the reaction between antigen and the constituent cooperating cells in the immune response seems to be largely dependent on the nature of the antigen. Serum protein antigens cannot elicit any response at all in the absence of T cells, whereas the response to pneumococcal polysaccharide SIII not only occurs in their absence but is increased, suggesting that the T cells, in this situation, have a suppressive effect (27). Depending, therefore, on the nature of the antigen being used, substances whose activity is orientated towards one kind of cell involved in the immune response can result in a degree of selectivity in immunopotentiation or immunosuppression. Such a selective immunopotentiation has been demonstrated in a model system in which thymectomized and normal CBA mice were immunized with a range of doses of sheep erythrocytes (SRBC). The data obtained were interpreted as showing that the potentiating effect of bacterial lipopolysaccharide (LPS) on the immune response to SRBC was orientated towards B lymphocytes and a polysaccharide of *Lentinus edodes* (lentinan) was orientated towards (helper) T lymphocytes (28, 29). *Bordetella pertussis* organisms (pertussis) were previously shown in a similar experimental model to be orientated towards both T and B lymphocytes (30), while some time before that it had been shown that pertussis acted on M cells (31). *Corynebacterium parvum* (Cp) is a likely candidate for an adjuvant mostly orientated towards M cells (32). An outline summary of this situation is presented in Table 1.

Although not much is known about the cellular orientation of mycobacterial adjuvants, there is some evidence that they react with T lymphocytes and possibly also B lymphocytes (21, 33). Immunization of guinea pigs with an adjuvant containing mycobacterial substances (complete Freund's adjuvant (CFA)) elicits a γG_1 and a γG_2 response, whereas the use of adjuvant without mycobacteria (IFA) elicits a largely γG_1 response (34, 35). In further experiments, Stone and

TABLE 1. Cellular Orientations of Various Adjuvants: Based on Experiments with Mice Immunized by Sheep Erythrocytes

Adjuvants	M	T	B
Cp	+	−	−
LPS	−	−	+
Lentinan	−	+	−
Pertussis	+	+	+

Asherson (*36*) showed that pre-immunization with alum-precipitated protein stimulated a largely γG_1 response and that guinea pigs so immunized failed to make a γG_2 response on subsequent immunization with antigen in CFA. They coined the term "immune deviation" for this phenomenon. CFA is known to be a good adjuvant of delayed hypersensitivity (*37*), which is one manifestation of T-lymphocyte immunity, although another form of T immunity (homograft rejection) seems to be unaffected.

At this point it seems relevant to pause to consider one of the possible fallacies in the interpretation just given. Take for instance, the interpretation that lentinan interacts directly with helper T-lymphocytes, stimulating them to help more numerously, vigorously, or even perhaps more lengthily. However compatible the data is with this simple explanation, a more complex, but perhaps equally valid effect may exist. The lentinan may, in fact, act solely on the B lymphocytes to make them more susceptible to the effects of T-lymphocyte help: this hypothetical effect on B lymphocytes would have to be different to the form of stimulation given by LPS.

One of the major problems is that in assaying the immune response, the measured end product is often several stages removed from the event being experimentally manipulated.

Adjuvant Action on Different Aspects of the Immune Response

In terms of selective immunopotentiation, not only the target cells need to be considered but also the particular branch of the immune response. There are two quite distinct aspects of the response which are significant here and will be outlined briefly.

1) An adjuvant may have a genuine potentiating effect but on a "control" rather than an "executive" branch of the immune response. Close scrutiny of the literature concerned with immunological adjuvants reveals that in many cases adjuvants can non-specifically suppress the immune response, especially if too high a dose is used. The timing of the injection of adjuvant can be very important, suppression occurring when the adjuvant is injected 12–36 hr before antigen (*28*). In contrast, low doses of immunosuppressive agents such as 6-mercaptopurine (*38*) or irradiation (*39*) can have significant potentiating effects. Treatment with anti-lymphocyte serum can result in potentiation of the response of mice to pneumococcal polysaccharide SIII (*27*), and a similar phenomenon was observed with the response to SRBC (*40*). These results could be explained by the presence of suppressor T-lymphocytes, and in these terms with certain antigens and adjuvants, suppressor rather than helper activity could be potentiated (*41*). Another example of adjuvant action on a control branch of the immune response has been demonstrated by White (*33*), where adjuvant treatment in the fowl can potentiate the production of antibodies with negative as well as positive feedback characteristics.

2) A second possible point of selective immunopotentiation could be at the level of the memory cell pool. In an immune response of mice to SRBC, lentinan was shown to have an adjuvant action orientated towards T lymphocytes (*28, 29*), but recent experiments using very low doses of SRBC (4×10^6) have failed to show

TABLE 2. Effect of Pertussis and Lentinan of the Day 6 PFC Response of Mice to 4×10^6 SRBC i.p.

Adjuvants	No. of PFC $\times 10^{-2}$/mouse	
	γM	γG_{2a}
Controls	289	50
Pertussis	113	38
Lentinan	176	14

i.p.: intraperitoneal injection.

TABLE 3. Secondary Response of Mice to SRBC Following Primary with 4×10^6 SRBC i.p. Either Alone (Controls) or with Pertussis or Lentinan

Adjuvants	No. of PFC $\times 10^{-2}$/mouse	
	γM	γG_{2a}
Controls	323	127
Pertussis	540	583
Lentinan	3,271	1,382

any increase of the primary plaque-forming cell (PFC) response. Pertussis was also shown to be orientated towards T cells with a dose of 4×10^7 SRBC (30). Similarly, pertussis has also failed to show an increased primary PFC response with 4×10^6 SRBC (see Table 2). When, however, the secondary response of these mice was examined 3 months later, those mice which had been primed in the presence of either of these two adjuvants showed considerably increased responses (Table 3). This would suggest that the potentiating effect under these conditions was on a memory cell pool, and by extrapolation from their known effects on the T cells one may speculate that this may be on the T-memory cells.

It is clear that all these points will have to be borne in mind in the planning of possible clinical applications of adjuvants or adjuvant-like factors. The use of adjuvants under circumstances where they result in immunosuppression or in contradistinction, immunosuppressive agents under circumstances where they result in immunopotentiation must be avoided. However, it could be advantageous when immunizing for future protection to use an adjuvant which has most of its potentiating effect on the memory pool.

Potentiation at the Level of the Lymphocyte

Adjuvants could potentiate an immune response by acting on lymphocytes in one (or more) of three ways: (1) increasing the amount of antibody produced by each cell, (2) increasing the amount of cell proliferation before or after induction by antigen, and (3) controlling the switch from tolerance to immune differentiation.

In experiments with mice immunized by SRBC, we have demonstrated adjuvant effects (LPS and pertussis) of over 10-fold both with respect to titres of circulatory antibody and the number of antibody (plaque)-forming cells (28, 42). Measurement of plaque size showed that any increase in amount of antibody produced per cell in adjuvant-treated mice was less than 30 percent greater than in controls. It is clear that most, if not all, the observed increase in amount of circulatory antibody was accountable to an increase in the number of antibody-producing cells. Subsequent experiments, using the isoelectric focusing (IEF) overlay technique, have shown that in a response to a low dose of SRBC pertussis potentiates the response mostly by increasing the amount of post-antigen proliferation (burst size) and perhaps also to a lesser extent increasing the number of antigen sensitive precursor cells which are induced to differentiate into producer cells (43). However, these experiments made use of an immunogenic antigen, and earlier work with a non-immunogen (soluble bovine-gamma globulin (BGG)) showed clearly not only that no response was elicited to BGG unless an adjuvant was administered within a few hours of the antigen, but also that non-immunogenic BGG induced a state of tolerance in which the animal became specifically refractory to the subsequent administration of highly immunogenic forms of the antigen. From this original observation a two-stimulus (signal) hypothesis for the immune response has been developed (44–48). In essence this hypothesis, which is, strictly speaking an encapsulation of the experimental facts, states that an ASC receiving a specific stimulus becomes tolerant unless, at the same time, it receives a non-specific (adjuvant-like) stimulus. The effector of this second stimulus can be adjuvant, polymerized or particulate antigen and perhaps also in some circumstances factors released by helper T lymphocytes

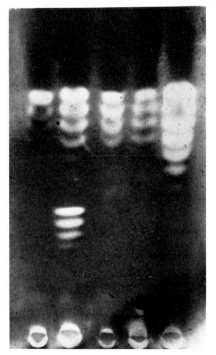

Fig. 2. γG_{2a} anti-SRBC spectrotypes in mice following transfer of primed spleen cells from a previously selected recipient. Bands were visualized by the IEF-overlay technique of Phillips and Dresser (53). The mice showing a response restricted to one spectrotype were used as a source of spleen cells to build up a pool for the experiment summarized in Table 4.

(49, 50), or even a cytotoxic attack by a T-lymphocyte "mistaking" a B-lymphocyte binding a foreign antigen for a foreign cell (51).

The action of adjuvants on primed cells may well be an entirely different phenomenon. Specific immunological unresponsiveness can only be induced in these cells by extremely high doses of antigen, and the non-immunogenic antigen dose which induced a state of tolerance in virgin cells serves as a good stimulus for producing an immune response in primed cells. In an adoptive transfer situation a very low dose of SRBC (4×10^4) will boost a γG_{2a} response in primed cells but will not induce a response of this subclass in virgin cells. We used such a system to compare the immunopotentiating effects of LPS at this dose of antigen with giving the same dose of antigen (without LPS) in 4 small aliquots at 2-day intervals. The population of "primed" spleen cells used for this experiment were selected on the basis of their production of a single antibody spectrotype and have been maintained over a number of generations by serial transplantation of spleen cells into irradiated syngeneic mice (52). In Fig. 2 we illustrate the γG_{2a} spectrotypes of donors of cells for this experiment visualized by the IEF-overlay technique of Phillips and Dresser (53): the mice showing a heterogeneous response were not used.

TABLE 4. A Comparison of the Effects of LPS with Antigen and of Repeated Antigen Stimulation on the Potentiation of the PFC Response of a Population of SRBC-primed Spleen Cells

Treatment	Integral γM PFC (days 5–21)$\times 10^{-3}$	Integral γG_{2a} PFC (days 5–21)$\times 10^{-3}$
4×10^4 SRBC (day 0)	154	61
4×10^4 SRBC$+50$ μg LPS (day 0)	67	67
1×10^4 SRBC (days 0, 2, 4, 6)	1,729	767

The results in Table 4 show that LPS had no potentiating effect at all on the response of these primed cells whereas giving the antigen at 2-day intervals, thereby ensuring its continual presence throughout the initial proliferative stage of the response, resulted in an increased PFC response of more than 10-fold. Thus, under these circumstances, LPS did not act as an immunopotentiating agent, whereas antigen (no more in total quantity than in controls) given as repeated stimuli had a very considerable potentiating effect.

One of the major mechanisms of immunopotentiation may therefore be seen as the result of cells being switched from a tolerance to an immunity pathway. In a more general context it may be considered that a "normal" antigen is a mixture of both antigenic and adjuvant stimuli, an immunogenic antigen being defined as one which contains intrinsic or closely attached adjuvant properties. The immunogenic portion of the antigenic preparation will induce a certain number of cells to enter a state of immune induction, the non-immunogenic portion simultaneously inducing a state of tolerance in other ASC. An adjuvant substance totally unrelated to the antigen (extrinsic adjuvanticity) will tip the balance, inducing many more cells to become immune than would in the absence of the adjuvant.

Immunocyte Differentiation: A Hypothesis

It seems reasonable to suppose that the immune mechanism has evolved from an archetypal process of cellular differentiation and that immunocyte differentiation will be similar in some basic ways to that seen in other kinds of cell. From the zygote onwards, development consists of cycles of cell division with points integral to the cycle where the future of descendant cells is decided. This concept of a progressive increase in the number of cell lines each with a progressively increasing restriction in ability to express the whole genome and consequently showing increased specialization is implicit in early epigenetic models (*54, 55*).

Thomas and colleagues (*56, 57*) have studied the murine mastocytoma line P815Y in synchronous *in vitro* culture. These cells continue to divide in favourable culture conditions unless they receive a growth inhibitory stimulus at a critical (switch) point during the cell cycle. A model of cell differentiation based on their work is illustrated in Fig. 3. Cells receiving the inhibitory stimulus switch from the inner pathway of continuous cycling to the outer pathway, where they continue to cycle through S, G_2, and M but then enter a terminal inactive state (G_0 or G_1). Since the cells are neoplastic it is possible that they contain within themselves their own "Go" signal, but non-neoplastic cell lines may require external signals to stimulate and direct them into one of these two pathways. Given a dependence on an internal (metabolic) switch point stimulus (SPS) it is possible to imagine a situation where cells stimulated to divide continue for several cycles of proliferative division. A neoplastic or "transformed" cell could be an example where the SPS is relatively stable. In a normal *in vivo* environment G_0 cells may remain alive and quiescent until receiving a mitotic stimulus, inducing them to enter the switch point and pass through the next differentiational gate. Figure 4 illustrates an application to immunocyte differentiation of the possible archetypal differentiation process just outlined. It is postulated that antigen gives a mitogenic stimulus to cells bearing a receptor of appropriate specificity. In the absence of an external SPS these cells enter a pathway of terminal differentiation which in this instance would repre-

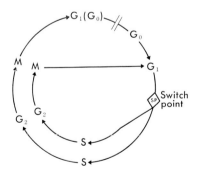

Fig. 3.   The Thomas and Lingwood model for the inhibition of cell division: based on data derived from experiments with murine mastocytoma (P815Y) *in vitro*. Under favourable culture conditions the cells are continually dividing along the inner "cycling" pathway shown above. Inhibition stimuli applied at the switch point divert dividing cells into the outer pathway where, after one further cycle of DNA synthesis and mitosis, the cells enter a terminal state.

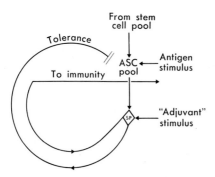

Fig. 4. The role of adjuvant substances in the tolerance-immunity "switch." Antigen is considered to be mitogenic acting on that specific ASC pool. In the absence of external stimuli it is considered that the antigen stimulated cells undergo a cycle of division and become tolerant (outer pathway). If, however, these antigen-stimulated cells receive an adjuvant stimulus at the switch point, either by an intrinsic property of the antigen or by an extrinsic adjuvant, then they enter a pathway where they are allowed to continue cycling and mature to antibody-forming cells.

sent the induction of a state of immunological tolerance. If ASC induced to divide, received an SPS, then these cells enter a pathway which can lead them to immune differentiation. We propose that adjuvants perform the role of an SPS. Having passed this initial switch point the cells may now have different susceptibilities to stimuli. They may cycle as in the Thomas inner pathway until they cease to receive an antigenic (mitogenic) stimulus or until an SPS to divert into another pathway is received: exhaustion of a non-replicating metabolite might be the source of this SPS. Alternatively, with each division cycle the daughter cells may be different from their immediate precursor, e.g., receptor density, and have different susceptibilities to the available stimuli (antigen, adjuvant, intracellular components, or intercellular factors such as T- or M-cell factors), until eventually they become terminal antibody producing cells. Memory cells which are likely to have a higher density of specific receptors than virgin cells (58) might arise as an integral part of this differentiational process possibly as the result of a response to repeated capping by excess post primary antigen, resulting in them passing through a receptorless stage during which they will be refractory to antigen.

It is not impossible that many mitogens described in the literature are not mitogenic at all, but stimuli which divert cells which have already received a "mitotic" stimulus (e.g., from environmental factors) into a pathway where a certain degree of proliferation is permitted. This may be the inner cycling pathway illustrated in Fig. 3. Our explanation would be compatible with the data of Quintans and Lefkovits (59), who show that LPS can activate antibody production in the absence of antigen but that maturation and antibody production occur after relatively few divisions: for significant clonal expansion antigen stimulation is also required. Our results documented in Table 4 also emphasize the need for antigen in stimulating proliferation of specific ASC.

Thymus-independent antigens have been shown to be "mitogenic" for B cells by Coutinho and Möller (60), who suggest that the mitogenic action of these antigens allows them to be capable of stimulating B cells independently of T lymphocytes. We propose that thymus-independent antigens contain such powerful SPS that they divert cells, mitogenically stimulated by the specific antigen portion, into a pathway of division and maturation where any potentially available T-cell help is ineffective.

REFERENCES

1. Claman, N. H., Chaperon, E. A., and Triplett, R. F. Thymus-marrow cell combination. Synergism in antibody production. Proc. Soc. Exp. Biol., *122*: 1167–1171, 1966.

2. Davies, A. J. S., Leuchars, E., Wallis, V., Marchant, R., and Elliott, E. V. The failure of thymus-derived cells to produce antibody. Transplantation, *5*: 222–231, 1967.

3. Taylor, R. B., Wortis, H. H., and Dresser, D. W. Production of class-specific immunoglobulin and antibody by thymectomized-irradiated mice bearing syngeneic and allogeneic thymus grafts. *In;* J. M. Yoffey (ed.), Lymphocytes in Immunology and Haemopoiesis, chap. 27, Arnold, London, 1967.

4. Rajewsky, K. and Rottländer, E. Tolerance specificity and the immune response to lactic dehydrogenase isoenzymes. Cold Spring Harbor Symp. Quant. Biol., *32*: 547–554, 1967.

5. Mitchison, N. A. Antigen recognition responsible for the induction *in vitro* of the immune response. Cold Spring Harbor Symp. Quant. Biol., *32*: 431–439, 1967.

6. Coutinho, A. and Möller, G. B cell mitogenic properties of thymus-independent antigens. Nature New Biol., *245*: 12–14, 1973.

7. Mosier, D. E. A requirement for two cell types for antibody formation *in vitro*. Science, *158*: 1573–1575, 1967.

8. Unanue, E. The regulatory role of macrophages in antigenic stimulation. Adv. Immunol., *15*: 95–165, 1972.

9. Mitchison, N. A. The carrier effect in the secondary response to hapten-protein conjugates. II. Cellular cooperation. Eur. J. Immunol., *1*: 18–27, 1971.

10. Cantor, H., Simpson, E., Sato, V. L., Fathman, C. G., and Herzenberg, L. A. Characterization of subpopulations of T lymphocytes. I. Separation and functional studies of peripheral T-cells binding different amounts of fluorescent anti Thy 1.2 (Theta) antibody using a fluorescence activated cell sorter (FACS). Cell. Immunol., 1975, in press.

11. Cantor, H. and Asofsky, R. Synergy among lymphoid cells mediating the graft-*versus*-host response. II. Synergy in graft-*versus*-host reactions produced by Balb/c lymphoid cells of differing anatomic origin. J. Exp. Med., *131*: 235–246, 1970.

12. Bucher, N. L. R. and Malt, R. A. Regeneration of Liver and Kidney, Little Brown & Co., Boston, 1971.

13. Uhr, J. W. and Möller, G. Regulatory effect of antibody in the immune response. Adv. Immunol., *8*: 81–128, 1968.

14. Henry, C. and Jerne, N. K. Competition of 19S and 7S antigen receptors in the regulation of the primary immune response. J. Exp. Med., *128*: 133–152, 1968.

15. Baker, P. J., Stashak, P. W., Amsbaugh, D. F., Prescott, B., and Barth, R. F. Evidence for the existence of two functionally distinct types of cells which regulate

the antibody response to type III pneumococcal polysaccharide. J. Immunol., *105*: 1581–1583, 1970.

16. Gershon, R. K. and Kondo, K. Cell interactions in the induction of tolerance: the role of thymic lymphocytes. Immunology, *18*: 723–737, 1970.

17. Ramon, G. Sur l'augmentation anormale de l'antitoxines chez les chevaux producteurs de sérum antidiptériques. Bull. Soc. Centr. Méd. Vét., *78*: 227–234, 1925.

18. Glenny, A. T., Pope, C. G., Waddington, H., and Wallace, U. Immunological notes XVII–XXIV. J. Pathol., *29*: 31–40, 1926.

19. Lederer, E. Le rôle immunitaire des mycobactéries. La Récherche, *4*: 1049–1058, 1973.

20. Freund, J. The response of immunised animals to specific and non-specific stimuli. *In;* A. M. Pappenheimer, Jr. (ed.), Nature and Significance of the Antibody Response, pp. 46–68, Columbia University Press, New York, 1953.

21. Allison, A. C. Effects of adjuvants on different cell types and interactions in immune responses. *In;* G. E. W. Wolstenholme and J. Knight (eds.), Immunopotentiation (Ciba Foundation Symposium), vol. 18, pp. 73–99, Elsevier / Excerpta Medica / North-Holland, Amsterdam / London / New York, 1973.

22. Taub, R. N., Krantz, A. R., and Dresser, D. W. The effect of localized injection of adjuvant material on the draining lymph node. I. Histology. Immunology, *18*: 171–186, 1970.

23. Dresser, D. W., Taub, R. N., and Krantz, A. R. The effect of localized injection of adjuvant material on the draining lymph node. II. Circulating lymphocytes. Immunology, *18*: 663–670, 1970.

24. Frost, P. and Lance, E. M. The relation of lymphocyte trapping to the mode of action of adjuvants. *In;* G. E. W. Wolstenholme and J. Knight (eds.), Immunopotentiation (Ciba Foundation Symposium), vol. 18, pp. 29–45, Elsevier / Excerpta Medica / North-Holland, Amsterdam / London / New York, 1973.

25. Smith, R. O. and Wood, W. B. Cellular mechanisms of antibacterial defense in lymph nodes. II. The origin and filtration effect of granulocytes in the nodal sinuses during acute bacterial lymphadenitis. J. Exp. Med., *90*: 567–576, 1949.

26. Florey, H. W. Inflammation. *In;* H. W. Florey (ed.), General Pathology, 4th ed., pp. 40–123, Lloyd-Luke, London, 1969.

27. Baker, P. J., Barth, R. F., Stashak, P. W., and Amsbaugh, D. F. Enhancement of the antibody response to type III pneumococcal polysaccharide in mice treated with antilymphocyte serum. J. Immunol., *104*: 1313–1315, 1970.

28. Dresser, D. W. and Phillips, J. M. The cellular targets for the action of adjuvants: T-adjuvants and B-adjuvants. *In;* G. E. W. Wolstenholme and J. Knight (eds.), Immunopotentiation (Ciba Foundation Symposium), vol. 18, pp. 3–28, Elsevier / Excerpta Medica / North-Holland, Amsterdam / London / New York, 1973.

29. Dresser, D. W. and Phillips, J. M. The orientation of the adjuvant activity of *Salmonella typhosa* lipopolysaccharide and lentinan. Immunology, *27*: 895–902, 1974.

30. Dresser, D. W. The role of T cells and adjuvant in the immune response of mice to foreign erythrocytes. Eur. J. Immunol., *2*: 50–57, 1972.

31. Unanue, E. R., Askonas, B. A., and Allison, A. C. A role of macrophages in the stimulation of immune responses by adjuvants. J. Immunol., *103*: 71–78, 1969.

32. Howard, J. G., Scott, M. T., and Christie, G. H. Cellular mechanisms underlying the adjuvant activity of *Corynebacterium parvum*: interactions of activated macrophages with T and B lymphocytes. *In;* G. E. W. Wolstenholme and J. Knight (eds.), Im-

munopotentiation(Ciba Foundation Symposium), vol. 18, pp. 101–120, Elsevier / Excerpta Medica / North-Holland, Amsterdam / London / New York, 1973.

33. White, R. G. Immunopotentiation by mycobacteria in complete Freund-type adjuvant as the failure of normal immunological homeostasis. In; G. E. W. Wolstenholme and J. Knight (eds.), Immunopotentiation (Ciba Foundation Symposium), vol. 18, pp. 47–72, Elsevier / Excerpta Medica / North-Holland, Amsterdam / London / New York, 1973.

34. White, R. G., Jenkins, G. C., and Wilkinson, P. C. The production of skin-sensitizing antibody in the guinea pig. Int. Arch. Allergy, 22: 156–165, 1963.

35. Benacerraf, B., Ovary, Z., Bloch, K. J., and Franklin, E. C. Properties of guinea-pig FS antibodies. I. Electrophoretic separation of two types of guinea-pig FS antibodies. J. Exp. Med., 117: 937–949, 1963.

36. Asherson, G. L. and Stone, S. H. Selective and specific inhibition of 24 hour skin reactions in the guinea-pig. I. Immune deviation: description of the phenomenon and the effect of splenectomy. Immunology, 9: 205–217, 1965.

37. White, R. G. Role of adjuvants in the production of delayed hypersensitivity. Brit. Med. Bull., 23: 39–45, 1967.

38. Chanmougan, D. and Schwartz, R. S. Enhancement of antibody synthesis by 6-mercaptopurine. J. Exp. Med., 124: 363–378, 1966.

39. Taliaferro, W. H. and Taliaferro, L. G. Effect of radiation on the initial and anamnestic IgM hemolysin responses in rabbits; antigen injection after X-rays. J. Immunol., 103: 559–569, 1969.

40. Anderson, H. R., Dresser, D. W., Iverson, G. M., Lance, E. M., Wortis, H. H., and Zebra, J. The effects of ALG on the murine immune response to sheep erythrocytes. Immunology, 22: 277–289, 1972.

41. Dresser, D. W. and Tao, T.-W. The immune response of mice to ϕX 174: the potentiation of B-cell immunity and the suppression of T-cell help by pertussis vaccine. Immunology, 28: 443–450, 1975.

42. Dresser, D. W., Wortis, H. H., and Anderson, H. R. The effect of pertussis vaccine on the immune response of mice to sheep red blood cells. Clin. Exp. Immunol., 7: 817–837, 1970.

43. Dresser, D. W., Phillips, J. M., and Pryjma, J. Aspects of the mechanism of adjuvant action. 4th Int. Convoc. Immunol., Buffalo, N. Y., 1974, pp. 191–200, Karger, Basel, 1975.

44. Dresser, D. W. The specific inhibition of antibody production. II. Paralysis induced in adult mice by small quantities of a protein antigen. Immunology, 5: 378–388, 1962.

45. Dresser, D. W. Specific inhibition of antibody production. IV. Standardization of the antigen-elimination test; immunological paralysis of mice previously immunized. Immunology, 9: 261–273, 1965.

46. Dresser, D. W. The immune response: circumvention and suppression. Proc. 4th Int. Congr. Pharmacol., 4: 192–202, 1970.

47. Bretscher, P. and Cohn, M. A theory of self-nonself discrimination. Science, 169: 1042–1049, 1970.

48. Bretscher, P. The control of humoral and associative antibody synthesis. Transplant. Rev., 11: 217–267, 1972.

49. Dutton, R. W., Falkoff, R., Hirst, J. A., Hoffmann, M., Kappler, J. W., Kettman, J. R., Lesley, J. F., and Vann, D. Is there evidence for a non-antigen specific dif-

fusable chemical mediator from the thymus-derived cell in the initiation of the immune response? Prog. Immunol., *1*: 355–367, 1971.

50. Schimpl, A. and Wecker, E. Replacement of T-cell function by a T-cell product. Nature New Biol., *237*: 15–17, 1972.

51. Kreth, H. W. and Williamson, A. R. A cell surveillance model for lymphocyte cooperation. Nature, *234*: 454–456, 1971.

52. Askonas, B. A., Williamson, A. R., and Wright, B. E. G. Selection of a single antibody-forming cell clone and its propagation in syngeneic mice. Proc. Natl. Acad. Sci. U.S., *67*: 1398–1403, 1970.

53. Phillips, J. M. and Dresser, D. W. Isoelectric spectra of different classes of anti-erythrocyte antibodies. Eur. J. Immunol., *3*: 524–527, 1973.

54. Waddington, C. H. Organisers and Genes, Cambridge Univ. Press, London, 1940.

55. Holtzer, H., Weintraub, H., Mayne, R., and Mochan, B. The cell cycle, cell lineages and cell differentiation. Contemp. Topics Dev. Biol., *7*: 229–256, 1973.

56. Thomas, D. B., Medley, G., and Lingwood, C. A. Growth inhibition of murine tumor cells, *in vitro*, by puromycin, [^{6}N]O$^{2\prime}$-dibutyryl-3′,5′-adenosine monophosphate or adenosine. J. Cell Biol., *57*: 397–405, 1973.

57. Thomas, D. B. and Lingwood, C. A. A model for cell cycle control: effects of thymidine on synchronous cell cultures. Cell, *5*: 37–44, 1975.

58. Klinman, N. The mechanism of antigenic stimulation of primary and secondary clonal precursor cells. J. Exp. Med., *136*: 241–260, 1972.

59. Quintans, J. and Lefkovits, I. Clonal expansion of lipopolysaccharide stimulated B lymphocytes. J. Immunol., *113*: 1373–1376, 1974.

60. Coutinho, A., Gronowicz, E., Bullock, W. W., and Möller, G. Mechanism of thymus-independent immunocyte triggering: mitogenic activation of B cells results in specific immune responses. J. Exp. Med., *139*: 74–92, 1974.

Discussion of Paper of Drs. Phillips and Dresser

DR. JERNE: Isn't it true that in certain situations an antigen is not required to stimulate a lymphocyte to begin producing antibody as, for example, by employing mitogens?

DR. DRESSER: Yes, Lefkovitz and Quintans, working at the Basel Institute for Immunology, have observed that with a polyclonal stimulant, such as LPS, one can elicit a response to SRBC. It is possible that SRBC and LPS share common determinants; however, LPS may indeed be stimulating a genuine response as appears to be true in other antigenic systems. In the Lefkovitz and Quintans experiments LPS alone leads to a proliferative response of two or three cycles of division, whereas the addition of antigen permits a proliferative response of up to seven or eight cycles.

In the context of the modified Thomas model LPS acts both as an antigen and as SPS, the antigenic portion of the LPS molecule acting as a specific (antigenic) mitogenic stimulus and the lipid A portion of the molecule acting as the SPS.

DR. JERNE: With reference to your study employing lentinan, couldn't you more directly demonstrate that it acts on T cells by showing that it is a T cell mitogen in the absence of antigen?

DR. DRESSER: I have not yet tried that experiment.

DR. NAKAHARA: There is something peculiar about the anti-tumor capacity of lentinan, *viz.*, it is effective against sarcoma-180 but not against other types of transplanted tumor. Can you offer an explanation for this tumor specificity?

DR. DRESSER: Lentinan is but one of a host of anti-tumor polysaccharides you and your colleagues have isolated. Sarcoma-180 is an unusual tumor in the immunological sense, since its growth is suppressed by humoral antibody. It was a paper from your Institute revealing that lentinan acted by potentiating T-cell immunity which led us to use it in the SRBC system in mice, where we also found it to act on T lymphocytes. However, an alternative interpretation of the existing data proposes that lentinan acts on B cells by rendering them more susceptible to the available T cell help. If this is correct, it is clear that this proposed activity of lentinan on B cells is very different from that of LPS.

DR. HOBBS: LPS is able to fix complement through the alternate pathway and thus provides a high source of C3b, which is probably the factor necessary for complement receptor function. B cells are known to have complement receptors, while T lymphocytes most probably do not. Can lentinan act in a similar way?

DR. DRESSER: I am not sure. However, using our SRBC system in mice we presented evidence in a paper delivered at the International Convocation on Immunology in Buffalo (1974) that C3 was not an important source of the "second stimulus" necessary for initiation of an immune response.

DR. NISHIOKA: Dr. Okuda, working in my laboratory, has shown that lentinan does have C3 activating activity, splitting it into C3a and C3b *via* the alternate pathway, as does LPS. C3b or C3d can lead to an antibody response in a T cell-dependent system. As the SRBC system you employed is T lymphocyte-dependent, did you attempt to compare the adjuvant activities of lentinan or LPS in a thymus-independent system as well?

DR. DRESSER: We have evidence which can be interpreted to show that the complement system is not essential for B cell triggering. I performed an experiment similar to the one presented here using the T-independent antigen pneumococcal polysaccharide (SIII) but I discovered that I had employed far too large a dose, and so must repeat it.

DR. DUKOR: I do not think that C3b has a direct role in B-cell activation, but it may have an important function in cooperative immune responses. A modulatory capacity of C3b in B-cell triggering may still be considered, however.

DR. ALEXANDER: Your terminology of antigen dose puzzles me. You seem to consider 4×10^9 SRBC a reasonable dose of antigen, when this must comprise over one-third of the total red cell volume of the mouse. Most investigators believe that adjuvants normally boost responses to rather small doses of antigen. What complications arise by injecting a mouse with virtually its own number of xenogeneic erythrocytes? I suspect that a variety of problems related to antigen clearance might appear. Also, is lentinan an adjuvant under the conditions in which one usually refers to such substances, *i.e.*, while employing a small amount of an antigen, possibly administered subcutaneously or intradermally?

DR. DRESSER: A dose of 4×10^9 SRBC is exceedingly large and can either kill unhealthy mice directly or healthy mice when administered with LPS. However, our experiments were designed to reveal something about the immune system rather than to serve as a clinical model. The effect of the adjuvants we have used seems to be dependent on antigen dose. At doses of 4×10^8 SRBC or higher, lentinan had little adjuvant effect, whereas at lower dose (4×10^7) there was an adjuvant effect on T cell help, and at lower doses still (4×10^6 or less) we have shown in preliminary experiments that lentinan has no adjuvant effect on a primary response but a dramatic effect on subsequent secondary responsiveness. It seems that B orientated adjuvants are more effective in the high antigen dose range.

DR. ALEXANDER: Shouldn't one employ a word other than adjuvant, then, to describe these phenomena, for when one thinks of the classic adjuvants such as Freund's and alum, they tend to work at low antigen doses, and do not assist in the presence of extremely high doses as you used?

DR. DRESSER: I agree that using the word "adjuvant" may be misleading: perhaps one should talk of "chemical immunopotentiators." I think that most of the classic adjuvants act in a way analogous to that presented in the final experiment I described, where repeated small doses of antigen had a greater effect than a single dose equivalent to the total of all the small doses. With depot adjuvants, the release of minute quantities of antigen over prolonged periods is probably a very important aspect; serving to mediate the adjuvant effect through the antigen and not *via* a direct chemical reaction between the material injected and the antibody producing cells.

HOST DEFENSE AGAINST CANCER AND ITS POTENTIATION, D. MIZUNO ET AL. (EDS.),
UNIV. OF TOKYO PRESS, TOKYO / UNIV. PARK PRESS, BALTIMORE, PP. 31-42, 1975

Selective Suppression of T-cell Activity in Tumor-bearing Host and Attempt for Its Improvement

Masayasu Kitagawa, Toshiyuki Hamaoka, Seiji Haba, Kiyoshi Takatsu, and Hiroaki Masaki

Institute for Cancer Research, Osaka University Medical School, Osaka, Japan

Abstract: The cellular site of immunosuppression in the tumor-bearing state was analysed with particular reference to thymus-derived (T) and bone marrow-derived (B) cell activities as measured by immune response to thymus-dependent and thymus-independent antigens (hapten-carrier conjugates).

The development of a T-cell activity as measured by helper function in induction of hapten-specific antibody response was markedly suppressed in mice bearing Ehrlich ascites tumor cells or pretreated with the cell-free ascitic fluid. On the other hand, the development of a B-cell activity as detected by the response to thymus-independent antigen was intact in the tumor-bearing state as compared with the control.

In adoptive secondary immune response to thymus-dependent antigen, the suppressed antibody response was observed when the recipient mice received inoculation of tumor cells or injection with cancerous ascites fluid prior to the primed lymphoid cell transfer but not when the recipient mice were rendered tumor-bearing after the lymphoid cell transfer.

It was also found that the redistribution of T cell, but not B cell, into spleen was suppressed in mice pretreated with cancerous ascites fluid.

The suppression of T-cell activity in either tumor-bearing mice or cancerous ascites fluid-treated mice could be reverted to the normal state by treatment with lentinan, a branched β-glucan, with anti-tumor activity against murine sarcoma 180 and the cell wall components from tubercle bacilli.

Specific immune response to tumor-specific antigen has been demonstrated by many investigators. A question arises as to why immunogenic tumor cells escape from host immune surveillance. It has been generally accepted as one of the reasons that the immune capacity of the tumor-bearing host is impaired.

Our previous study has demonstrated that mice bearing several transplantable tumors including Ehrlich ascites tumor and sarcoma 180 showed markedly suppressed immune responses to the primary and secondary antigenic stimulation (*1–3*). The suppression of the immune response could be clearly reproduced by the treatment of either nuclear components of tumor cells or cell-free cancerous ascites fluid (*2*). Toxohormones which were originally discovered by Nakahara and Fukuoka (*4*) and known as catalase-depressing substance showed also strong immunosuppressive activity (*3*). The present paper investigated the cellular site of immune suppression in the tumor-bearing host with particular reference to T- and B-cell activities.

Suppressed Development of T-cell Activity in Tumor-bearing State

In the first experiment, the influence of the tumor-bearing state on T-cell activity was estimated. Helper function in the induction of anti-hapten antibody response was used as an indicator of T-cell activity according to the method described previously (*5*). Briefly, T-cell donor mice were immunized with thymus-dependent antigen (bacterial α-amylase (BαA) derived from *Bacillus subtilis*) and B-cell donor mice were immunized with a DNP-heterologous protein conjugate. The lymphoid cells from both donor mice of T- and B-cells were transferred into sublethally irradiated recipient mice. The helper T-cell activity was measured

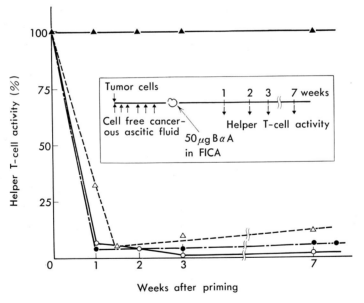

FIG. 1.   The suppressed development of helper T-cell activities on various periods after carrier priming in tumor-bearing and cancerous ascites fluid-treated mice. Experimental group of mice received either with inoculation of 10^7 Ehrlich ascites tumor cells or with daily intraperitoneal (i.p.) injection of 1 ml of cancerous ascites fluid for 6 days and for 3 days prior to the carrier priming, respectively. The helper T-cell activity developed on 1, 2, 3, and 7 weeks after the carrier priming were compared to that of non-treated control mice and expressed on a percent basis to the control level. ▲ normal; △ tumor-bearing; ● ascites×6 (−6∼−1 days); ○ ascites×3 (−3∼−1 days).

by the capacity to induce an anti-DNP antibody response in the recipient mice upon stimulation with DNP-BαA. Four groups of T-cell donor mice were investigated as follows. The first group served as control. The second group was inoculated subcutaneously with 10^7 Ehrlich ascites tumor cells, and the third and fourth groups received intraperitoneally daily injection of 1 ml of cancerous ascites fluid for 6 days and for 3 days prior to the immunization, respectively. The helper T-cell activity of experimental groups developed 1, 2, 3, and 7 weeks after carrier priming was compared with that of the control and compared on a percent basis to the control helper activity. As shown in Fig. 1, the development of helper T-cell activities 1, 2, 3, and 7 weeks after carrier priming was almost completely suppressed in both tumor-bearing and ascitic fluid-treated groups.

Normal Development of B-cell Activity in Tumor-bearing State

In the next experiment, in order to estimate B-cell activity in tumor-bearing state, DNP-dextran and DNP-*Salmonella* Milwaukee were used as thymus-independent antigens. The thymus independency of these antigens was confirmed by the fact that an anti-DNP antibody response could be induced by these antigens on almost a comparable level in both normal and anti-θ plus complement-treated spleen cells. This was sharply contrasted to the response to the thymus-dependent antigen DNP-BαA, which was completely abrogated by the treatment of anti-θ plus complement. Two sets of 3 groups of mice were used. The 1st group was control. The 2nd and 3rd groups were either inoculated with tumor cells or treated intraperitoneally with 1 ml of cancerous ascites fluid for 7 days, respectively and were then immunized with DNP-*Salmonella* Milwaukee or DNP-dextran. For comparison, another two sets of 3 groups were immunized with DNP-horse erythrocyte (HRBC) and DNP-BαA, respectively.

The anti-DNP responses in mice were assayed by counting anti-DNP plaque-forming cells (PFC) in spleen at their peak of responsiveness according to the method of Cunningham (6). As shown in Fig. 2, anti-DNP responses by DNP-*Salmonella* as well as DNP-dextran were not suppressed or even higher in tumor-beaing or cancerous ascites fluid-treated groups as compared with the control mice. These results were sharply contrasted with the cases of DNP-HRBC and DNP-BαA immunization, where, as shown in the lower part of Fig. 2, the anti-DNP antibody response in the tumor-bearing and ascitic fluid-treated groups were markedly suppressed as compared with the control group.

From these results, we can clearly conclude that the B-cell activity was not suppressed in the tumor-bearing state and that the suppressed immune response to thymus-dependent antigens as observed in the Ehrlich ascites fluid-treated and tumor-bearing mice was due to selective impairment of T-cell activity. It must be noticed, however, that thymus-dependent and -independent antigens correspond to macrophage-dependent and -independent antigens, respectively. A possibility remains to be solved that the function of macrophage may be primarily impaired in the tumor-bearing state.

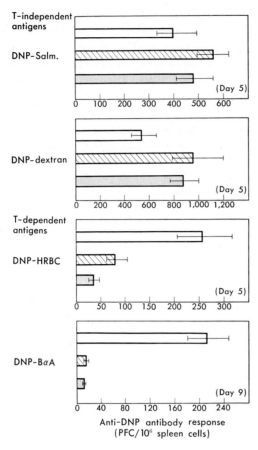

FIG. 2.   The normal development of B-cell activity and the suppressed development of T cell activity in the tumor-bearing state. In each set of 3 groups of mice, the 1st group was control, the 2nd one was inoculated with 10^7 Ehrlich ascites tumor cells 7 days before the antigenic stimulation and the 3rd one was treated i.p. once a day with 1 ml of cancerous ascites fluid for 7 days before antigenic stimulation. The 1st and 2nd sets of mice were immunized with thymus-independent antigens, DNP-*Salmonella* (Salm.) and DNP-dextran, respectively and the 3rd and 4th sets of mice with thymus-dependent antigens, DNP-HRBC and DNP-BαA, respectively. The anti-DNP antibody-forming cells in spleens were measured 5 days later for the 1st, 2nd, and 3rd sets and 9 days later for the 4th set of mice. □ normal; ▨ tumor-bearing; ▨ ascites-treated.

Effect of Timing of Tumor Cell Inoculation or Cancerous Ascites Fluid Treatment on T-cell Activity

The reasons why the T-cell activity is selectively suppressed in the tumor-bearing state under the present conditions are not clear yet. Recently, it was found, however, that the T-cell activity was not suppressed when the recipient mice were first transferred cells primed with thymus-dependent antigen and then rendered tumor-bearing. As can be seen in groups IV and V in Table 1, when normal recipient mice were transferred on day 0 with DNP-BαA-primed cells, and inoculated with

TABLE 1. Effect of Timing of Tumor Inoculation or Ascitic Fluid Injection into Recipient Mice on the Adoptive Secondary Antibody Response to Thymus-dependent Antigen

| Exp. group | Experimental protocol | | | | Anti-DNP antibody response on day 15 (PFC/spleen) |
	Tumor-bearing state on day	Primed cells transferred on day 0	Tumor-bearing state on day	Antigenic stimulation on day 8	
I	—		—		8,723 (1.23)[a]
II	Tumor inoculation (−7 day)		—		397 (1.33)
III	Ascites injection (−7 ~ −1 days)	DNP-BαA-primed cells (i.v.)	—		581 (1.33)
IV	—		Tumor inoculation (+1 day)	100 μg of DNP-BαA (i.p.)	6,179 (1.02)
V	—		Ascites injection (+1 ~ +7 days)		4,996 (1.20)
VI			—	DNP-BαA primed cells (i.v.) (+8 day)	63,585 (1.28)
VII			Tumor inoculation (+1 day)		14,840 (1.23)
VIII			Ascites injection (+1 ~ +7 days)		3,066 (1.60)

i.v.: intravenously.   i.p.: intraperitoneally.   [a] Number in parentheses represents standard error (SE).

TABLE 2. Suppression of Development of Helper T-cells and Antibody-forming Cell Precursor (AFCP) in Mice Treated with Cell-free Ehrlich Ascites Fluid

| Helper cell donor treated with | Antibody response on day 7 | |
	Anti-DNP PFC per spleen	Anti-BαA PFC per spleen
Saline	81,600	45,600
Tumor-bearer (1 × 10⁷)	7,200	1,920
Cancerous ascitic fluid		
6 days before Ag[a] (1 ml × 6)	3,360	9,600
3 days before Ag (1 ml × 3)	1,440	1,920
3 days before Ag (1 ml × 3)	53,760	20,160

Donor mice were immunized with BαA 21 days before the cell transfer.   [a] Antigenic stimulation.

tumor cells on day 1 or treated with cancerous ascites fluid on days 1 to 7, then stimulated with DNP-BαA on day 8, the anti-DNP antibody responses of those groups IV and V were not significantly suppressed as compared with the group I as control and sharply contrasted with the suppressed groups II and III, which had been inoculated with tumor cells or treated with ascitic fluid, respectively, prior to the cell transfer. It was also found, as shown in Table 2, that the helper T-cell development was not significantly suppressed when the cancerous ascites fluid was given after the primary antigenic stimulation. As a control, treatment of recipient mice with serum from normal mice prior to antigenic stimulation did not show any suppression of T-cell development, as shown in Table 3. These results suggest that the T cells once populated in the immune organ may not be significantly

TABLE 3. Comparison of the Effect of Ehrlich Ascites Fluid and Normal Mouse Serum of Development of Helper T-cells and AFCP in Mice

Helper cell donor treated with	Primary response on day 10 in donor mice	Antibody response on day 7 in recipient mice	
	Anti-BαA PFC per 10^6 cells	Anti-DNP PFC per spleen	Anti-BαA PFC per spleen
Control	192.0	48,000	10,800
Ascites 1 ml	57.0	1,920	960
Normal serum 1 ml	107.3	49,920	8,640

Ehrlich ascites fluid and normal mouse serum were given into helper T-cell donor mice 3 days prior to the primary antigenic stimulation with BαA.

influenced by the tumor-bearing state. In other words, the T cells may be strongly influenced when transferred into a tumor-bearing recipient. This possibility was strongly supported by the results shown in the next experiment.

Selective Suppression of T-cell Redistribution in Spleens of Cancerous Ascites Fluid-pretreated Recipients

The recipient mice were treated with daily injections of cancerous ascites fluid for 7 days, heavily X-irradiated and then inoculated with 10^8 spleen cells primed either with BαA or DNP-keyhole limpet hemocyanin (KLH). Seven days later, total cell numbers recovered in spleens were counted. The numbers of T and B cells were determined by their sensitiveness to anti-θ and anti-B-cell sera using a dye exclusion test. It is evident from Table 4 that in cancerous ascites fluid-treated mice the recovery of T cells in spleen was about one third of that of T cells in spleen of the control mice, although the recovery of B cell in both groups was almost comparable. Thus, it is likely that selective suppression of T-cell activity observed in the

TABLE 4. Redistribution of T and B Cells in the Spleens of Ascites Fluid Pretreated Recipients

Exp. No.	Donor cells	Recipient	Total cell No. recovered on day 7 ($\times 10^{-6}$)	T cells		B cells	
				% cells killed by anti-θ serum plus complement (range)	T cell No. recovered ($\times 10^{-6}$)	% cells killed by anti-B serum[a] plus complement (range)	B cell No. recovered ($\times 10^{-6}$)
I	BαA- primed spleen	Normal	160	28.1(25.9–29.7)	44.9	17.7(15.5–19.7)	33.0
		Ascites	100	15.0(11.3–18.5)	15.0	42.9(39.7–45.0)	42.9
II	DNP-KLH- primed spleen	Normal	110	33.2(30.8–36.6)	36.5	26.7(25.7–27.3)	29.3
		Ascites	73	17.0(15.0–19.6)	12.0	43.3(36.4–49.0)	31.6
	No cell transfer	Normal	<4				

Recipient mice were treated with daily injection of cancerous ascites fluid for 7 days. Spleen cells (1×10^8) were injected i.v. to 800R X-irradiated recipients and 7 days later the redistributed T- and B- cells into spleen were counted. [a] Anti-B serum was supplied from Dr. T. Masuda (Kyoto Univ.).

tumor-bearing host is due to a failure in the trapping of T cells into immune organ and in the effective interaction with B cells.

Recovering Effect of Lentinan and Cell Wall Skeleton of Tubercle Bacilli on the Suppression of T-cell Development in Tumor-bearing State

The immunodeficiency, especially the suppressed T-cell activity in the tumor-bearing host, may cause failure in discrimination of antigenic tumor cells from normal cells and may cause a failure in induction of immune resistance against tumor growth. It is, therefore, necessary to attempt to recover or prevent from the immunosuppression of the tumor-bearing state, in order to approach a radical immunotherapy of neoplastic disease.

The anti-tumor polysaccharide, lentinan, which is a glucan with molecular weight of approximately one million, has been isolated from *Lentinus edodes* and shown a pronounced anti-tumor effect against the transplantable murine tumor, sarcoma 180 by Chihara *et al.* (*7, 8*). Thus, lentinan was expected to recover or prevent from the suppression of helper T-cell activity in a tumor-bearing host. This possibility was tested as follows.

Normal or cancerous ascites fluid-pretreated mice were immunized with 50 μg BαA in Freund's incomplete adjuvant. Nine days after priming, the helper T-cell activities developed in both groups were measured by the capacity to induce anti-DNP antibody response to DNP-KLH-primed B-cells upon DNP-BαA stimulation. As shown in Table 5, helper T-cell development was clearly suppressed in the cancerous ascites fluid-treated animals. However, when the ascitic fluid-injected animals were daily treated with 50 μg of lentinan for 7 days prior to and after the priming, the level of helper T-cell development was at almost the same level as the normal

TABLE 5. Reversed Effect of Lentinan on the Suppression of Helper T-cell Development in Tumor-bearing State

| Exp. No. | Helper T-cell donor[a] treated with | | Helper activity tested on day | B cells | Anti-DNP antibody response on day 7[b] (indirect PFC/spleen) |
	Ascitic fluid	Lentinan			
1	—	—	Day 9 after priming	DNP-KLH-primed cells	336,000 (1.24)[c]
	0.5 ml×3 (−3~−1 day)	—			32,640 (1.10)
	0.5 ml×3 (−3~−1 day)	50 μg×7 (−3~+3 day)			288,000 (1.20)
	—	50 μg×7 (−3~+3 day)			76,800 (1.24)
2	—	—	Day 25 after priming	DNP-TAA-primed cells	60,480 (1.11)
	1 ml×1 (−3 day)	—			15,920 (1.23)
	1 ml×1 (−3 day)	50 μg×10 (−3~+6 day)			67,170 (1.17)

[a] Helper T-cell donors were immunized with 50 μg BαA in Freund's incomplete adjuvant on day 0 and treated with ascitic fluid or lentinan on the time schedule as indicated.   [b] The data are expressed as geometric means of 5 animals.   [c] Number in parentheses represents SE.

TABLE 6. Effect of Cell Wall Components of Tubercle Bacilli on Development of Helper T-cells and AFCP in Cancerous Ascites Fluid-treated Mice

Donor mice treated with	Primary response in donor mice	Antibody response on day 7 in recipient mice	
	Anti-BαA PFC per 10^6 spleen cells	Anti-DNP PFC per spleen	Anti-BαA PFC per spleen
None	408.0	31,200	4,680
CW	357.4	127,200±9,600	21,360
Ascitic fluid	55.6	3,600±1,690	720
Ascitic fluid+paraffin oil	70.6	10,500± 900	2,400
Ascitic fluid+CW	84.7	29,600±6,974	4,320
Ascitic fluid+CWS	68.0	55,200±9,600	7,920

The donor mice of helper T-cell were treated twice with 1 ml of Ehrlich ascitic fluid 3 and 2 days prior to BαA-immunization. The cell wall component (200 μg) of tubercle bacilli was given i.v. twice 3 days before and simultaneously with the carrier priming. Nine days later, the carrier-primed cells were transferred together with the DNP-specific B-cells into recipient mice for assay of helper T-cell activity. CW: cell wall fraction. CWS: cell wall skeleton from tubercle bacilli. These substances were given in form of oil in water (9).

mice. Very interestingly, however, treatment with lentinan, as the above schedule of normal animals, does not augment but rather inhibits the development of helper T-cell activity. Basically the same result was also observed in the 2nd experiment. In this experiment, the dose of ascitic fluid was decreased and the duration of lentinan treatment was prolonged than Exp. 1, and a clearer restoration of T-cell activity was produced. Thus, lentinan was clearly effective in the protection or recovery of hosts from the ascitic fluid-induced T-cell suppression, although sole administration of lentinan failed to augment normal T-cell activity.

The cell wall and cell wall skeleton were prepared from tubercle bacilli and found to be effective on suppression of tumor growth as well as regression of established tumor by Yamamura et al. (9). The suppressed T-cell activity in the cancerous ascites fluid-treated mice could be also reverted to the control level by treatment with these cell wall components from tubercle bacilli as shown in Table 6. It should be noticed that the cell wall components, unlike lentinan, showed strong potentiating activity for helper T-cell development in normal mice. Therefore, the mechanism for immune potentiation with lentinan may be different from that with the cell wall components of tubercle bacilli.

Further study is now under way to elucidate whether or not the suppressed repopulating ability of T cells in the tumor-bearing state is recovered with these immunopotentiators and what role the helper T-cell plays in tumor immunity. A preliminary experiment concerning the latter problem shows that the helper T-cell enhances the generation of effector T-cell against tumor in the same manner as it does that of B cell.

ACKNOWLEDGMENTS

This work was supported in part by Grants-in-Aid for Scientific Research from the Ministry of Education and from the Ministry of Health and Welfare of Japan.

The authors are indebted to Dr. G. Chihara and Dr. G. Hamuro for providing lentinan, Dr. Y. Yamamura and Dr. I. Azuma for providing cell wall components of tubercle bacilli, Dr. T. Masuda for providing antiserum specific for mouse B-cell, and Miss R. Yamada for her valuable assistance to prepare this manuscript.

REFERENCES

1. Takatsu, K., Hamaoka, T., Yamashita, U., and Kitagawa, M. Suppressed activity of thymus-derived cell in tumor-bearing host. Gann, *63*: 273–275, 1972.
2. Masaki, H., Takatsu, K., Hamaoka, T., and Kitagawa, M. Immunosuppressive activity of chromatin fraction derived from nuclei of Ehrlich ascites tumor cells. Gann, *63*: 633–635, 1972.
3. Kitagawa, M., Hamaoka, T., Takatsu, K., Haba, S., Yamashita, U., and Masaki, H. Disturbance of immune surveillance in tumor-bearing host. GANN Monograph on Cancer Research, *16*: 45–52, 1974.
4. Nakahara, W. and Fukuoka, F. Toxic cancer tissue constituent as evidenced by its effect on liver catalase activity. Japan. Med. J., *1*: 271–277, 1948.
5. Hamaoka, T., Takatsu, K., and Kitagawa, M. Antibody production in mice. IV. The suppressive effect of anti-hapten and anti-carrier antibodies on the recognition of hapten-carrier conjugate in the secondary response. Immunology, *21*: 259–271, 1971.
6. Cunningham, A. J. and Szenberg, A. Further improvements in the plaque technique for detecting single antibody-forming cells. Immunology, *14*: 599–600, 1968.
7. Chihara, G., Maeda, Y. Y., Hamuro, G., Sasaki, T., and Fukuoka, F. Inhibition of mouse sarcoma-180 by polysaccharide from *Lentinus edodes* (BERK) SING. Nature, *222*: 687–688, 1969.
8. Maeda, Y. Y., Hamuro, J., Yamada, Y., Ishimura, K., and Chihara, G. The nature of immunopotentiation by the anti-tumor polysaccharide lentinan and the significance of biogenic amines in its action. *In;* G. E. W. Wolstenholme and J. Knight (eds.), Immunopotentiation (Ciba Foundation Symposium), vol. 18, pp. 259–286, Elsevier / Excerpta Medica / North-Holland, Amsterdam / London / New York, 1973.
9. Yamamura, Y., Azuma, I., Taniyama, T., Ribi, E., and Zbar, B. Suppression of tumor growth and regression of established tumor with oil-attached mycobacterial fractions. Gann, *65*: 179–181, 1974.

Discussion of Paper of Drs. Kitagawa et al.

DR. JERNE: Have you tested this tumor ascites fluid *in vitro* in a system such as the Mishell-Dutton culture?

DR. KITAGAWA: No, we have not, but Dr. Urushizaki and his co-workers at Sapporo Medical College have demonstrated a repressed responsiveness of normal lymphocytes to phytohemagglutinin (PHA) when treated with serum from cancer patients *in vitro*. Also, Dr. Suzuki and his co-workers at Okayama University have shown that the ability of lymphoid cells to kill a certain tumor and to produce macrophage migration inhibitory factor (MIF) was suppressed when combined with a toxohormone preparation *in vitro*, although responsiveness to PHA remained intact.

DR. NAKAHARA: From your studies, it appears that factors released from tumor cells may account for the depressed immune responsiveness of tumor-bearing animals. In this regard, did you attempt to restore the immune potential of such animals by surgical extirpation of their tumors? For, Greenstein showed that tumor removal abolished the toxohormone effect.

DR. KITAGAWA: We have not attempted such an experiment but would like to try it in the future according to your suggestion. I expect that the suppressed immune responsiveness of tumor-bearers would be recovered after removal of their neoplasms, since the suppressive effect of cancerous ascites fluid and toxohormone seems to be transient.

DR. HALPERN: In your system, the Ehrlich ascites tumor is allogeneic. Did you record similar results in a syngeneic system? Secondly, there is certainly a great quantity of tumor cell membranes in the ascitic fluid, originating from shedding of such constituents by growing cells and from dead cells. Is there a possibility of antigenic competition accounting for the results you obtained?

DR. KITAGAWA: So far, we have tested only a few syngeneic system, in which the immunosuppression was much less than that observed in allogeneic systems, such as Ehrlich ascites tumor and sarcoma 180. However, even in the allogeneic system, the degree of immunosuppression varied from tumor to tumor.

Antigenic competition is ruled out by the experimental results shown in Table 1, where primed cells were transferred into X-irradiated recipients, inoculated with tumor cells or treated with the ascites fluid for one week, and then stimulated with the secondary antigen. Immunosuppression was here not seen (Groups IV and V). Tumor inoculation or ascites treatment of such recipients prior to adoptive cell transfer and subsequent stimulation with antigen could completely abrogate the secondary immune response (Groups II and III). If antigenic competition is relevant for this suppression, an inhibitory effect would be expected in the former cases (Groups IV and V) after compared with the latter cases (Groups II and III). Also, the ascites fluid retains its immunosuppressive activity following ultracentrifugation or passage through a milipore filter, which removed a large amount of particulate matter.

DR. FROST: We have also used syngeneic tumor ascitic fluid, and it is just as effective as the allogeneic fluid. However, we have also used inflammatory fluid induced by proteose-peptone or Fuller's earth (diatomaceous earth), and this substance is as effective as the tumor ascitic fluid. The effects may therefore not be due to tumor factor but rather something present in inflamed peritonea in general. One of the controls that should be included in such experiments must be fluid derived from the inflamed peritonea of otherwise normal syngeneic animals.

DR. T. HAMAOKA (Institute for Cancer Research, Osaka University Medical School, Osaka):   As controls we used both normal mouse serum and complete Freund's adjuvant-induced peritoneal exudates from normal mice, and neither exhibited any immunosuppressive activity.

DR. AMOS: You may be observing the immunosuppressive effect of a virus, and I think Dr. Frost's use of an inflammatory ascites fluid wouldn't necessarily rule this out. Dr. Hatler and I once transferred skin from cancer patients to normal individuals and obtained an extraordinary prolongation of survival; a number of scientists have carried out similar skin grafting experiments in mice bearing Ehrlich ascites tumors, noting variable results which are to some extent dependent on the particular Ehrlich ascites tumor being employed. You state that you had ultracentrifuged your ascites fluid. Was this at a sufficient rate and time to be able to be reasonably assured that any virus particles were removed?

DR. T. HAMAOKA: The ascites fraction obtained following ultracentrifugation at 105,000 g for 2 hr showed a strong immunosuppressive effect. I think this indicates that virus contamination does not appear to be a relevant mechanism for immunosuppression.

DR. KITAGAWA: Dr. Yamazaki and his collaborators* at the National Institute of Health, Tokyo, fractionated cell-free Ehrlich ascites fluid by Diaflo ultrafiltration to obtain 3 fractions with immunosuppressive activity. One fraction had a very low molecular weight, of some 10,000 to 1,000 daltons. This may also eliminate a participation of virus in the immunosuppression.

* Yamazaki, H., Nitta, K., and Umezawa, H., Gann, *64*: 83, 1973.

DR. FACHET: In your experiments, lentinan seems to have a striking effect on T cells, stimulating the regeneration of immune responsiveness. Have you attempted to break T cell tolerance to T-dependent antigens with lentinan? Such an investigation may prove to be relevant in delineating the mechanism of its action.

DR. KITAGAWA: We haven't as yet defined the details of the mechanism of the potentiating activity of lentinan. But lentinan may not directly activate the depressed ability of T cells to help B cells in ascitic fluid-treated mice. Since the activated T cell does not express its helper function when transferred into recipients pretreated with ascitic fluid, it is rather possible that some tumor product, such as toxohormone, coats the T cells, thereby interfering with splenic and lymph node trapping of these cells. Lentinan in some manner may correct this dysfunction, as evidenced by selective disturbance of T-cell redistribution in ascitic fluid-treated mice.

DR. JERNE: Is there any relationship between your ascites cell-free extract and one described recently in the Proc. Natl. Acad. Sci. U.S. by F. Jacob and others working at the Pasteur Institute*? It is secreted by tumor cells and inhibits the immune response.

* Fauve, R. M., Hevin, B., Jacob, H., Gaillard, J. A., and Jacob, F. Proc. Natl. Acad. Sci. U.S., *71*: 4052, 1974.

DR. KITAGAWA: We haven't enough data to be able to compare our factor with theirs. Our immunosuppressive material derived from Ehrlich ascites tumor cells is exclusively localized in the nuclei of the tumor cells and released from the tumor cells into ascites fluid or blood of tumor-bearing mice, probably when the tumor cells are destroyed *in vivo*. It is interesting that an anti-inflammatory compound released from tumor cells has a molecular weight of 1,000 to 10,000.

DR. ALEXANDER: I believe that one shouldn't discuss factors secreted by tumor cells as if such products were formed by all neoplastic cells. The immunosuppressive effect of some transplanted tumors is indeed real. However, for primary cancers this phenomenon is invariably absent. In man, immunosuppression is only a very late sequelae of cancer; early in the course of the disease it is not realized. Similarly, primary induced tumors in experimental animals that have not been transplanted do not give an immunosuppressive effect, these animals having normal responses to sheep erythrocytes as well as normal homograft rejection (see Alexander *et al.*, Proc. Roy Soc., *B174*: 237, 1969). When one transplants tumors, the immune potential of the host then begins to vary. I always assumed that the explanation Dr. Amos just offered, namely, it depends upon when and where the animal is infected by a virus, was the ultimate cause of this variation. I therefore think this immunosuppression is most likely a transplantation artifact, as I know of no studies in which a primary tumor not involving the reticuloendothelial system has been significantly immunosuppressive.

HOST DEFENSE AGAINST CANCER AND ITS POTENTIATION, D. MIZUNO ET AL. (EDS.),
UNIV. OF TOKYO PRESS, TOKYO / UNIV. PARK PRESS, BALTIMORE, PP. 43-53, 1975

Lymphocyte-mediated Cytotoxicity: Mechanisms and Relationship to Tumor Immunity[*1]

K. T. Brunner, F. Plata,[*2] D. M. Vasudevan, and J.-C. Cerottini

Department of Immunology, Swiss Institute for Experimental Cancer Research and Lausanne Unit of Human Cancer Immunology, Ludwig Institute for Cancer Research, Lausanne, Switzerland

Abstract: Destruction of tumor cells *in vitro* by immune lymphoid cells may be based on several mechanisms, *i.e.*, (a) direct killing by sensitized cytotoxic thymus-dependent lymphocytes (CTL); (b) antibody-dependent killing by normal lymphoid cells carrying receptors for the Fc portion of IgG molecules: and (c) cell-mediated lysis by macrophages "armed" or activated by soluble factors released by sensitized T cells following interaction with antigen. In the present report, studies will be described which were aimed at the analysis of the role of CTL *in vitro* and *in vivo*. Two different approaches were used.

First, attempts were made to increase cytotoxic activities of immune cell populations by incubating and separating CTL from other irrelevant lymphoid cells. A combination of preincubation and separation techniques led to a considerable increase in cytotoxic activities of lymphoid cell populations, allowing the detection of CTL in spleens of C57BL/6 mice bearing syngeneic EL4 lymphoma cells. Second, *in vitro* generation of CTL was studied using mixed lymphocyte-tumor cell cultures (MLTC). Under appropriate culture conditions, CTL were formed in MLTC containing normal C57BL/6 spleen cells and irradiated RBL-5 lymphoma cells or moloney sarcoma virus (MSV)-induced sarcoma cells. Moreover, it was found that generation of CTL *in vitro* was at least 10-fold higher when spleens from mice carrying or having rejected an MSV-induced tumor were used instead of normal spleens as the source of responding cells, suggesting the presence of increased numbers of CTL precursors in the former animals. Together, these results suggest that two approaches should be used in attempts to evaluate the immune status of tumor-bearing individuals. Lymphoid cell populations should be tested for CTL using various cell purification procedures to obtain cell subpopulations enriched in effector cells. CTL precursors should be sought using methods for generation of CTL in

---

[*1] Supported by grants from the Swiss National Foundation.
[*2] Chargé de Recherches à l'Inserm, France.

MLTC. The relevance of *in vitro* findings to resistance to tumor growth will be discussed.

In attempts to understand the mechanisms leading to resistance against tumor growth, many recent studies have focussed on the *in vitro* analysis of humoral and cell-mediated immune responses to tumor-associated antigens. Following the demonstration that lymphocytes of immune individuals may be cytotoxic for target cells carrying the sensitizing membrane-bound antigens, the *in vitro* assay of lymphocyte-mediated cytotoxicity (LMC) was widely used to measure cell-mediated immunity to grafts and tumors. Also, it was tempting to assume that cytotoxicity of sensitized lymphocytes constituted the main mechanism of tumor immunity. However, further studies have shown that a number of important problems remain to be solved. In particular, it has now become clear that *in vitro* destruction of tumor cells by immune lymphoid cells may be based on several mechanisms, *i.e.*, on (a) direct killing by sensitized cytotoxic thymus-dependent lymphocytes (CTL), (b) antibody-dependent killing by normal mononuclear non-T lymphocytes (K cells) which carry receptors for the Fc portion of the IgG molecule, and (c) cell-mediated lysis by macrophages "armed" or activated by soluble factors released by sensitized T cells following interaction with antigen (*1*).

Little information is at present available concerning the significance of these *in vitro* mechanisms in terms of tumor immunity *in vivo*. Furthermore, it is obvious that the *in vitro* demonstration of LMC using whole lymphoid cell populations from tumor-bearing individuals gives little information about the type of effector cell involved, and cell separation and identification procedures are necessary to identify the cytotoxic mechanism. In the few studies where such procedures were applied, it was found that the relative role of the different effector mechanisms depended on the assay system used, the time of immunization or state of tumor growth, the source of immune lymphocytes, and other factors.

In order to analyse more closely the role of CTL *in vitro* and *in vivo*, recent studies in our laboratory have concerned with the separation, the physico-chemical characterization and the quantitative *in vitro* assay of CTL formed in the primary and secondary *in vivo* and *in vitro* response to alloantigens (*2–4*) and tumor antigens (*5, 6*). The present report summarizes studies of (a) the separation and identification of CTL in the EL4 mouse lymphoma system, (b) the analysis of LMC in the moloney sarcoma virus (SMV) tumor system, and (c) the primary and secondary *in vitro* generation of tumor specific CTL in the SMV system. Furthermore, the problem of the relevance of the *in vitro* findings to resistance to tumor growth will be discussed.

Separation and Identification of CTL in the EL4 Mouse Lymphoma System

In syngeneic tumor systems it is often difficult to detect cytotoxic lymphocytes, presumably due to low effector cell frequencies and/or inhibitory factors. The possibility to separate CTL from irrelevant cells in order to increase cytotoxic activities

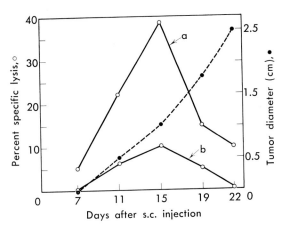

FIG. 1. Cytolytic activity of preincubated or BSA-gradient separated spleen cells of mice bearing a growing EL4 tumor. Spleen cells of C57BL/6 mice were collected at different time intervals after subcutaneous (s.c.) injection of 10^4 EL4 lymphoma cells and their cytolytic activity assayed, (a) after 24-hr preincubation, and (b) after 24-hr preincubation followed by BSA-gradient separation of low density (<1.08 g/cm^3) cells, against ^{51}Cr-labeled EL4 target cells at a spleen cell to target cell ratio of 100:1 (24-hr incubation). No cytotoxic activity could be detected with spleen cells tested at time of collection (results not shown). ○ percent specific lysis; ● tumor diameter (cm).

of immune cell populations was suggested by studies in allograft systems. They had shown that early in the immune response, CTL were predominantly large cells (7, 8) of low density which could be separated from other cells by simple density gradient or velocity sedimentation procedures (9, 10).

In attempts to apply these findings to a weak syngeneic tumor system, spleen cells from C57BL/6 mice immunized by two intraperitoneal injections of irradiated (4,000 R) EL4 lymphoma cells were separated into a low and a high density fraction on a bovine serum albumin (BSA) density gradient. Cytotoxicity tests using a ^{51}Cr-release assay showed that the low density fraction containing 15–20% of the total cell number had a 5-fold increased cytotoxic activity as compared with the initial cell population (5). A comparable increase in activity was noted when immune peritoneal cells were tested following removal of phagocytic cells. Similarly, preincubation of immune spleen cells for 24 hr led to increased cytotoxic activities for reasons which are still not clear, and a combination of preincubation followed by density gradient separation led to a 30 to 100-fold increase. In an extension of these studies it was found that the application of these preincubation and separation techniques also allowed the detection of CTL in spleens of EL4 tumor bearing mice, i.e., in a situation where it was not possible to detect cytotoxic lymphocytes in the direct ^{51}Cr-release assay (Fig. 1).

Treatment of immune spleen or peritoneal cells with anti-θ serum and C in order to selectively remove T cells completely abolished cytotoxicity, whereas passage through Ig-anti-Ig coated columns to remove surface membrane Ig carrying cells (bone marrow-derived cells (B cells)) and cells carrying Fc receptors (K cells) had no effect. These tests demonstrated the T-cell nature of the effector cells (5).

LMC in the MSV Tumor System

Mice injected with MSV form a sarcoma at the site of virus inoculation which may undergo complete regression within 2–3 weeks. Tumor regression is accompanied by the development of resistance to challenge with MSV. The tumor hosts form antibodies which react with membrane-bound antigens associated with MSV-induced tumors, and which are cytotoxic in the presence of complement or in the presence of normal lymphoid cells (K cells).

Studies of LMC in MSV immune mice showed a complex picture with the following characteristics. When assayed by the microcytotoxicity assay of Takasugi and Klein (*11*), cytotoxic activity of spleen cells was detectable within a few days after MSV injection, disappeared at the time of maximal tumor size, and then reappeared and persisted for several weeks after tumor regression (*12, 13*). The characterization of the effector cells indicated that both T-cell and non-T-cell cytotoxicity was involved before and shortly after tumor regression (*13, 14*). Late after regression, however, non-T cells only appeared to be responsible for the activity detected with this particular assay system.

When assayed by a ^{51}Cr-release test, cytotoxic activity was also detected within a few days after MSV injection, but it reached a peak at the time of maximal tumor size and then gradually declined (*15, 16*). Lymphoid cells collected late after complete regression of the tumor had no activity. Characterization of the effector cells showed that T cells only were responsible for the cytotoxic activity (*16, 17*) detectable with this assay system.

It is thus apparent that conflicting results may be obtained when the same lymphoid cell population is tested for LMC using two different assay systems.

In Vitro Generation of MSV Tumor-specific CTL

The formation of CTL with specificity for alloantigens can be readily induced in mixed lymphocyte cultures (MLC) *in vitro*. In recent studies in our laboratory

TABLE 1. Generation of CTL in Primary and Secondary MLTC as a Function of Time after MSV Inoculation

Origin of spleen cells in MLTC (days after MSV)	Lytic activity of MLTC cells: percent specific ^{51}Cr release from RBL-5 target cells in 3 hr at MLTC cell to target cell ratios of					
	100	30	10	1	0.1	Lytic units/culture
Normal	35	23	11	3	2	4
Immune (5 days)	85	57	33	5	2	39
Normal	66	44	15	2	3	8
Immune (14 days)	100	97	79	20	4	217
Normal	44	27	15	2	0	4
Immune (64 days)	82	75	72	17	1	155

Spleen cells from C57BL/6 mice collected at various times after MSV injection (immune cells) or spleen cells from uninjected C57BL/6 mice (normal cells) were mixed with X-irradiated RBL-5 lymphoma cells at a ratio of 25:1 (MLTC), incubated for 6 days and then assayed for lytic activity against ^{51}Cr-labeled RBL-5 target cells *in vitro*. Lytic units/culture were determined as described previously (*2*).

it was found that the MLC response of spleen cells from mice immunized 2–3 months previously with an allograft led to over 5-fold higher CTL activities than the MLC response of normal lymphocytes (2). This secondary type *in vitro* cell-mediated immune response was presumably based on the presence of increased numbers of CTL precursors (memory cells) in the spleens of the immune animals. Furthermore, a qualitative difference in the responsiveness of normal and immune spleen cells was suggested by the observation that immune cells responded almost as well to subcellular alloantigen preparations as to intact irradiated spleen cells, whereas normal spleen cells responded only to intact cells (18).

When similar experiments were carried out in the syngeneic MSV tumor system, it was found that CTL able to lyse ^{51}Cr-labeled Rauscher virus-induced RBL-5 leukemia cells were formed in cultures of C57BL/6 spleen cells and irradiated RBL-5 cells (mixed lymphocyte-tumor cell culture (MLTC)). Moreover, it could be dmeonstrated that the generation of CTL was at least 10-fold higher when spleens from mice carrying or having rejected an MSV-induced tumor were used as the source of responding cells (6), suggesting the presence of increased numbers of CTL in these animals. The results of an experiment in which the generation of CTL in primary and secondary MLTC was followed as a function of time after MSV inoculation are presented in Table 1.

It can be seen from these results that an increased, secondary type response could be observed with spleen cells collected as early as 5 days and as late as 64 days after MSV inoculation.

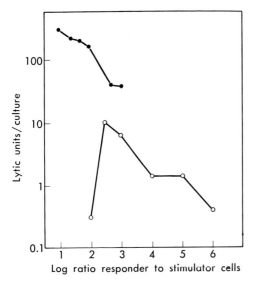

FIG. 2.   Generation of CTL in secondary MLTC as a function of the ratio of stimulator to responder cells. MLTC were prepared by mixing spleen cells of C57BL/6 mice collected 26 days after rejection of an MSV-induced tumor (responding cells) with X-irradiated RBL-5 lymphoma or MSV-BL/6 sarcoma cells (stimulating cells) at various ratios. The MLTC were incubated for 6 days and the resulting cell population tested for cytolytic activity against ^{51}Cr-labeled RBL-6 target cells in a 3-hr assay. Lytic units/culture were determined as described elsewhere (2).

TABLE 2. Lytic Activity against ^{51}Cr-labeled MSV-BL/6 Target Cells of CTL Generated in Secondary MLTC Using Either the RBL-5 Lymphoma or the MSV-BL/6 Sarcoma as a Source of Stimulator Cells

Stimulating cells used in secondary MLTC	Lytic activity of secondary MLTC cells: percent specific ^{51}Cr release from MSV-BL/6 sarcoma target cells in 24 hr at MLTC cell to target cell ratios of			
	30	10	3	1
None	2	3	4	2
RBL-5 lymphoma	87	73	56	31
MSV-BL/6 sarcoma	71	36	20	1

Spleen cells from C57BL/6 mice collected following rejection of a tumor induced 26 days previously with MSV were mixed at ratios of 25:1 with X-irradiated (4,000 R) RBL-5 cells or at 300:1 with MSV-BL/6 cells in MLTC and incubated for 6 days. The cytolytic effect of the MLTC cells was then tested on ^{51}Cr-labeled MSV-BL/6 target cells at the ratios indicated.

The cytolytic activity of the *in vitro* generated CTL was demonstrable not only against RBL-5 target cells, but also against MSV-induced sarcoma cells, using both the ^{51}Cr-release test and the microcytotoxicity assay. Similarly, both RBL-5 lymphoma and MSV-BL/6 sarcoma cells were effective as stimulator cells in secondary MLTC, although at different optimal ratios (Fig. 2), inducing the formation of CTL which readily lysed ^{51}Cr-labeled MSV-BL/6 target cells (Table 2).

Studies of the specificity of target cell lysis by the primary and secondary MLTC cells showed that the reactivity appeared to be directed against surface antigens common to Rauscher virus- and Graffi virus-induced lymphoma cells and MSV-induced sarcoma cells (6).

As discussed before, mice which were resistant to MSV challenge late after rejection of an MSV tumor contained no detectable CTL in the spleen, while the present studies demonstrated secondary type MLTC responses suggesting the presence of increased numbers of CTL precursors as late as 64 days after MSV inoculation (Table 1). These findings draw attention to the fact that in attempts to evaluate the immune status of tumor-bearing individuals, immune lymphoid cell populations should not only be tested for CTL with the most sensitive methods available, perhaps including cell purification procedures as described above, but also for the presence of precursor or memory T-cells.

Relevance of In Vitro Findings to Resistance to Tumor Growth

Taken together, the studies so far described have shown that at least 3 LMC mechanisms observed *in vitro* may play a role in tumor immunity, namely killing by CTL, by antibody and K cells, and by immune non-T cells. Whether lysis by immune non-T-lymphoid cells is related to antibody-forming cells and K cells remains to be established. In addition, our studies now draw attention to the fact that memory T cells may be present in immune lymphoid cell populations and may be restimulated *in vitro* (or *in vivo*) to form CTL. (Complement dependent lysis by antibody is not being considered in this context).

To assign a definite *in vivo* function to a mechanism observed *in vitro*, one approach consists in studying the activity of a well-defined cell population following transfer into animals which are normally or artificially depleted of a given cell type. As shown above, separation procedures based on physico-chemical or immunological properties are available and may be useful to prepare cells enriched in a given cell category.

In the MSV tumor system, both serum (*19, 20*) and lymphoid cells from immune mice have been shown to confer protection *in vivo* (*19, 21–23*). Since the cytotoxicity assays of spleen cells from MSV immune mice described earlier had shown that late after tumor rejection the effector cells of LMC belonged to the non-T-lymphoid cells, it appeared possible that antibody and K cells were active in the cell transfer experiments. However, cell separation studies demonstrated that only T cells from immune spleens were able to protect irradiated recipients (*23*). As shown by our studies, immune spleen cells also contained increased numbers of CTL precursors, and it appears possible that these transferred memory cells had mediated protection, presumably by rapidly differentiating into CTL. This hypothesis is also supported by the finding that immune spleen cells restimulated *in vitro* in MLTC were able to confer resistance to mice injected with murine leukemia virus-induced leukemia cells (*24*). These MLTC populations contained a relatively large number of CTL, and it is tempting to speculate that protection was related to the direct action of these effector cells. However, immune T cells may also contain helper cells required for IgG antibody formation, and T cells which produce mediators acting on macrophages. Further studies are therefore required to more clearly define the relative importance of the various *in vitro* mechanisms of lymphocyte-mediated cytotoxicity for resistance to tumor growth.

REFERENCES

1. Cerottini, J.-C. and Brunner, K. T. Cell-mediated cytotoxicity, allograft rejection, and tumor immunity. Adv. Immunol., *18*: 67–132, 1974.
2. Cerottini, J.-C., Engers, H. D., MacDonald, H. R., and Brunner, K. T. Generation of cytotoxic T lymphocytes *in vitro*. I. Response of normal and immune mouse spleen cells in mixed leukocyte cultures. J. Exp. Med., *140*: 703–717, 1974.
3. MacDonald, H. R., Engers, H. D., Cerottini, J.-C., and Brunner, K. T. Generation of cytotoxic T lymphocytes *in vitro*. II. Effect of repeated exposure to alloantigens on the cytotoxic activity of long-term mixed leukocyte cultures. J. Exp. Med., *140*: 718–730, 1974.
4. MacDonald, H. R., Cerottini, J.-C., and Brunner, K. T. Generation of cytotoxic T lymphocytes *in vitro*. III. Velocity sedimentation studies of the differentiation and fate of effector cells in long-term mixed leukocyte cultures. J. Exp. Med., *140*: 1511–1521, 1974.
5. Vasudevan, D. M., Brunner, K. T., and Cerottini, J.-C. Detection of cytotoxic T lymphocytes in the EL4 mouse leukemia system: Increased activity of immune spleen and peritoneal cells following preincubation and cell fractionation procedures. Int. J. Cancer, *14*: 301–313, 1974.
6. Plata, F., Cerottini, J.-C., and Brunner, K. T. Primary and secondary *in vitro* generation of cytolytic T lymphocytes in the murine sarcoma virus system. Eur. J. Immunol., *5*: 227–233, 1975.

7. MacDonald, H. R., Phillips, R. A., and Miller, R. G. Allograft immunity in the mouse. II. Physical studies of the development of cytotoxic effector cells from their immediate progenitors. J. Immunol., *111*: 573–589, 1973.

8. Greenberg, A. H. Fractionation of cytotoxic T lymphoblasts on Ficoll gradients by velocity sedimentation. Eur. J. Immunol., *3*: 793–797, 1973.

9. Pelet, J., Brunner, K. T., Nordin, A. A., and Cerottini, J.-C. The relative distribution of cytotoxic lymphocytes and of alloantibody-forming cells in albumin density gradients. Eur. J. Immunol., *1*: 238–242, 1971.

10. Shortman, K., Brunner, K. T., and Cerottini, J.-C. Separation of stages in the development of the T cells involved in cell-mediated immunity. J. Exp. Med., *135*: 1375–1391, 1972.

11. Takasugi, M. and Klein, E. A microassay for cell-mediated immunity. Transplantation, *9*: 219–227, 1970.

12. Lamon, E. W., Skurzak, H. M., and Klein, E. The lymphocyte response to a primary viral neoplasm (MSV) through its entire course in Balb/c mice. Int. J. Cancer, *10*: 581–588, 1972.

13. Plata, F., Gomard, E., Leclerc, J.-C., and Levy, J. P. Comparative *in vitro* studies on effector cell diversity in the cellular immune response to murine sarcoma virus (MSV)-induced tumors in mice. J. Immunol., *112*: 1477–1487, 1974.

14. Lamon, E. W., Wigzell, H., Klein, E., Andersson, B., and Skurzak, H. M. The lymphocyte response to primary moloney sarcoma virus tumors in Balb/c mice: Definition of the active subpopulations at different times after infection. J. Exp. Med., *137*: 1472–1493, 1973.

15. Leclerc, J.-C., Gomard, E., and Levy, J. P. Cell-mediated reaction against tumors induced by oncornaviruses. I. Kinetics and specificity of the immune response in murine sarcoma virus (MSV)-induced tumors and transplanted lymphomas. Int. J. Cancer, *10*: 589–601, 1972.

16. Herberman, R. B., Nunn, M. E., Lavrin, D. H., and Asofsky, R. Effect of antibody to θ antigen on cell-mediated immunity induced in syngeneic mice by murine sarcoma virus. J. Natl. Cancer Inst., *51*: 1509–1512, 1973.

17. Plata, F., Gomard, E., Leclerc, J. C., and Levy, J. P. Further evidence for the involvement of thymus-processed lymphocytes in syngeneic tumor cell cytolysis. J. Immunol., *111*: 667–671, 1973.

18. Engers, H. D., Cerottini, J.-C., and Brunner, K. T. Generation of cytotoxic T lymphocytes *in vitro*. V. Response of normal and immune mouse spleen cells to subcellular alloantigens. J. Immunol., *115*: 356–360, 1975.

19. Fefer, A. Immunotherapy and chemotherapy of moloney sarcoma virus-induced tumors in mice. Cancer Res., *29*: 2177–2183, 1969.

20. Pearson, G. R., Redmon, L. W., and Bass, L. R. Protective effect of immune sera against transplantable moloney virus-induced sarcoma and lymphoma. Cancer Res., *33*: 171–178, 1973.

21. Hellström, I., Hellström, K. E., Pierce, G. E., and Fefer, A. Studies on immunity to autochthonous mouse tumors. Transplant. Proc., *1*: 90–94, 1969.

22. Fefer, A. Immunotherapy of primary moloney sarcoma virus-induced tumors. Int. J. Cancer, *5*: 327–337, 1970.

23. Gorczynski, R. M. Evidence for *in vivo* protection against murine-sarcoma virus-induced tumors by T lymphocytes from immune animals. J. Immunol., *112*: 533–539, 1974.

24. Plata, F. Unpublished.

Discussion of Paper of Drs. Brunner et al.

DR. JERNE: Would you further define K cells?

DR. BRUNNER: K cells have not as yet been fully classified. They appear to be non-adherent mononuclear cells capable of lysing antibody coated target cells. They are most probably lymphoid cells distinct from T and B lymphocytes, although a few studies suggest they are B cells, *i.e.*, immunoglobulin carrying cells. In experiments involving antibody-dependent cell mediated killing of chicken erythrocytes, effector cells consist of monocytes and granulocytes as well as K cells, while human red blood cells are lysed by monocytes and granulocytes only. A common denominator of this type of effector cell is the presence of receptors for the Fc portion of the IgG molecule.

DR. HALPERN: In your separation and purification procedure to obtain a lymphocyte population enriched in cytotoxic cells, you discarded the high density fractions. Have you looked at the cytotoxicity of the cells which you removed?

DR. BRUNNER: We have thus far only examined the phenomenon of increased cytotoxicity following preincubation of the low density cell fraction alone or of the entire lymphocyte population which, of course, includes the high density fractions containing small lymphocytes. Preincubation of the light density fraction resulted in a sharp decrease in activity, whereas similar treatment of the entire population revealed a marked increase. We concluded that the high density fraction, which contains the cells we usually discard, includes precursor cells which may be activated by preincubation.

DR. HALPERN: We, as well as other investigators, have noted inhibitory interactions between lymphocytes and macrophages. Might this serve as an explanation for the fact that when one adds the cytotoxicity of the high density and low density cell population as measured separately in our laboratory, the sum is lower than the effect of each individual fraction?

DR. BRUNNER: By simple density gradient separation of spleen cells, we fortuitously were able to select out a population, comprising 15–20% of the total and located in the low density region, which contained a relatively high frequency of effector cells. This low density population also contained the macrophages, and it is therefore difficult to explain your observation by their inhibitory effect.

DR. HOBBS: Experiments which O. Fakhri and I performed using the mouse plasmacytoma model may offer an explanation for the observation that the sum of individual immune activities was less than a given fraction. In this system we established heterologous rat attack on the mouse tumor, without the generation of T cell-mediated cellular immunity in the rat. Only 5 macrophages per tumor cell are required for effective killing, while 14 K cells, which are non-immune, non-adherent, lymphoid-like cells, are required for good cytotoxicity. However, a mixture of these two effector cell populations is not as good as either alone, perhaps because there is a limited amount of cell surface to which a tumor cell can attach.

DR. AMOS: In partial confirmation of some of your results, we found an extraordinarily high concentration of suppressor cells in the spleens of animals that had been intraperitoneally immunized with EL4 ascites tumor which is known to carry virus. We also observed insensitivity of lymphocytes to the target tumors produced by Rous sarcoma virus (RSV). Is the cell operative in your cultures a T cell or can it possibly be a B cell functioning *via* antibody production? Also, have you demonstrated the specificity of these effector cells?

DR. BRUNNER: In the Moloney sarcoma virus system we have shown that the effector cells are T cells by using anti-θ serum plus complement as well as column separation techniques. Determination of specificity in the MSV system is complex in that the antigen is not clearly defined. We have demonstrated specificity by employing three types of MSV associated cells along with two unrelated control tumor cell lines, one syngeneic to C57BL/6, namely the EL-4 tumor used in the present system, and the P815 mastocytoma, which has DBA/2 histo-compatibility. Neither of the latter two served as target cells for the lymphocytes sensitized in primary or secondary mixed leukocyte tumor-cell cultures.

DR. M. HOZUMI (National Cancer Center Research Institute, Tokyo):   Do you have any proposals concerning the details of the mechanism of target cell killing by lymphocytes? Have substances responsible for this cytotoxicity been isolated?

DR. BRUNNER: Direct contact between the target and effector cells appears to be necessary, and no demonstration of any active principle released by lymphocytes in sufficient concentrations to be cytotoxic has yet been offered. If some factor is released by cytotoxic lymphocytes it must be so specific that it only kills the appropriate target cells and not itself or a syngeneic bystander cell. A cytotoxic T lymphocyte can apparently kill another cytotoxic T lymphocyte, but it cannot commit suicide.

DR. F. SENDO (Cancer Institute, Hokkaido University School of Medicine, Sapporo): You showed that there is an increased number of precursors of cytotoxic cells in the tumor-bearing host. Why don't these cells differentiate into effectors? Also, did you check the activity of the culture medium in which spleen cells from the tumor-bearing animals were preincubated?

DR. BRUNNER: The reason why these precursor cells do not differentiate into cytotoxic lymphocytes may be because of suppressor mechanisms in the tumor-bearing mice or because these cells are saturated with antigen or complexes which inhibit this differentiation. Preliminary results with supernatants from our preincubation cultures have revealed an inhibitory effect in only some experiments.

DR. Y. KINOSHITA (Osaka City University School of Medicine, Osaka): Using lymph node cells obtained from Wistar rats injected with freeze-thawed Walker carcinosarcoma cells we were able to isolate two populations of lymphocytes by a combination of discontinuous density gradient centrifugation and a column packed with absorbent cotton. Our results published in the J. Natl. Cancer Inst., 1974, differ from yours in that the effector lymphocytes, assayed by microscopic observation and a ^{51}Cr release method, were here enriched in the highest density fraction. T cells from peripheral lymphoid tissues were more numerous in the high than low density populations. We proposed that, shortly after the last sensitization, some T cells transform into blastoid cells of low density and then further differentiate to form small lymphocytes, which have high cytotoxic activity and segregate in the higher densities. I, therefore, believe you have separated effector lymphocytes at the stage of blastoid cells or larger cells, while we performed this separation at the end of the maturation pathway.

DR. BRUNNER: In our experiments we took advantage of the fact that early in the immune response the cytotoxic lymphocyte is a low density large lymphoblast which will later transform into a small lymphocyte with higher density but is still cytotoxic. It is purely operationally that we segregated out the low density fraction to obtain a population with increased cytotoxic activity. I fully agree that cytotoxic lymphocytes exist in the high density fraction also, as well as precursor cells. Thus, depending on which type of cell you want, you can locate these effector cells in either fraction. It also depends on the system used for testing cytotoxic activity, as in the microplate assay, which usually requires a 48-hr incubation period, and even in course of the shorter lytic assays, differentiation may occur. Therefore, one may find most of the cytotoxic activity in high density cells either because they have had time to differentiate into cytotoxic lymphocytes, or because they already possess a high level of effector activity.

HOST DEFENSE AGAINST CANCER AND ITS POTENTIATION, D. MIZUNO ET AL. (EDS.),
UNIV. OF TOKYO PRESS, TOKYO / UNIV. PARK PRESS, BALTIMORE, PP. 55-65, 1975

Dissociation between Delayed Hypersensitivity and Cytotoxic Activity against Syngeneic or Allogeneic Tumor Grafts

Kikuo Nomoto, Mikio Sato, Yasutsugu Yano, Kazuto Taniguchi, and Kenji Takeya

Department of Microbiology, School of Medicine, Kyushu University, Fukuoka, Japan

Abstract: Relationship between delayed hypersensitivity and cytotoxicity against cellular antigens was studied in syngeneic and allogeneic hosts. A methylcholanthrene (MCA)-induced sarcoma of a C57BL/6 mouse was used as immunogen and as target cells. 1) In syngeneic C57BL/6 mice, cytotoxic activity of lymphocytes developed only after immunization with viable tumor cells (VTC) as demonstrated by *in vivo* neutralization test. Delayed hypersensitivity developed only after immunization with tumor cells in complete Freund's adjuvant (CFA) as demonstrated by migration inhibition test. 2) When syngeneic mice had been treated with tumor cells in CFA (T-CFA) previously, cytotoxic lymphocytes were raised after the booster with VTC. 3) In allogeneic C3H/He mice, cytotoxic lymphocytes were raised also only after immunization with VTC. On the other hand, delayed hypersensitivity developed not only after immunization with T-CFA, but also after immunization with VTC, although the former induced more efficiently delayed hypersensitivity than did the latter. 4) AKR mice were immunized with MCA tumor cells. Their spleen cells were mixed with MH134 tumor cells for *in vivo* neutralization test. When spleen cells were obtained from the mice immunized with VTC, growth of bystander MH134 tumor was inhibited. Spleen cells of the mice immunized with T-CFA could not inhibit growth of MH134 tumor.

These results suggest the possibility of dissociation between delayed hypersensitivity and cytotoxicity against cellular antigens. These results indicate also that development of cytotoxic activity depends entirely upon the existence of VTC as immunogen.

Cell-mediated immunity includes several types of reactions of which expressions are entirely different from each other. Typical patterns of cell-mediated immunity may be classified into three types, namely, homograft rejection, delayed hypersensitivity, and protective immunity against intracellular parasites, such as *Mycobacteria*, *Salmonella*, *Brucella*, and *Listeria*. Homograft rejection has been found to depend primarily upon the activity of cytotoxic lymphocytes. Delayed hypersensitivity includes several types of skin reactions all of which are evoked by cellular infiltration at the site of antigen injection. Tuberculin type and Jones-Mote type of sensitivity and contact sensitivity belong to this category. Tuberculin type has been assumed to be the most typical pattern of delayed hypersensitivity. In this type of skin reaction, the majority of infiltrating cells are macrophages and the minority are small lymphocytes. Protective immunity against intracellular parasites depends upon the inhibitory effect of activated immune macrophages on the intracellular proliferation of such bacteria. All the reactions have proved to depend upon thymus-derived sensitized lymphocytes in the antigen-specific steps in their elicitation.

In many experiments or clinical cases, two of these three categories develop concurrently, for example, protective immunity and delayed hypersensitivity in infection with intracellular parasites as mentioned above, or cytotoxic activity and delayed hypersensitivity in homograft reaction.

In this series of our studies, experiments have been designed to know whether these reactions have to be ascribed to the functions of the same population of sensitized lymphocytes or to the functions of the different subpopulations of sensitized lymphocytes. In this communication, we would like to present our studies on the relationship between cytotoxic activity and delayed hypersensitivity against tumor specific antigens or allogeneic antigens.

Nomoto, one of the authors, started the studies in this communication 6 years ago in Yale University under the support of Dr. Waksman, Dr. Gershon, and Dr. Greene. An allotransplantable lymphoma of a golden hamster was presented as a material by them (1). When the lymphoma cells were grafted subcutaneously into inbred MHA hamsters or outbred golden hamsters, tumor grew progressively and induced immunity concomitantly (2). A large number of mononuclear cells were detected around and within the grafts, of which the majority consisted of macrophages and the minority consisted of small lymphocytes (3). The study in Yale University suggested that macrophages were accumulated as the result of delayed hypersensitivity and that lymphocytes exerted cytotoxic effect on lymphoma cells. In other words, cytotoxic activity and delayed hypersensitivity developed concurrently (4).

In Japan, we had to change the hosts from MHA hamsters to outbred golden hamsters which were purchased from a local breeder. In these golden hamsters, the lymphoma grew progressively and raised concomitant immunity as well as in MHA hamsters. However, only a few macrophages could be detected around the grafts. In the golden hamsters in our country, thus, tumor-bearing state induced cytotoxic activity but not delayed hypersensitivity as demonstrated by a migration inhibition test or a peritoneal macrophage disappearance test. These results suggested a possible dissociation between cytotoxic activity and delayed hypersensitivity against cellular antigens (5). Unfortunately, the extent of antigenic difference between the hosts and grafts was not quantitatively definite, since the lymphoma had been derived from an outbred golden hamster and the hosts were outbred golden hamsters.

In the studies presented in this paper, a methylcholanthrene (MCA)-induced sarcoma of female C57BL/6 origin was chosen as an antigen. This tumor proved to have a tumor-specific antigen of a substantial degree. C57BL/6 mice were used as syngeneic hosts, in which tumor-specific antigen might be recognized as a foreign antigen. C3H/He and AKR mice were used as allogeneic hosts, in which H-2 antigens and a tumor-specific antigen might be recognized as foreign antigens.

Immune Response after Primary Immunization in Syngeneic Hosts

Tumor cells 5×10^6 in saline viable tumor cells (VTC), in complete Freund's adjuvant (CFA) or in incomplete Freund's adjuvant (IFA) were subcutaneously injected into the right flanks of female C57BL/6 mice. Tumors grew progressively after the inoculation of viable tumor cells (VTC), but not after the injection of tumor cells in CFA(T-CFA) or in IFA(T-IFA). Cytotoxic activity and delayed hypersensitivity were examined 12 days after immunization (Tables 1–3).

The mixed solution of 5% starch and 5% proteose-peptone was injected intraperitoneally on day 9 and peritoneal exudate cells (PEC) were harvested 72 hr later. PEC were added to VTC in the ratios of 3 to 1 or 10 to 1 and the mixtures were subcutaneously inoculated into the C57BL/6 mice which had received 600 R of whole body irradiation (Table 1). Tumor growth was read 8 days later. In this *in vivo* neutralization test, tumor growth was inhibited by the addition of the PEC from the mice immunized with VTC, namely tumor-bearing mice. PEC from non-treated controls, the mice immunized with T-CFA, or those immunized with T-IFA did not exhibit inhibitory effect on tumor growth.

TABLE 1. Neutralization Test with PEC in Syngeneic System

| Treatment on day 0 | Tumor cells ($\times 10^5$) to PEC | | | |
| | 1 : 3 | | 1 : 10 | |
	No. of tumor growth/total	Tumor size (mm²)	No. of tumor growth/total	Tumor size (mm²)
None	11/20	22.1	19/36	13.0
VTC	2/20	5.3	1/20	0.5
T-CFA	13/19	25.4	10/19	20.0
T-IFA	ND	ND	13/18	13.0

C57BL/6 — 12 days — PEC + tumor cells — 600 R — 8 days

Immunization with tumor cells (5×10^6)

ND : not determined.

Cytotoxic activity of the PEC was completely depleted by the treatment with anti-θ antiserum and complement.

VTC 5×10^6 were subcutaneously inoculated into 4 groups, namely, non-treated control and groups treated in such ways as mentioned above (day 12). Tumor growth was read 8 days after the rechallenge test (day 20) (Table 2). Tumor

TABLE 2. Rechallenge Test with VTC on Day 12 after Immunization in C57BL/6

Treatment on day 0	Tumor growth on day 20 (8 days after rechallenge)	
	No. of tumor growth/total	Tumor size (mm^2)
None	28/34	55.6
VTC	2/20	11.9
T-CFA	16/17	58.0
T-IFA	13/16	68.1

C57BL/6 — 12 days — 8 days

Immunization with tumor cells (5×10⁶)   Rechallenge with tumor cells (7×10⁶)

TABLE 3. Migration Inhibition Test with PEC Harvested 12 Days after Immunization in C57BL/6

Treatment on day 0	Percent migration in the presence of membrane antigen	Migration area Ag(+)/Ag(−)
None	153.0±28.3[a]	18.4/12.0
VTC 5×10⁶	156.7±21.9	13.0/ 8.3
T-CFA	87.4± 7.6	13.0/14.8
T-IFA	152.3±16.5	18.3/12.0

[a] $\dfrac{\text{An average migration area in the presence of antigen}}{\text{An average migration area in the absence of antigen}} \times 100.$

growth was inhibited only in the mice which had been immunized with VTC and were rendered in tumor-bearing state.

Migration inhibition test was performed using the PEC harvested on day 12 after immunization (Table 3). Sonicated antigen of tumor cells was used as the test antigen. The addition of sonicated tumor antigen inhibited migration, when PEC were obtained from the mice immunized with T-CFA. The addition of sonicated tumor antigen promoted migration, when PEC were obtained from other groups.

In the syngeneic system, thus, cytotoxic activity developed only after immunization with VTC and delayed hypersensitivity developed only after immunization with T-CFA.

Appearance of Cytotoxic Activity and Delayed Hypersensitivity after the Booster Immunization in Syngeneic Hosts

Booster immunization with VTC, T-CFA, or T-IFA was performed in the C57BL/6 mice which had received VTC, T-CFA, or T-IFA. Primary immunization, booster immunization, and examinations of cytotoxicity and delayed hypersensitivity were done, respectively on day −20(−14), day −10(−7) and day 0. PEC were harvested on day 0 for the examinations from the groups treated in various ways. The results are summarized in Table 4.

TABLE 4. Dependency of Cytotoxicity on the Presence of Viable Tumor Grafts

Day −20 (−14)	Day −10 (−7)	Cytotoxicity on day 0	Delayed hypersensitivity
None	VTC	+	−
T-CFA	None	− (suppression)	++
"	VTC	+	−
T-IFA	None	−	−
"	VTC	+	−
VTC	None	+	−
"	T-CFA	+⊥	+
"	"	+⊥	−

Cytotoxic activity was detected in the PEC from the groups which were rendered in tumor-bearing state as results of primary or booster injection with VTC, namely, (none → VTC), (T-CFA → VTC), (T-IFA → VTC), (VTC → none), (VTC → T-CFA), and (VTC → T-IFA) mice. These results showed that development of cytotoxic activity depended entirely upon the existence of VTC as immunogen.

Delayed hypersensitivity was detectable in the mice which had received VTC in primary immunization and T-CFA in booster. On the contrary, delayed hypersensitivity was diminished after booster with VTC in the mice which had received T-CFA in primary immunization and had raised delayed hypersensitivity once. The mechanisms of such mutual regulation between cytotoxicity and delayed hypersensitivity remain to be determined in future studies.

Immune Response after Primary Immunization in Allogeneic Hosts

C3H/He mice were used as hosts and an MCA sarcoma of C57BL/6 origin was used as an antigenic tumor. Cytotoxic activity was examined by *in vivo* neutralization

TABLE 5. Neutralization Test with Spleen Cells in Allogeneic Mice

Treatment on day 0	Tumor cells (5×10^5) to spleen cells			
	1 : 5		1 : 25	
	No. of tumor growth/total	Tumor size (mm²)	No. of tumor growth/total	Tumor size (mm²)
None	14/15	54.0	12/15	24.8
VTC 5×10^6	0/16	0	0/16	0
T-CFA	15/16	42.1	15/16	26.3
T-IFA	13/13	45.8	13/13	36.6

C3H/He ──10 days──► Spleen cells + tumor cells ──► 600 R C3H/He ──10 days──►

Immunization with tumor of C57BL/6

TABLE 6. Migration Inhibition Test with PEC Harvested 10 Days after Immunization in C3H/He

Treatment on day 0	Percent migration in the presence of antigen	Migration area Ag (+)/Ag (−)
None	110.5± 4.4[a]	14.5/13.1
VTC	86.6±15.6	28.4/32.8
T-CFA	42.5±10.9	23.7/55.9
T-IFA	114.1±15.0	19.2/16.8

[a] $\dfrac{\text{An average migration area in the presence of antigen}}{\text{An average migration area in the absence of antigen}} \times 100.$

test 10 days after immunization (Table 5). Spleens were used as sources of cytotoxic lymphocytes. VTC 5×10^5 were added to spleen cells in the ratios of 1 to 5 or 1 to 25 and the mixtures were injected subcutaneously into the C3H/He mice which had received 600R of whole body irradiation. Tumor growth was recorded 10 days later. Tumor growth was suppressed by the addition of the spleen cells from the mice immunized with VTC. Inhibitory effect on tumor growth could not be detected in the spleen cells from the non-treated controls, the mice immunized with T-CFA, or those immunized with T-IFA.

Migration inhibition test was done with the PEC harvested 10 days after immunization (Table 6). Migration was inhibited remarkably in the presence of sonicated tumor antigen, when the PEC were obtained from the mice immunized with T-CFA. Migration inhibition of a substantial degree was detected in the presence of the antigen, when the PEC were obtained from the mice immunized with VTC.

With respect to the development of cytotoxic activity, stimulation with viable tumor grafts was required in allogeneic as well as syngeneic hosts. However, delayed hypersensitivity was raised by immunization not only with T-CFA but also with VTC in allogencic hosts. Delayed hypersensitivity could not be induced by immunization with VTC in syngeneic hosts, as mentioned above.

Indirect Target Cell Destruction in Allogeneic Hosts

AKR mice were immunized with MCA tumor cells of C57BL/⁶ origin. Spleen and lymph node cells were harvested 7 days after immunization with VTC in saline or T-CFA. A portion of the lymphoid cells were used for *in vitro* direct cytotoxicity test as control. Lymphoid cells 5×10^7 were added to cultured MCA tumor cells 5×10^5. Three days later, VTC were counted (Table 7). Cytotoxic activity was detected only in the spleen cells harvested from the mice immunized with VTC.

A portion of the lymphoid cells were used for *in vivo* test of indirect cytotoxicity. MH134 hepatoma cells of C3H origin were used as bystander target cells. Lymphoid cells 5×10^7/ml were added to MH134 cells 5×10^5/ml. Sonicated MCA tumor antigen was added to one half of individual groups but not to the other half. Three-tenths milliliter of the mixed cell suspensions was subcutaneously injected into the AKR mice which had received 600 R of whole body irradiation. Suppressive effect on the growth of bystander MH134 tumors was detected in the spleen cells obtained

TABLE 7. Comparison between Direct and Indirect Target Cell Destruction

Treatment on day 0	Direct target cell destruction against MCA tumor	Indirect target cell destruction against MH134 tumor	
		Sonicated Ag (+)	Sonicated Ag (−)
None	100%[a]	21/25 (84)[b]	ND
VTC	22	8/34 (24)	2/18 (11)
T-CFA	82	22/23 (86)	ND

Ag (+): antigen present. Ag (−): antigen absent. ND: not determined.
[a] Percent viability. [b] Number of tumor growth/total number of mice. Number in parentheses represents %.

TABLE 8. Summarized Results in Syngeneic and Allogeneic Systems

Immunization	Tumor cells	Responses		
		Direct cytotoxicity	Indirect cytotoxicity	Delayed hypersensitivity
MCA-syngeneic	VTC	+	(−)[a]	−
	T-CFA	−	(−)	+
	T-IFA	−	(−)	−
MCA-allogeneic	VTC	++	+	+
	T-CFA	−	−	++
	T-IFA	−	−	−

[a] Negative results were obtained in a preliminary experiment.

from the mice immunized with VTC but not in those from the mice immunized with T-CFA (Table 7). Cytotoxic activity was detected not only in the presence of sonicated immunizing antigen but also in the absence of the antigen.

The treatment with anti-θ antiserum and complement eliminated completely the direct and indirect cytotoxic activity from the lymphoid cells harvested from the mice immunized with viable tumor cells.

All the results in this communication are summarized in Table 8.

DISCUSSION

Delayed skin reactions against allogeneic cellular antigens were reported to be elicited in guinea pigs (6), hamsters (7), and rats (8) after allografting. Since the establishment of migration inhibition test as an *in vitro* correlate of delayed hypersensitivity by George and Vaughan (9), delayed hypersensitivity was studied extensively on allografts, tumor-isografts or autochthonous tumors. Migration inhibition test has been advanced as a sensitive method to detect allograft rejection in an early stage in guinea pigs (10), rats (11), and mice (12, 13). Delayed hypersensitivity was found to become positive in human tumors as demonstrated by skin reaction (14), migration inhibition (15), or syngeneic guinea pig MCA tumors as demonstrated by skin reaction (16). These results suggest that delayed hypersensitivity and cytotoxic activity might be ascribed to the same population of sensitized lymphocytes or at least cytotoxic activity was accompanied by delayed hypersensitivity. In our present results, immunization with viable allogeneic tumor cells raised not only cytotoxic activity but also delayed hypersensitivity.

In our experiments, immunization with syngeneic tumor cells raised cytotoxic activity but not delayed hypersensitivity. However, delayed hypersensitivity was raised against syngeneic tumor antigen, when the mice were immunized with T-CFA. Moreover, cytotoxic activity did not develop after immunization with syngeneic T-CFA. These results seem to support the concept that cytotoxic activity and delayed hypersensitivity are ascribable to the different subpopulations of sensitized lymphocytes. Tigelaar and Gorzynski reported results suggesting that separable populations of thymus-dependent (T) cells were involved in mediating cytotoxic activity and migration inhibitory activity against allogeneic mastocytoma cells (17). In their experiments, cytotoxic activity was found to reside in spleen-seeking and small lymphocyte-rich population, while migration inhibitory activity was found to reside in lymph node-seeking and large lymphocyte-rich population. Loewi and Temple also reported dissociated development between cytotoxic activity and delayed hypersensitivity against chicken erythrocytes in guinea pigs (18).

Appearance of cytotoxic activity depended entirely on the existence of antigenic stimulation by live tumor grafts in both syngeneic and allogeneic hosts. The existence of T-CFA did not interfere with cytotoxic activity raised by syngeneic viable tumor grafts as primary or secondary immunization. We have as yet no decisive explanation on the mechanism whereby viable tumor grafts raise cytotoxic activity.

Booster with syngeneic viable tumor cells interfered with delayed hypersensitivity which had been induced once by immunization with tumor cells in CFA as primary immunization (Table 4). This result may suggest the possibility that cytotoxic lymphocytes and effector lymphocytes in delayed hypersensitivity respond to the common antigen. Mutual regulation between both types of cell-mediated immunity will be studied on the basis of this finding.

In indirect target cell destruction, cytotoxic activity was detected in the lymphoid cells from the mice immunized with allogeneic VTC. In this system, cytotoxic lymphocytes and bystander target cells acquired contact only through mechanical one. The addition of the sonicated antigen of immunizing tumor cells was not required for the expression of cytotoxicity against bystander target cells. Cytotoxic activity was not detectable in both the presence and the absence of sonicated immunizing antigen, when the lymphoid cells were harvested from the mice immunized with allogeneic T-CFA. The mechanism of indirect cytotoxicity in this paper may be different from the mechanism on which indirect target cell destruction by purified protein derivative (PPD)-sensitized lymphocytes depend (19).

Cytotoxic lymphocytes proved to be thymus-derived in both direct and indirect target cell destruction. Cytotoxic activity was diminished by the treatment with anti-θ antiserum and complement not only in syngeneic but also in allogeneic system, at least, against an MCA tumor of C57BL/6. However, in other systems reported by many investigators, destruction of allogeneic or syngeneic tumor cells depends upon cytotoxic activity of activated macrophages (*20–22*) or antibody-dependent cell-mediated cytotoxicity (*23–25*).

In vivo systems such as ours include many problems in terms of antigen modification, relative sensitivity of the methods for detection, and others. In spite of such problems, attempts to separate each type of cell-mediated immunity seem to be required for further development of immunobiological studies on this subject.

REFERENCES

1. Greene, H. S. M. and Harvey, E. K. The inhibitory influence of a transplanted hamster lymphoma on metastasis. Cancer Res., *20*: 1094–1100, 1960.
2. Gershon, R. K., Carter, R. L., and Kondo, K. On concomitant immunity in tumor-bearing hamsters. Nature, *213*: 674–676, 1967.
3. Carter, R. L. and Gershon, R. K. Studies on homotransplantable lymphomas in hamsters. I. Histologic responses in lymphoid tissues and their relationship to metastasis. Am. J. Pathol., *49*: 637–655, 1966.
4. Nomoto, K., Gershon, R. K., and Waksman, B. H. Role of nonimmunized macrophages in the rejection of an allotransplanted lymphoma. J. Natl. Cancer Inst., *44*: 739–749, 1970.
5. Nomoto, K., Yamada, H., Muraoka, S., and Takeya, K. The role of sensitized lymphocytes and macrophages in cell-mediated immunity against tumor grafts. GANN Monograph on Cancer Research, *16*: 89–98, 1974.
6. Brent, L., Brown, J. B., and Medawar, P. B. Quantitative studies on tissue transplantation immunity. VI. Hypersensitivity reactions associated with rejection of homografts. Proc. Roy. Soc., Ser. B, *156*: 187–209, 1962.
7. Ramseir, H. and Billingham, R. E. Delayed cutaneous hypersensitivity reactions and transplantation immunity in Syrian hamsters. Ann. N. Y. Acad. Sci., *120*: 379–392, 1964.
8. Strelilein, J. W. and Billingham, R. E. Cutaneous hypersensitivity reaction to cellular isoantigens in rats. J. Exp. Med., *126*: 455–473, 1967.
9. George, M. and Vaughan, J. H. *In vitro* cell migration as a model for delayed hypersensitivity. Proc. Soc. Exp. Biol. Med., *111*: 514–521, 1963.
10. Al-Askari, S. and Lawrence, H. S. *In vitro* studies on transplantation immunity. II. The migration inhibition in homograft reactions in guinea pigs. Cell. Immunol., *6*: 292–299, 1973.
11. Eidemiller, L. R. and Bell, P. R. F. Migration inhibition and homograft rejection in rats. Transplantation, *13*: 5–8, 1972.
12. Friedman, H. Cellular immunity of mice to skin allo-grafts assessed by direct and indirect macrophage inhibition reactions *in vitro*. Transplantation, *11*: 288–294, 1971.
13. Al-Askari, S., David, J. R., Lawrence, H. S., and Thomas, L. *In vitro* studies on homograft sensitivity. Nature, *205*: 916–917, 1965.
14. Bluming, A. Z., Vogel, C. L., Siegler, J. L., and Kiryabwire, J. W. M. Delayed cutaneous sensitivity reactions to extracts of autologous malignant melanoma: A second look. J. Natl. Cancer Inst., *48*: 17–24, 1972.
15. Hilberg, R. W., Balcerzak, S. P., and LoBuglio, A. F. A migration inhibition-factor assay for tumor immunity in man. Cell. Immunol., *7*: 152–158, 1973.
16. Holmes, E. C., Reisfeld, R. A., and Morton, O. L. Delayed cutaneous hypersensitivity to cell-free tumor antigens. Cancer Res., *33*: 199–202, 1973.

17. Tigelaar, R. E. and Gorzynski, R. M. Separable populations of activated thymus-derived lymphocytes identified in two assays for cell-mediated immunity to murine tumor allografts. J. Exp. Med., *140*: 267–289, 1974.

18. Loewi, G. and Temple, A. Cytotoxicity of immune guinea-pig cells. I. Investigation of a correlation with delayed hypersensitivity and a comparison of cytotoxicity of spleen, lymph node and peritoneal exudate cells. Immunology, *23*: 559–567, 1972.

19. Ruddle, N. H. and Waksman, B. H. Cytotoxic effect of lymphocyte-antigen interaction in delayed hypersensitivity. Science, *157*: 1060–1062, 1967.

20. Granger, G. A. and Weiser, R. S. Homograft target cells: Specific destruction *in vitro* by contact interaction with immune macrophages. Science, *145*: 1427–1429, 1964.

21. Bennet, B. Specific suppression of tumor growth by isolated peritoneal macrophages from immunized mice. J. Immunol., *95*: 656–664, 1965.

22. Grant, C. K. and Alexander, P. Nonspecific cytotoxicity of spleen cells and the specific cytotoxic action of thymus-derived lymphocytes *in vitro*. Cell. Immunol., *14*: 46–51, 1974.

23. MacLennan, I. C. M. and Loewi, G. Effect of specific antibody to target cells on their specific and non-specific interactions with lymphocytes. Nature, *219*: 1069–1070, 1968.

24. Perlmann, P., Perlmann, H., and Biberfeld, P. Specifically cytotoxic lymphocytes produced by preincubation with antibody-complexed target cells. J. Immunol., *108*: 558–561, 1972.

25. Tucker, D. F., Dennert, G., and Lennox, E. S. Thymus-derived lymphocytes as effectors of cell-mediated immunity to syngeneic and allogeneic transplants in the rat. J. Immunol., *113*: 1302–1312, 1974.

Discussion of Paper of Drs. Nomoto et al.

Dr. JERNE: You have clearly demonstrated that the cells responsible for delayed hypersensitivity are different from cytotoxic cells, but can you separate them when present in the same population, perhaps on the basis of morphologic criteria?

Dr. NOMOTO: We were unsuccessful in separating these two cell fractions by density gradient centrifugation, and there did not appear to be distinct morphologic differences by which they can be distinguished.

Dr. HALPERN: We have been able to afford a high degree of protection in an allogeneic system by intraperitoneal immunization of mice with tumor cells, somewhat modified by heating, administered in CFA. Have you noted similar results in other syngeneic or allogeneic systems?

Dr. NOMOTO: We utilized another allogeneic system in which administration of tumor cells in CFA could indeed raise cytotoxic activity.

In Vitro and In Vivo Effects of Immunosuppressive and Toxic Material Produced and Released by Cancer Cells*

J. C. Kennedy

Division of Cancer Research of the Department of Pathology, Queen's University and the Kingston General Hospital, Kingston, Ontario, Canada

Abstract: Certain types of murine cancer cells produce and release biologically active non-particulate material which is able to reproduce both *in vitro* and *in vivo* at least some of the effects of the cancer cells from which the material was obtained. The addition of progressively increasing numbers of such cancer cells to cultures containing syngeneic mouse spleen cells and sheep erythrocytes at first stimulates and then strongly inhibits the *in vitro* hemolytic plaque-forming cell (PFC) response. Exactly the same pattern of response is obtained if preparations of supernatant from the cancer cell cultures are substituted for the cancer cells. This cancer cell culture supernatant material can also inhibit thymidine incorporation by phytohemagglutinin-stimulated spleen cells, plaque formation by hemolytic PFC obtained from immunized mice, and proliferation of human fibroblasts. When injected into normal mice, the cancer-derived material causes immunodepression of a degree similar to that observed in mice bearing large tumors containing the corresponding type of cancer cells. Moreover, the mechanisms responsible for the immunodepression in both cases appear to have certain similarities. Just as injection of a non-immunosuppressive dose of carbon tetrachloride (CCl$_4$) can lead to immunodepression in mice bearing tumors which are too small to be immunosuppressive by themselves, so also immunodepression can be produced in mice pre-treated with CCl$_4$ and then injected with a non-immunosuppressive dose of the cancer-derived material. It is therefore suggested that the non-specific immunodepression associated with the presence of large tumors is caused by soluble material produced and released by the malignant cell component of those tumors. It is also suggested that the biologically active cancer-derived material is ordinarily metabolized, excreted, or otherwise rendered harmless by some mechanism which can be damaged by CCl$_4$.

* This work was supported by the National Cancer Institute of Canada.

Basic Concepts and Models

The normal relationship between a cancer and its host is a state of war. Each of the combatants is equipped with "offensive weapons" capable of killing or damaging his opponent, and each also has "purely defensive" protective mechanisms which can prevent or repair damage caused by enemy attacks. This paper will present and discuss evidence that one of the offensive weapons possessed by certain types of cancer cells is a soluble material which is non-specifically toxic to a variety of different cell types. Consequently, it is capable of causing a variety of different local and systemic effects, including the localized suppression of various host defense mechanisms which takes place in the immediate environment of a tumor, and the non-specific systemic immunodepression which is often found in association with advanced cancer. Evidence that the host defenses include a "purely defensive" mechanism capable of metabolizing or excreting the cancer toxin will also be presented. It must be emphasized that although this mechanism is not capable of killing a single cancer cell, it may be of critical importance in the complex relationship between a cancer and its host, since it can prevent circulating cancer toxin from damaging the immune system and thereby destroying the host's chief offensive weapon against cancer.

Our present working model for this particular aspect of the tumor-host relationship may be summarized as follows. The first few malignant cells which appear during the development of a toxin-producing cancer are highly susceptible to destruction if detected by cells of immune system. However, if they escape destruction until the developing cell mass is large enough to saturate their local environment with an immunosuppressive concentration of the cancer toxin, then the cancer will become practically invulnerable to immunological attack unless the strength of that attack can be increased by additional stimulation of the immune system. As the tumor continues to increase in size, it releases progressively larger amounts of toxin per unit time. At first the toxin causes little systemic damage, since a host protective mechanism which is capable of metabolizing or excreting the toxin maintains its serum concentration at relatively low levels, but eventually the output of the toxin becomes so great that the maximum capacity of the protective mechanism is exceeded. At this point in the natural history of the disease, the concentration of toxin in the circulation quickly rises to a level at which it can produce harmful effects, and the clinical state of the cancer patient suddenly deteriorates with the rapid development of immunodepression, multiple secondaries, severe wasting of muscles and fatty tissue, various metabolic abnormalities, and eventually death. On the basis of this model, it can be predicted that exposure of a cancer patient or tumor-bearing animal to any agent capable of damaging the mechanism which metabolizes or excretes the cancer toxin may precipitate sudden deterioration in the clinical situation and acceleration of the natural course of the disease.

Non-specific Immunodepression Associated with Cancer

Different types of malignant disease may result in very different patterns of immunodepression. However, if we eliminate from consideration all malignancies involving cells of the marrow and lymphoid organs, and all ascitic cancers, we are left with a much more homogeneous situation. Typically, the immunodepression associated with solid tumors is rather late in onset, and appears in association with other systemic signs and symptoms of malignancy. What is the cause of this non-specific immunodepression? There appear to be five reasonable possibilities. First, malignant cells might compete with cells of the immune system for a limited supply of essential nutrients. Second, non-specific stress resulting from the presence of a large tumor might induce the host to produce immunosuppressive quantities of steroid hormones. Third, material released by damaged host or tumor cells might induce the liver to increase production of α-2 globulin, a known immunosuppressive material whose serum levels are often increased in cancer patients. Fourth, the chronic antigenic stimulation caused by constant release of tumor material into the circulation might induce the immune system to produce immunoregulatory cells or factors capable of causing non-specific immunodepression. Fifth, the cancer cells themselves might produce non-specifically immunosuppressive material and release it into the general circulation. These mechanisms are not necessarily mutually exclusive, and it is possible that all five may have some part in producing cancer-associated immunodepression.

The suggestion that localized cancers may secrete biologically active material which is responsible for various systemic abnormalities often found in association with cancer was first made by Greenstein and Andervont (1) in 1942. Since that time, the excellent pioneering work of Nakahara and others (2–14) has demonstrated that material capable of causing a variety of biological effects when injected into animals can be extracted from many different kinds of tumors. Many others (15–32) have reported that immunosuppressive material is often present in the body fluids of cancer patients or animals bearing tumors, and there have also been several reports (33–35) that pure cultures of cancer cells produce material which shows biological activity when tested in vitro against a variety of other types of cells. However, it should be noted that material extracted from tumors growing in vivo is not necessarily derived from the malignant cell component of those tumors, and immunosuppressive material obtained from serum, peritoneal fluid, or urine may be of host rather than tumor origin. Consequently, we adopted the following experimental approach to the question of whether or not the non-specific immunodepression found in association with certain solid tumors is caused by material produced and released by the malignant cells. First, we selected a tumor (SaD2-AG, a methylcholanthrene-induced fibrosarcoma) which does not produce immunodepression until quite late in the course of the disease. This is the usual pattern found in human patients with cancers other than those of the marrow and reticuloendothelial system. Second, we used only pure cultures of the cancer cells being tested rather than cells obtained from tumors. In this way we avoided any possibility that what we were studying was derived from the reactive host cells which are present in large numbers in many different kinds of tumors (36, 37). We also could be sure that our preparations of cancer cells were not coated with any host-derived material, such as immunoglobulins, or contaminated by bacteria, fungi, or mycoplasma. Third, we did not attempt to isolate immunosuppressive material from the cancer cells by chemical procedures but instead collected and tested the supernatants from cultures of healthy cancer cells, in the hope that material obtained in such a way might be similar to whatever material is released by cancer cells *in vivo*. The technique used to prepare the supernatants has been described in detail elsewhere (*38*). The important points to be noted are that these preparations contained no serum and no viruses, and the nutrients which had been used up during culture of the cancer cells were replaced. The effects of the fibrosarcoma cells and fibrosarcoma culture supernatants were compared both *in vitro* and *in vivo*. In both situations we were able to demonstrate that the immunodepression produced by the cancer cell culture supernatants and that produced by the cancer cells themselves shared certain characteristics. While such similarities do not prove beyond question that immunosuppressive material similar to that produced by the fibrosarcoma cells *in vitro* is responsible for the immunodepression caused by fibrosarcomas *in vivo*, it does appear to be the most reasonable explanation for the data.

In Vitro Effects of Fibrosarcoma Cells and Culture Supernatants

Figure 1 combines data from representative experiments involving four different test systems. One system involved Marbrook (*39*) cultures containing a fixed number of mouse spleen cells, sheep erythrocytes (SRBC), and either various numbers of heavily irradiated cancer cells or various concentrations of cancer cell supernatant material. The anti-sheep plaque-forming cell (PFC) responses were

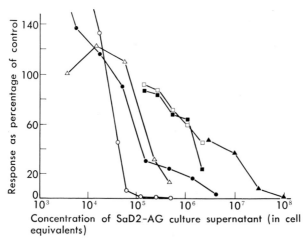

FIG. 1.   *In vitro* effects of fibrosarcoma cells and culture supernatants. Various amounts of SaD2-AG culture supernatants were added to spleen cell cultures containing SRBC (PFC response assayed on day 3, ●), spleen cell cultures containing PHA (thymidine incorporation measured on day 3, △), human fibroblast cultures in log-phase growth (total viable cells counted on day 6, ▲), and pre-formed PFC from the spleens of mice immunized with SRBC 4 days previously (PFC assayed after 30-min incubation at 37°C, ■; or 1 hr at 0°C, □). PFC response of spleen cell cultures in presence of various numbers of irradiated SaD2-AG cells (○).

assayed 3 days later. As reported previously (*38*), the addition of very small numbers of cancer cells or comparable amounts of cancer cell "toxin" resulted in stimulation of the *in vitro* PFC responses; somewhat larger doses of cancer cells or toxin produced strong inhibition. Although not illustrated in Fig. 1, the addition of comparable numbers of syngeneic fibroblasts or comparable amounts of fibroblast culture supernatant did not produce inhibition (*38*).

The cancer cell culture supernatant material is measured in "cell equivalents." The number of cell equivalents in the total volume of supernatant removed from a culture of cancer cells after 24 hr of incubation is the total number of cells in that culture. Various dilutions of the concentrated supernatant are then expressed as appropriate fractions of the total number of cells from which the stock supernatant was obtained. It is of considerable interest that the *in vitro* PFC response inhibition curves for intact cancer cells are so similar to those obtained by the use of cancer cell culture supernatants expressed in terms of cancer cell equivalents.

Figure 1 also includes an inhibition curve for thymidine incorporation into spleen cells stimulated by phytohemagglutinin (PHA). Various concentrations of cancer cell culture supernatant were added to cultures containing a fixed number of mouse spleen cells and PHA; thymidine incorporation was measured 3 days later. The resulting thymidine incorporation inhibition curve is very similar to the curves showing inhibition of *in vitro* PFC responses.

Both *in vitro* PFC responses and stimulation of thymidine incorporation by PHA involve cell proliferation and depend upon normal thymus-derived cell (T cell) function. However, the cancer toxin also has an effect upon non-dividing bone marrow-derived cells (B cells). Tubes containing various concentrations of fibrosarcoma cell culture supernatant and spleen cells from mice injected with SRBC 4 days previously were held at either 37°C for 30 min or 0°C for one hour, and then assayed for PFC. In both cases the number of PFC detectable decreased as the concentration of cancer toxin with which they were incubated increased, probably as a result of interference with protein production or secretion rather than cell lysis, since the plaques were not lost suddenly during the period of incubation but instead became progressively smaller until finally they vanished. It should be noted that the messenger RNA which is responsible for the formation of antibody is quite stable; consequently, it appears likely that the cancer toxin acts either at the level of the ribosomes or upon the protein secretory mechanism. In this regard it is of interest that the presence of a Walker 256 rat carcinoma, which is a good source of toxohormone (*13*), is associated with decreased ability of polyribosomes from the gastrocnemius muscle to incorporate amino acids into protein (*40*).

The activity of the fibrosarcoma culture supernatant material is not limited to cells of the immune system, and consequently it should not be thought of as a chalone or as a normal immunoregulatory factor which happens to be produced in excess by certain types of cancer cells. As illustrated in Fig. 1, the addition of SaD2-AG culture supernatants to human fibroblasts during exponential growth can greatly increase the doubling time of the cultures. Actual lysis of the fibroblasts may be observed after 3 to 6 days of culture with SaD2-AG supernatants. It appears possible that this *in vitro* effect on fibroblasts of material produced and released by cancer cells may be of some significance *in vivo*. The normal reaction of a host to a benign tumor is to surround it with a connective tissue capsule which walls it off from normal tissue. Such a capsule never develops about a malignant tumor. If cancer cells can produce a high local concentration of material capable of preventing the proliferation of fibroblasts, the failure of host defenses to encapsulate malignant tumors with connective tissue is hardly surprising.

The biologically active material present in SaD2-AG culture supernatants is also effective against macrophages. Dr. Dennis Blakeslee, a member of our cancer research group in Kingston, has been studying the effect of both SaD2-AG cells and SaD2-AG culture supernatants on the ability of activated macrophages to kill SaD2-AG cells. He has found that activated macrophages readily kill SaD2-AG cells if the cancer cells are present in low concentrations; at higher concentrations, the SaD2-AG cells inhibit macrophage activity and eventually kill the macrophages. The inhibitory and lethal effect of the SaD2-AG cells on the activated macrophages appears to be mediated by soluble material produced and released by the cancer cells. These *in vitro* findings may explain another failure of the host defenses against cancer. Although approximately 50% of the cells in many malignant tumors (including SaD2-AG) are macrophages rather than cancer cells (*36, 37*) these macrophages do not appear to kill many of their malignant neighbours. This might be expected if the high concentrations of cancer cells present in a tumor can locally inhibit the cancer-killing activity of macrophages *in vivo* as well as *in vitro*.

Recently it was reported that at least certain types of murine malignant cells release material which can prevent the migration of macrophages and the development of inflammatory reactions in the immediate vicinity of injected cancer cells (*41*). Others (*33–35*) have reported that human cancer cell lines also may produce and release material which can inhibit DNA synthesis by a variety of different types of cells, including fibroblasts. Consequently, the possibility must be considered that many different types of malignant cells release material whose biological activity shows little tissue or species specificity, and that this material is responsible for the ability of a cancer to erode through normal tissue, the failure of the host to encapsulate the tumor with connective tissue, the inhibition of various types of immunological and inflammatory reactions in the immediate vicinity of the tumor, and various systemic abnormalities often associated with large but still localized tumors.

In Vivo Effects of Fibrosarcoma Cells and Culture Supernatants

Figure 2 (upper) summarizes data from an experiment which illustrates the effect on *in vivo* PFC responses of SaD2-AG fibrosarcomas of various ages. Four groups of age-matched mice were injected with SRBC at each time point and assayed for splenic PFC 4 days later: normal controls; normal mice injected subcutaneously with 0.1 ml of carbon tetrachloride (CCl_4) 24 hr previously; fibrosarcoma-bearing mice; and fibrosarcoma-bearing mice injected with CCl_4 as described above. Figure 2 (lower) illustrates the affect on *in vivo* PFC responses of injecting various doses of SaD2-AG culture supernatant 2 hr before injection of the SRBC.

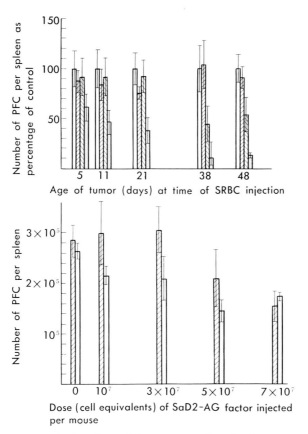

FIG. 2. *In vivo* effects of fibrosarcoma cells and culture supernatants. Upper: SRBC injected into normal mice, tumor-bearing mice, and normal and tumor-bearing mice injected subcutaneously with 0.1 ml CCl_4 24 hr previously. Splenic PFC assayed 4 days later. ☐ normal controls; ▨ CCl_4 alone; ▧ SaD2-AG tumor alone; ▥ CCl_4+SaD2-AG tumor. Lower: SRBC injected into normal mice, mice injected 24 hr previously with 0.1 ml CCl_4, mice injected 2 hr previously with various doses of cancer cell culture supernatant, and mice injected with both the CCl_4 and the cancer cell culture supernatant. ▨ no CCl_4; ☐ plus CCl_4.

Both normal mice and mice injected with 0.1 ml of CCl_4 24 hr previously were tested at each dosage level. Comparison of the results of these two experiments shows several striking similarities between the effects of SaD2-AG tumors and the effect of injections of SaD2-AG culture supernatants on *in vivo* PFC responses. In both cases the resulting immunodepression is dose-dependent; only large (old) tumors and only large doses of supernatant material cause immunodepression in mice not pre-treated with CCl_4. Moreover, in both cases the nature of the immunodepression produced is such that it can be potentiated by administration of a non-immunosuppressive dose of CCl_4. By itself, a subcutaneous injection of 0.1 ml of CCl_4 24 hr prior to SRBC injection has little effect on the subsequent splenic PFC response. In a series of 14 consecutive experiments involving a total of 102 mice in each group, dividing the PFC responses of mice injected with this standard dose of CCl_4 by those of the untreated age-matched controls produced a ratio of 1.06 to 1. However, when this same non-immunosuppressive dose of CCl_4 was injected into mice bearing utmors or given injections of cancer toxin too small to be immunosuppressive by themselves, definite immunodepression resulted. Although these similarities between the *in vivo* effects of SaD2-AG tumors and injections of material produced *in vitro* by SaD2-AG cells does not prove beyond question that the immunodepression observed in mice bearing large SaD2-AG tumors is caused by the *in vivo* release of similar material, such a mechanism appears to explain most readily data of the type presented above.

Mechanisms Responsible for the Potentiating Effect of CCl_4

The *in vivo* data presented in Fig. 2 is compatible with a large number of alternative explanations. Since we know from *in vitro* experiments (see Fig. 1) that the cancer toxin can affect cells other than those involved in immune responses, we must consider the possibility that the *in vivo* immunodepression which follows the injection of an adequate dose of cancer toxin (see Fig. 2, lower) may be caused by either a direct toxic effect upon cells of the immune system or an indirect effect secondary to damage elsewhere. For example, material released by toxin-damaged tissue may be toxic to cells of the immune system, or it may induce the liver to produce increased amounts of α-2 globulin, a material known to be immunosuppressive. Alternatively, the cancer toxin may damage detoxifying and excretory organs, such as the liver or kidneys, with a consequent build-up of metabolic waste products of normal body processes to immunosuppressive levels or a decreased ability to metabolize or excrete the cancer cell toxin. Moreover, the various alternatives noted above are not necessarily mutually exclusive. Since similar alternatives must be

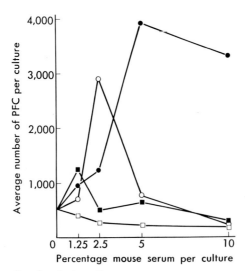

FIG. 3.   *In vitro* effects of serum from CCl_4-treated donors. Donors bled 1, 2, or 3 days after subcutaneous injection of 0.1 ml CCl_4. Various concentrations of serum added to cultures containing mouse spleen cells and SRBC; PFC assayed 3 days later. ● day 1 serum; ○ day 2 serum; ■ day 3 serum; □ normal control.

considered as possible consequences of a dose of CCl₄ large enough to cause liver and kidney damage, there were initially a large number of possible explanations for the ability of CCl₄ to potentiate the immunosuppressive effects of either injections of cancer cell toxin or malignant tumors growing *in vitro*. Some of these possibilities now appear to have been eliminated. Figure 3 presents typical data from an experiment designed to find out whether or not an injection of the standard dose of CCl₄ results in an increase in circulating immunosuppressive material of any kind. Various dilutions of serum obtained from normal mice, or from mice injected with the standard dose of CCl₄ 1, 2, or 3 days prior to bleeding, were added to Marbrook tubes containing a fixed number of mouse spleen cells and SRBC. Anti-sheep PFC were assayed after 3 days of culture. As usual, the higher concentrations of serum from the normal donors were somewhat immunosuppressive. In contrast, the serum from donors injected with CCl₄ one day prior to bleeding was strongly stimulatory at these same concentrations. The amount of stimulation produced by the serum from the CCl₄-treated donors decreased progressively as the time interval between injection of CCl₄ and bleeding increased. Consequently, no evidence was obtained to support the suggestion that an injection of CCl₄ large enough to damage liver and kidneys results in immunosuppressive serum levels of α-2 globulin, tissue breakdown products, or metabolic waste. It is of interest that in all of the *in vivo* experiments described previously (see Fig. 2), the SRBC were injected 24 hr after the administration of the CCl₄, a time when the serum is most stimulatory to PFC responses *in vitro*. This stimulatory effect of the serum from CCl₄-treated donors may explain observations that the administration of CCl₄ 6 hr before the injection of antigen leads to enhanced primary immune responses (*42–44*).

The *in vivo* immunosuppressive effects of CCl₄ and cancer toxin are not simply additive. Figure 4 illustrates the splenic PFC responses of mice immunized against SRBC 24 hr after they had been injected with various doses of CCl₄. The standard dose, used in all of the experiments described above, is 0.1 ml CCl₄ per mouse. Note that twice that dose was given without producing any detectable immunodepression, although the standard dose always causes immunodepression if the

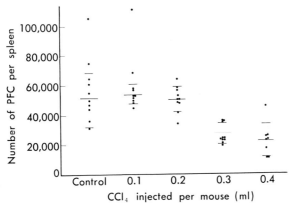

Fɪɢ. 4.   Effect of CCl₄ on *in vivo* PFC responses. Various doses of CCl₄ injected subcutaneously 24 hr before SRBC injection, and splenic PFC assayed 4 days later.

recipient also bears a tumor or has been given an adequate but non-immunosuppressive dose of cancer toxin. Now if the data of Fig. 2 are again examined, it can be seen that 3×10^7 cell equivalents of cancer toxin did not produce any detectable immunodepression in normal animals, although 1×10^7 cell equivalents caused immunodepression when given to animals previously injected with the standard non-immunosuppressive dose of CCl_4. The non-additive features are even stronger when the effect of SaD2-AG tumors of various sizes (ages) is examined. Immunodepression resulted when the standard dose of CCl_4 was injected into mice bearing non-immunosuppressive tumors from 5 to 21 days old, although the 5 day tumors were so small that they could not be detected by palpation while the 21 day tumors were all larger than 1 cm in diameter. Such a relationship between two toxic factors cannot be explained on the basis of simple addition of toxicity, even if a detection threshold excluding suboptimal damage is postulated. Some form of synergism must be involved.

Evidence for the Existence of Host Defenses against Cancer Toxin

One possible explanation for the observation that a non-immunosuppressive dose of CCl_4 can act synergistically with a non-immunosuppressive dose of cancer toxin to produce definite immunodepression is that the CCl_4 acts by damaging some mechanism which otherwise would have detoxified, adsorbed, or excreted much of the cancer toxin. Evidence that such a mechanism exists was obtained through experiments in which various doses of SaD2-AG cancer toxin were injected into normal mice and into mice injected 24 hr previously with the standard dose of CCl_4. The results were quite consistent. An injection of 3×10^7 or more cell equivalents of cancer toxin into normal mice resulted in a definite change in their behaviour and appearance, characterized by greatly decreased spontaneous activity, a hunched posture, ruffled fur, and (at the higher doses) diarrhea and mild respiratory distress. The first signs of abnormal behaviour appeared 2 to 10 min after injection of the cancer toxin, and reached a peak after about 30 min. Thereafter the mice began to recover, and 24 hr later they could not be distinguished in appearance from completely normal mice or from mice given only CCl_4. It is apparent that the cancer toxin injected into these mice was quickly rendered harmless in some way—perhaps merely by being used up in reactions with the host cells, but perhaps also by some mechanism involving excretion, adsorption, or metabolic degradation of the cancer toxin.

For the first hour following the injection of cancer toxin into CCl_4-treated mice, the strength and timing of the resulting clinical effects could not be distinguished from those produced by injection of a similar amount of cancer toxin into normal mice. There was a short delay, followed by the first appearance of abnormalities, a rapid rise to maximum intensity, and the beginning of a slow return toward normal. However, with the CCl_4-treated mice, the return to normal was extremely prolonged, with all of the mice still definitely sick 24 hr after the injection of the cancer toxin. Some never recovered; out of a total of 29 mice which were pre-treated with CCl_4 and then given between 3×10^7 and 7×10^7 SaD2-AG cell equivalents of cancer toxin, 10 died 48 to 72 hr later. The survivors were still sick after 48 hr, but appeared to be back to normal after 72 hr. It seems then that the SaD2-AG supernatant material is toxic to both normal and CCl_4-treated mice, but the CCl_4-treated mice are much less capable of recovering from its harmful effects. The most reasonable explanation for these observations is that mice possess some mechanism which can metabolize or excrete the cancer toxin, and that this mechanism can be damaged by administration of CCl_4.

Many questions still remain to be answered. Identification of the mechanism responsible for defending the host against the harmful effects of the cancer toxin has a high priority; both liver and kidneys are prime suspects, since the dose of CCl_4 used in the experiments described above can cause damage to both. Identification of the nature of the cancer toxin and the biochemical mechanisms by which it causes its harmful effects is also of potential clinical value. A third question of major importance has to do with the possibility that infection of tumors by non-oncogenic viruses of certain types may induce the cancer cells to produce the toxin. If such is the case, treatment directed against the virus infection may produce significant clinical benefit. Finally, the effect on the clinical course of cancer of exposure to halogenated hydrocarbons other than CCl_4 must be examined, since such chemicals are very common in all industrialized societies.

REFERENCES

1. Greenstein, J. P. and Andervont, H. B. The liver catalase activity of tumor-bearing mice and the effect of spontaneous regression and of removal of certain tumors. J. Natl. Cancer Inst., *2*: 345–355, 1942.
2. Nakahara, W. and Fukuoka, F. A toxic cancer tissue constituent as evidenced by its effect on liver catalase activity. Japan. Med. J., *1*: 271–277, 1948.
3. Nakahara, W. and Fukuoka, F. Toxohormone: A characteristic toxic substance produced by cancer tissue. Gann, *40*: 45–69, 1949.
4. Nakahara, W. and Fukuoka, F. Purification of toxohormone. A second study on toxohormone, a characteristic toxic substance produced by cancer tissues. Gann, *41*: 47–55, 1950.
5. Fukuoka, F. and Nakahara, W. Mode of action of toxohormone. A third study on toxohormone, a characteristic toxic substance produced by cancer tissue. Gann, *42*: 55–67, 1951.
6. Fukuoka, F. and Nakahara, W. Toxohormone and thymus involution in tumor-bearing animals. A fourth study on toxohormone, a characteristic toxic substance produced by cancer tissue. Gann, *43*: 55–62, 1952.
7. Hoshizima, H. Studies on the mechanism of toxohormone function. Gann, *49*: 171–176, 1958.
8. Nakahara, W. and Fukuoka, F. The newer concept of cancer toxin. Adv. Cancer Res., *5*: 157–177, 1958.
9. Kampschmidt, R. F., Adams, R. E., and McCoy, T. A. Some systemic effects of toxohormone. Cancer Res., *19*: 236–239, 1959.
10. Nakahara, W. A chemical basis for tumor-host relations. J. Natl. Cancer Inst., *24*: 77–86, 1960.

11. Raymond, M. J. Some effects of tumor growth upon rat muscle protein metabolism. Ph.D. Thesis, Univ. of St. Andrews, Scotland, 1972.

12. Masaki, H., Takatsu, K., Hamaoka, T., and Kitagawa, M. Immunosuppressive activity of chromatin fraction derived from nuclei of Ehrlich ascites tumor cells. Gann, *63*: 633–635, 1972.

13. Goodlad, G. A. J. and Raymond, M. J. The action of the Walker 256 carcinoma and toxohormone on amino acid incorporation into diaphragm protein. Eur. J. Cancer, *9*: 139–145, 1973.

14. Kitagawa, M., Hamaoka, T., Takatsu, K., Haba, S., Yamashita, U., and Masaki, H. Disturbance of immune surveillance in tumor-bearing host. GANN Monograph on Cancer Research, *16*: 45–52, 1974.

15. Fuchigami, A., Umeda, M., and Uno, T. Effect of the urine extract of cancer patients on liver catalase in mice. Gann, *47*: 295–297, 1956.

16. Saxen, E. and Penttinen, K. Host factors and cancer. Cell culture studies. Acta Pathol. Microbiol. Scand., *54* (Suppl. 153): 75–79, 1962.

17. Astaldi, G., Costa, G., and Airo, R. Phytohemagglutinin in leukemia. Lancet, *I*: 1394, 1965.

18. Saxen, E. and Penttinen, K. Differences in the effect of individual human sera on cell cultures. J. Natl. Cancer Inst., *35*: 67–73, 1965.

19. Ito, T., Fujiwara, M., and Hirai, T. Effect of the serum of patients with malignant tumors on HeLa cell cultures. Gann, *57*: 605–612, 1966.

20. Trubowitz, S., Masek, B., and Rosario, A. Del. Lymphocyte response to phytohemagglutinin in Hodgkin's disease, lymphatic leukemia and lymphosarcoma. Cancer, *19*: 2019–2023, 1966.

21. Parthenis, A. and Stone, D. Some morphological differences in HeLa cell cultures when grown in the presence of normal or cancer sera. Brit. J. Cancer, *21*: 218–227, 1967.

22. Silk, M. Effect of plasma from patients with carcinoma on *in vitro* lymphocyte transformation. Cancer, *20*: 2088–2089, 1967.

23. Hersh, E. M. and Irwin, W. S. Blastogenic responses of lymphocytes from patients with untreated and treated lymphomas. Lymphology, *2*: 150–160, 1969.

24. Gatti, R. A., Garrioch, D. B., and Good, R. A. Depressed PHA responses in patients with non-lymphoid malignancies. *In ;* J. Harris (ed.), Proceedings of Fifth Leukocyte Culture Conference, pp. 339–358, Academic Press, New York, 1970.

25. Sample, W. F., Gertner, H. R., and Chretien, P. B. Inhibition of phytohemagglutinin-induced *in vitro* lymphocyte transformation by serum from patients with carcinoma. J. Natl. Cancer Inst., *46*: 1291–1297, 1971.

26. Gatti, R. A. Serum inhibitors of lymphocyte responses. Lancet, *I*: 1351–1352, 1971.

27. Field, E. J. and Caspary, E. A. Lymphocyte sensitization in advanced malignant disease: A study of serum lymphocyte depressive factor. Brit. J. Cancer, *26*: 164–173, 1972.

28. Chan, P. L. and Sinclair, N. R. St. C. Immunologic and virologic properties of chemically and γ-irradiation-induced thymic lymphomas in mice. J. Natl. Cancer Inst., *48*: 1629–1640, 1972.

29. Brooks, W. H., Netsky, M. G., Normansell, D. E., and Horwitz, D. A. Depressed cell-mediated immunity in patients with primary intracranial tumors. J. Exp. Med., *136*: 1631–1647, 1972.

30. Yamazaki, H., Nitta, K., and Umezawa, H. Immunosuppression induced with cell-free fluid of Ehrlich carcinoma ascites and its fractions. Gann, *64*: 83–94, 1973.
31. Steward, A. M. Tuberculin reaction in cancer patients, "Mantoux Release," and lympho-suppressive-stimulatory factors. J. Natl. Cancer Inst., *50*: 625–632, 1973.
32. Glasgow, A. H., Nimberg, R. B., Menzoian, J. O., Saporoschetz, I., Cooperband, S. R., Schmid, K., and Mannick, J. A. Association of anergy with an immunosuppressive peptide fraction in the serum of patients with cancer. New Engl. J. Med., *291*: 1263–1267, 1974.
33. Smith, R. T., Bausher, J. A. C., and Adler, W. H. Studies of an inhibitor of DNA synthesis and a non-specific mitogen elaborated by human lymphoblasts. Am. J. Pathol., *60*: 495–504, 1970.
34. Round, D. E. A growth-modifying factor from cell lines of human malignant origin. Cancer Res., *30*: 2847–2851, 1970.
35. Anderson, R. J., McBride, C. M., and Hersh, E. M. Lymphocyte blastogenic responses to cultured allogeneic tumor cells *in vitro*. Cancer Res., *32*: 988–992, 1972.
36. Marshall, A. H. E. and Dayan, A. D. An immune reaction in man against seminomas, dysgerminomas, pinealomas, and the mediastinal tumors of similar histological appearance. Lancet, *II*: 1102–1104, 1964.
37. Evans, R. Macrophages in syngeneic animal tumors. Transplantation, *14*: 468–473, 1972.
38. Wong, A. O. B., Mankovitz, R., and Kennedy, J. C. Immunosuppressive and immunostimulatory factors produced by malignant cells *in vitro*. Int. J. Cancer, *13*: 530–542, 1974.
39. Marbrook, J. Primary immune response in culture of spleen cells. Lancet, *II*: 1279–1281, 1967.
40. Goodlad, G. A. J. and Clark, C. M. Activity of gastrocnemius and soleus polyribosomes in rats bearing the Walker 256 carcinoma. Eur. J. Cancer, *8*: 647–651, 1972.
41. Fauve, R. M., Hevin, B., Jacob, H., Gaillard, J. A., and Jacob, F. Antiinflammatory effects of murine malignant cells. Proc. Natl. Acad. Sci. U.S., *71*: 4052–4056, 1974.
42. Paronetto, F. and Popper, H. Enhanced antibody formation in experimental acute and chronic liver injury produced by carbon tetrachloride or allyl alcohol. Proc. Soc. Exp. Biol. (N.Y.), *116*: 1060–1064, 1964.
43. Popper, H., Paronetto, F., and Schaffner, F. Immune processes in the pathogenesis of liver disease. Ann. N.Y. Acad. Sci., *124*: 781–799, 1965.
44. Triger, D. R. and Wright, R. Studies on hepatic uptake of antigen. II. The effect of hepatotoxins on the immune response. Immunology, *25*: 951–956, 1973.

Discussion of Paper of Dr. Kennedy

DR. BRUNNER: The reduction in the number of PFC per spleen which you obtained using your supernatant material was very small, amounting to a decrease from 3×10^5 PFC in control animals to 2×10^5 PFC in the treated groups. I wonder whether it is valid to refer to such a small diminution as an immunosuppressive effect?

DR. KENNEDY: It is a relatively minor reduction, certainly, but that's the degree of reduction we obtained in all of our experiments, both those involving injection of supernatant material and those involving *in vivo* tumors. The fact that the number of cell equivalents of supernatant material required to produce this degree of immunosuppression is at least ten fold less than the minimum number of cells required for a tumor to be immunosuppressive is probably accounted for by the fact that we injected the supernatant material as a bolus rather than over an extended period of time.

DR. FROST: You apparently assume that a reduction in PFC response to SRBC is the equivalent of total immunosuppression, as that is the only criterion present to define the immune potential in your system. Have you tried treating mice with your factor and then challenging them with tumor doses that normally do not view? If one administers immunosuppressive substances to animals one can sometimes observe tumor growth using a tumor inoculum which would otherwise be rejected.

DR. KENNEDY: We have examined the rate of tumor progression and formation of secondaries in animals bearing solid tumors, and found that administration of CCl_4 accelerated the formation of secondaries. Animals injected with Friend virus developed large leukemic spleens more quickly when given CCl_4.

DR. FROST: But CCl_4 is extremely toxic to animals and may have a variety of effects.

DR. KENNEDY: We were able to double and even triple our standard dose of CCl_4 with only minor effects on immunological reactivity.

DR. FROST: If one accepts the surveillance hypothesis of tumor rejection, one might infer from your discussion that while tumors continuously arise, they become clinically evident only if they can produce some toxic factor, rather than because the host's immune system is already suppressed or initially defective. Do you agree?

DR. KENNEDY: Not necessarily. I believe that the state of immunocompetence of the host, which can be depressed by such circumstances as infection with certain common viruses, may sometimes determine whether or not a tumor will become established. In order to survive in an immunocompetent host the tumor must quickly establish a certain critical mass, perhaps aided by the production of an immunogenicity. In addition, the anatomical location in which the tumor arises may be important in determining its survival.

DR. JERNE: How extensively have you characterized your factor? Is it a protein?

DR. KENNEDY: Thus far we have only a rough characterization. It is retained by Amicon membranes which pass molecules smaller than 10,000, and on gel filtration columns it appears to separate into two peaks of approximately 30,000 and 60,000 daltons. We suspect that it is a component of cell membrane, since it has some biological effects similar to a cell membrane glycoprotein some of our associates have purified.

DR. JERNE: Your factor could thus be similar to diphtheria toxin, which also acts on ribosomes. Is your factor antigenic?

DR. KENNEDY: We are planning to test its antigenicity after modifying its toxicity.

DR. Y. IKAWA (Cancer Institute, Japanese Foundation for Cancer Research, Tokyo): Is your factor effective in accelerating the growth of other types of neoplasm?

DR. KENNEDY: The factor stimulated the growth of L1210 and Friend virus leukemia cells. These malignant cells do not produce much, if any, soluble immunosuppressive material.

DR. NAKAHARA: The immunosuppressive factors discussed by you and Dr. Kitagawa are reminiscent of our work with toxohormone, a substance produced by tumor cells and released into the circulation to produce immunodepressive effects and enzymatic disturbances in the host. We probably can't say we're working on the same substance, but we're surely working on the same principle. Our crude toxohormone fractions also produce a marked atrophy of the thymus, which in light of your recent work would appear to be the most likely basis for its effects on the immune response.

DR. HOBBS: Between 1959 and 1961, Tombs in Westminster and Restler in the U.S. found that α_1-glycoproteins extracted from tumors provoked a large α_2-globulin response in the liver when injected into normal animals. It is important to know whether CCl_4 can prevent such an α_2-globulin response, and I think that in small doses it can. If you repeat your experiments adding your immunosuppressive factor together with serum from CCl_4-treated animals, you could determine whether it is the lack of production of this macroglobulin which permits your factor to exert its effect.

DR. KENNEDY: Serum from mice given CCl_4 at various intervals before bleeding, serum from mice bearing tumors, and serum from mice bearing tumors and given CCl_4 were tested for *in vitro* immunosuppressive effects. The serum from the mice given only CCl_4 was stimulatory rather than immunosuppressive; serum from tumor-bearing mice was somewhat immunosuppressive, but less so than serum from tumor-bearing mice also given CCl_4. Exactly what the immunosuppressive material is and whether it originates from the host or the tumor has not yet been determined.

DR. HOBBS: A cleaner experiment designed to determine if there is a plasma factor produced by the liver that serves to counter your toxic factor would be simply to take plasma from CCl_4-treated animals and add it separately with your factor and note if it will permit inhibition of PFC *in vitro*.

HOST DEFENSE AGAINST CANCER AND ITS POTENTIATION, D. MIZUNO ET AL. (EDS.),
UNIV. OF TOKYO PRESS, TOKYO / UNIV. PARK PRESS, BALTIMORE, PP. 83-96, 1975

Complement System and Tumor Immunity

Kusuya NISHIOKA

Virology Division, National Cancer Center Research Institute, Tokyo, Japan and Institute of Medical Science, University of Tokyo, Tokyo, Japan

Abstract: Immunochemical analysis of complement cascade flowing in the immune system revealed the central function of C3 in the complement system interacting with other cellular and humoral factors competent in the host defense mechanism. Based on these facts, elevation of the complement system observed in the tumor-bearing host can be explained as compensatory increase in the host with depressed state of the cell-mediated immune system to maintain the defense mechanism against cancer. Therefore, immunopotentiation through stimulation of the complement system, especially C3, was attempted. Antitumor effect of *Corynebacterium* infection or administration of antitumor polysaccharides are in line with this concept and, moreover, direct activation of C3 by tumor cell membrane was observed.

The concepts of C3 central function and complement compensation are further supported by analysis of phylogeny and genetic maps of 4 immune systems, *i.e.*, C3 system, cell-mediated system, immunoglobulin system, as well as C142 system.

Complement System and Other Immune Systems in Host Defense

Since the first description of complement (*1*) as a heat-labile component present in the serum and responsible for bactericidal action of immune serum, much attention has been paid to its essential role in host defense system. By 1960 complement had emerged as a complex comprising 4 factors which act sequentially: C1, C4, C2, and C3. Among them, C3 was considered to be a serum factor(s) which reacts with cobra venom (*2*), yeast (*3*), and C142 (*4*). Based on the comprehensive outline and experimental method established by Mayer (*5*) on immune hemolysis and by Nelson (*6*) and Nishioka (*7*) on immune adherence, 6 new components were discovered (*8–11*) and 9 distinct proteins recognized in the complement system. They were designated as C1, C4, C2, C3, C5, C6, C7, C8, and C9 by the WHO immunology unit in 1968 (*12*). Components of a second mechanism of the complement system were described and initiating factor (IF), properdin (P), C3 proactivator (C3PA) (B), C3 activator ($\overline{\text{B}}$), C3PA convertase ($\overline{\text{D}}$) characterized

(*13*). Consequently, the essential roles of the complement system in fundamental immune mechanisms have been elucidated immunochemically. During the past decade and a half, extensive studies have been carried out by many investigators in different laboratories on the isolation, purification, reaction mechanism, and submolecular fragmentation of each complement component. Physicochemical characters of components in the complement system have all been determined with regard to sedimentation constant, electrophoretic mobility, isoelectric points and molecular weight (*13, 14*).

The immunological surveillance system in the host has been shown to be composed of 4 main systems through phylogenical, immunochemical, as well as immunogenetical studies, *i.e.*, C3 shunt or alternate complement pathway (IF, P, B, D, C3–C9), cell-mediated immunity (mainly through lymphocytes), immunoglobulin-mediated system and classical pathway of complement system (IgG, IgM, C1–C9). In the past decade, there has been a general tendency to focus attention mainly on the role of the lymphocyte-mediated system in tumor immunology. However, this covers only one-fourth of host defense mechanisms in general. Recent studies in complement research have contributed to understanding the host defense mechanism on a more fundamental basis through analyses of the classical complement pathway as well as the alternate complement pathway. The results demonstrate that the complement system does work synergistically with other immune systems, especially with immune systems composed of immunoglobulins, lymphocytes, macrophages, granulocytes, erythrocytes, and platelets (*14*). The so-called cell-mediated immune system and humoral immune system act synergistically in the immune

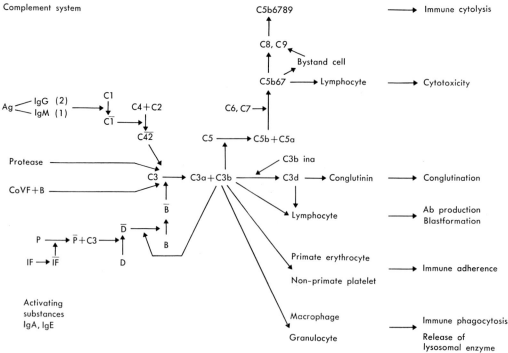

Fig. 1.   Interaction of complement system with cellular and humoral factors.

surveillance system and the present status of interaction of each complement component with other immune systems can be schematized as in Fig. 1.

One of the most remarkable achievements in basic immunology in recent years was the discovery of genetic regulation of immune reaction. Human histocompatibility antigen (HLA) is considered to be closely related to human immune regulation genes, and genetic regulation of C2 is considered to be associated with HLA (15). In the mouse system, the Ir-1 gene has been known to regulate immunoglobulin and to be present in IX linkage No. 17 chromosome linked with H-2 histocompatibility genes. In addition to this, Demant *et al.* showed the role of the H-2 linked Ss-Slp region in the control of mouse complement (16). More recently, genetic linkage of C3 regulation and H-2 was described by Ferreira and Nussenzweig (17). Also the rate of appearance of complement receptor lymphocytes is shown to be controlled by a gene linked to H-2D regions (18).

These observations, as well as the pattern of complement reaction reacting with other immunological systems suggest that all these different immunological systems, especially immunoglobulin- and lymphocyte-mediated systems, are integrated together with the complement system in the host defense system.

Central Function of C3 in Immune Reaction

As schematized in Fig. 1, we have considered that C3 plays a central function in various immune systems through complement pathways. The initial step is activation of non-activated native C3 into C3b (activated form) and C3a (anaphylatoxin).

This reaction can be induced by 4 different reactions.

1)   Antigen immunoglobulin complex (two molecules of IgG or one molecule of IgM specifically bound to the antigen site) binds Cl followed by formation of C42a complex in the region close to the antibody Cl-binding site. C42a is considered to be C3 convertase and split C3 into C3b and C3a.

2)   IF is activated by various polysaccharides (zymosan, inulin, lipopolysaccharides from Gram-negative bacterias, possibly by lentinan or tumor cell membrane) and by IgA or IgE. Activated IF ($\overline{\text{IF}}$) then reacts with P, and $\overline{\text{D}}$ is considered to be activated through reaction with native C3 resulting in formation of C3PA convertase ($\overline{\text{D}}$). Substrate of $\overline{\text{D}}$ is C3PA (B), and C3PA is split into GAG and C3 activator ($\overline{\text{B}}$). Native C3 is then activated by $\overline{\text{B}}$ and is split into C3a and C3b.

3)   Activation of C3 into C3b and C3a can also be induced by cobra venom factor (CoVF) B complex.

4)   Proteases directly activate C3 into formation of C3b and C3a.

Once C3 is activated, activated C3b is located on the surface of antigen. C3b present on the antigen surface interacts with (a) various cellular factors and (b) serum factors.

a)   Reactions with cellular factors are summarized as follows.

1)   C3b reacts with primate erythrocytes or non-primate platelets. This results in immune adherence reaction and we consider that this is also a kind of host defense mechanism as first described by Nelson (6).

2)   C3b also reacts with macrophages and granulocytes resulting in immune phago-cytosis of antigen particles. When the antigen particles are larger than phagocyting cells, this results in release of the lysosomal enzyme of the phagocyting cells (*19*). Through this reaction, these cells attack larger target antigen cells such as tumor cells.

3)   The lymphocytes interact with C3b on the antigen surface. This reaction is considered to be associated with antibody production in the T-B cooperative system (*20*). This is not observed in thymus (T)-independent antibody production system. Also, lymphoblast formation due to specific immune reaction such as tuberculin reaction or fungi infection was observed (*21*). This phenomenon was not observed in non-specific and non-immunological reactions such as drug-induced stimulation.

b)   Reaction with serum factors are as follows.

1)   Once activated C3b is formed, C3b is destroyed by C3b inactivator (*22*), which is present in normal serum. This results in formation of C3d, in parallel with loss of reactivities with macrophage, granulocytes, primate erythrocytes, non-primate platelets or C5 in sequential reaction of complement. In contrast to other cellular systems, the reactivity of C3d with B lymphocytes remains, *i.e.*, B lymphocytes give both receptors for C3b and C3d while other phagocyting cells and immune adherence reacting cells have only C3b receptor (*23, 24*). Also C3d obtains new reactivity with conglutinin, a kind of serum protein present in bovine. Conglutina-tion is due to this reaction (*25*).

2)   In complement cascade pathway, C3b reacts with C5 and splits native C5 into C5b and C5a. C5a has anaphylatoxin and chemotactic activities and is released into fluid phase, while C5b binds to the antigen surface followed by reaction with C6, C7 to form C5b67 complex. C5b67 complex is known to react with C8 and C9 resulting in destruction of membrane of antigen cell. This is the prototype of complement-mediated immune cytolysis.

3)   Before loosing binding activity, C5b67 complex can also bind to the surface of adjacent cells which have not been sensitized by antibody, and preceding comple-ment components and reactive lysis of this bystand cell can be induced after reac-tion of C8 and C9 (*27*).

4)   In addition to this complement-mediated lysis, when C5b67 complex is formed, cytotoxicity of antigen cells is induced after reaction with lymphocytes (*26*).

Complement Level in Tumor-bearing Host

To analyse the role of complement in tumor-immune mechanism, the first step is to observe the complement level in the tumor-bearing host. In many cases, elevated level of whole complement activity or complement component activity was described in the sera of experimental tumor-bearing animals or in the sera of patients with neoplastic diseases as reviewed in (*14*). Also, cobra venom induce B, C3–C9 hemolytic activity of the complement system increased in the tumor-bearing host (*28*).

Three possibilities can be considered with regard to elevation of the comple-ment system in the tumor-bearing host. First, the elevated complement system acts

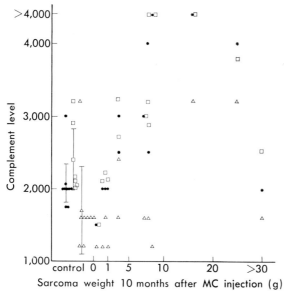

FIG. 2.   Relation of complement level and size of MCA-induced tumor.   ● CIA_{50}; □ C4;
△ C3.

against the function of cell-mediated immunity and results in a decrease of host
defense against cancer. Second, there is no relation between complement level and
host defense including cell-mediated immunity. Third, the complement system compensates the deficient state of cell-mediated immunity in the tumor host and the
elevated complement system acts to maintain the host defense even when cell-
mediated immunity is impaired. Based on the function analysis of the complement
system, synergistically working with cell-mediated immunity and immunoglobulin
systems as described above, we took the third possibility as our working hypothesis,
i.e., elevation of the complement system means manifestation of compensation of the
complement system in the impaired state of the cell-mediated system. This hypothesis
comes from the following observations.

As shown in Fig. 2 (*29*), complement level in the sera of rats bearing methylcholanthrene (MCA)-induced tumor was determined 10 months after subcutaneous
injection of 10 mg MCA in olive oil. Experimental animals which developed tumors
larger than 2.8 g showed increased levels of complement as determined by immune
adherence (CIA_{50}) as compared with the control group and groups with tumors
smaller than 1.0 g or the tumor-negative group. Up to 25 g, CIA_{50} levels showed
increases in parallel with the size of the tumor. C4 levels showed increases parallel
with CIA_{50} and C3 also increased in rats with tumors larger than 10 g. However,
when tumor size exceeded 30 g, CIA_{50}, C3, and C4 levels fell to normal level. This
observation coincides with previous observations that complement level increased
in many of the cases of experimental and human tumors.

Complement level of splenectomized rats was compared with non-splenectomized rats in the course of dimethylaminoazobenzene (DAB) feeding to induce

TABLE 1.   Tuberculin Reaction in Lung Cancer Patients

	Lung cancer metastasis (−)	Lung cancer metastasis (+)	Non-cancer control
Negative	28.6%	30%	5.3%
5−10 mm	0	32	10.6
>10 mm	71.4	38	84.1
Total No.	14	50	56

hepatoma. Higher complement levels were observed at 4- and 6-month feedings with DAB in splenectomized rats as compared with non-splenectomized rats (29).

These observations can be explained as follows. Experimental animals with large MCA-induced tumors or in splenectomized rats fed with DAB to induce hepatoma are considered to be in a state of decreased cell-mediated immunity and the level of the complement system is elevated to compensate for depressed cellular immunity. It is conceivable that the integrity of immune systems essential for host defense against cancer is maintained through these reactions.

As a marker of cell-mediated immunity, tuberculin reaction in lung cancer patients was measured comparing the level of the complement system (30). As first described by Prof. Ishibashi (31), tuberculin reactivity was depressed in lung cancer patients. As shown in Table 1, 62% of lung cancer with metastasis showed depressed tuberculin reaction as compared with 28.6% of lung cancer without metastasis and 15.9% in non-cancer control. As shown in Fig. 3, in a follow-up study of lung cancer, tuberculin reactivity decreased in parallel with the development of lung cancer in most of the cases. Complement level (CH_{50}) in these lung cancer patients as determined by immune hemolysis was plotted against tuberculin reactivity of the patients as graded −(0–5 mm), ±(5–10 mm), +(>10 mm), and ++(>10 mm, strong induration). As shown in Fig. 4, CH_{50} level in all these cases showed normal level (32.0–43.2 CH_{50}) irrespective of tuberculin reactivity.

Size of solid type of lung cancer as determined by X-ray examination was

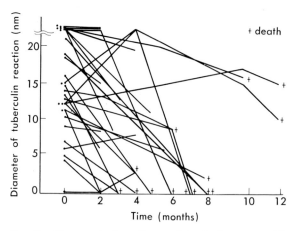

FIG. 3.   Change of tuberculin reactivity in the course of lung cancer development.

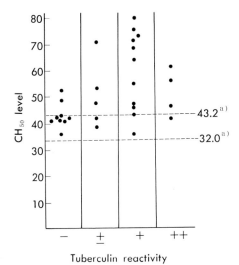

FIG. 4. Tuberculin reaction and complement level in lung cancer patients. [a] Normal range of CH_{50} level.

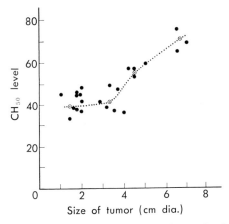

FIG. 5. Relation of serum complement level and size of lung cancer.

plotted against CH_{50} level (Fig. 5). Complement level increased in parallel with size of tumor showing the same tendency as we observed in the case of rat MCA-induced tumor. These observations demonstrate that the complement system remains intact when the cell-mediated immune system is depressed in the course of cancer development and support the third possibility that the complement system compensates for the depressed cell-mediated immunity to maintain the defense mechanism in the tumor-bearing host.

Potentiation of Complement System to Increase Host Defense against Tumor

Synergistic action of the complement system with other humoral and cellular factors involved in host defense mechanism has been elucidated and the possibility

TABLE 2.   Effect of *Corynebacterium* Injection on Tumor Growth of Transplanted Rat Ascites Hepatoma AH130

Hepatoma	*Coryne*. inject.	Numbers of rats		Survival days
		Transplant.	Survived	
AH130 3×10^6	7 days before +	10	8	8 8
	transplant. −	7	0	7 7 7 10 10 15 17
AH130 3×10^6	Simultaneous transplant.	5	1	9 9 9 10
	1 day after transplant.	5	0	7 9 9 10 11
AH130 3×10^6	Preinject. serum	5	1	7 10 14 14
mixed with	Postinject. serum	5	0	8 8 9 9 10

of compensatory increase of the complement system in a tumor-bearing host with a depressed cell-mediated immune system is shown as described above. Therefore, if we could stimulate activity of the complement system in the host in an intact immunological state, increase of host defence against cancer could be expected. A strain of *Corynebacterium* isolated from our rat colony was shown to increase complement level, especially C3, 7 days after injection of *Corynebacteria* (*29*). Seven days after injection of *Corynebacterium*, complement level was determined and 3×10^6 of AH130 rat ascites hepatoma cells were injected, and survival days and development of tumor growth were determined. It is significant that rats with increased levels of complement and C3 at the time of tumor inoculation survived without take of AH130. This phenomenon was reexamined by increasing the number of rats and the results are shown in Table 2. Eight out of 10 rats injected with *Corynebacterium* 7 days previously did not develop tumors after 3×10^6 of AH130 inoculation. All 7 rats in the control group without *Corynebacterium* injection died 7 to 17 days after tumor inoculation.

Corynebacterium suspension was injected simultaneously or one day after transplantation of 3×10^6 AH130 tumor cells. In both cases, no significant resistance induction was observed and the possibility of direct cytotoxic effect of *Corynebacterium* to AH130 is excluded. Two pools of rat sera were prepared from rats at the stage of preinjection of *Corynebacterium* and 7 days after the injection with *Corynebacterium*. After heating at 56°C for 30 min, 1 ml of these sera was mixed with 3×10^6 tumor cells and injected into 5 rats respectively. Only one rat out of 5 inoculated with AH130 mixed with preinjection sera survived without tumor growth and all the 5 rats received 3×10^6 AH130 mixed with postinjection sera and died with tumor growth of AH130. Therefore, antibody produced after *Corynebacterium* injection did not have any neutralizing effect on AH130 tumor growth, excluding the possibility of cross-reacting antibody against AH130 and *Corynebacterium*. Resistance induction against AH130 is more likely due to an increased level of the complement system in rats at the time of inoculation, that is, 7 days after *Corynebacterium* injection. Although we have not yet tested other strains of *Corynebacterium* infection, it is quite possible that the complement system, which is considered to be a kind of acute phase protein (*32*) might participate in in-

TABLE 3. Conversion of C3 and Host-mediated Antitumor Activity of Polysaccharide

Polysaccharide	Loss in C3 hemolytic activity (%)	Skin reaction	Tumor inhibition ratio	
			mg/kg/day	%
EA3[a]	92	⧺	5	96
			1	82
CM-EA3[a]	82	⧺	5	52
EA5[a]	59	⧻	5	98
			1	84
CM-EA5[a]	22	+	5	
HA3[b]	89	⧺	5	75
			1	80
CM-HA3[b]	3	±	5	54
HA5[b]	48	⧻	5	91
			1	37
HA52[b]	70	+	5	94
			1	70
HA53[b]	<1	+	5	5
			1	−10
HA6[b]	36		5	64
			1	39
Lentinan[c]	96	⧺	1	100
Pachyman[d]	44	⧻	5	0
Pachymaran[d]	68	⧺	5	86
CM-pachymaran[d]	9		5	39
Scleroglucan[e]	73	⧻	3	89
Dextran T-2000	6	±		
GVB	0			

Polysaccharides were obtained from: [a] *Flammulina velutipes* ; [b] *Pleurotus ostreatus* ; [c] *Lentinus edodes* ; [d] *Polia cocos* ; [e] *Schizophyllum commune*. GVB: gelatin veronal buffer.

duction of potentiation of resistance against cancer by other strains of *Coryne-bacterium* (*33*).

Various antitumor polysaccharides also have C3-activating activity resulting in C3b and C3a formation. C3a can be measured by anaphylatoxin activity and the split into C3b and C3a can be expressed as reduction of C3 hemolytic activity in fresh guinea pig serum after reaction with polysaccharides. As shown in Table 3 (*34*) all polysaccharides which had more than 50% C3-splitting activity (EA3, EA5, HA3, HA52, lentinan or scleroglucan) had a high inhibition ratio of the tumor growth of sarcoma 180 transplanted in mice and the polysaccharides which had moderate C3-splitting activity had moderate antitumor activity. Carboxymethylated (CM) polysaccharides had a very much lower level of C3 splitting than original polysaccharides. The antitumor activity of CM polysaccharides was also lower than that of the original ones, but the difference was less (*34*). These results indicate that all polysaccharides which have tumor inhibitory action, possibly including zymosan, had C3-splitting activity *in vitro*, and some qualitative correlation with antitumor

TABLE 4. Percentage of Rosette-forming Cells with Human Erythrocytes after Treatment with C4-deficient Guinea Pig Serum

Cell	Reaction medium		
	GVB^{2+} (%)	Mg^{2+} EGTA-GVB (%)	EDTA-GVB (%)
OAT	48	70	1
Daudi	81	88	3
P3HR-1	54	59	1
Raji	26	28	0

activities indicates a possible relationship with the host-mediated tumor inhibition *in vivo*.

C3 can be activated directly by tumor cell membrane and C3 was generated through C3 shunt alternate pathway (*35*). This was clearly shown by rosette formation due to immune adherence reaction of human erythrocytes to activated C3b site produced on the cell membrane of OAT cells (cell line from lung cancer), Daudi cells, P3HR1 cells and Raji cells (cell lines from African Burkitt lymphoma) after reaction with complement (Table 4). This was confirmed by measurement of C3b site formed on the tumor cell membrane by ^{125}I-labelled $F(ab')_2$ antibody against C3. Activation of C3 system leading to the reaction with humoral factors and cellular factors resulting in tumor cell membrane damage can be initiated by tumor cell membrane itself and it will be worthwhile to consider the presence of such a defense mechanism in the tumor-host relationship.

Phylogeny and Immunogenetics of the Complement System in Host Defense Immune Mechanism

Collaborating and synergistic action of complement system with immunoglobulin system (IgG, IgM, IgA, IgE), and cell-mediated immunity (lymphocytes, macrophage, granulocytes, erythrocytes, or platelets) is illustrated in Fig. 1, on the basis of immunochemical analysis of the sequential reaction of complement. Experimental and clinical observations of complement system in tumor-bearing host as well as potentiating effect of host defense against cancer through activation of the complement system indicate a possible new way for immunopotentiation through enhancing the complement system integrating cellular and humoral immune systems.

Schematic representation of phylogenical study of immune systems and immune regulation gene analysis is shown in Fig 6. C3 system is considered to start from invertebrates (*36*), performing the most fundamental function of all immune systems. Complement regulation genes are situated in the central area in No. 17 chromosome gene system linked to Ss-Slp regions (*16, 17*). Cell-mediated immunity system started from echinodermata (star fish) (*37*) and its control gene is considered to be located in the right peripheral side in No. 17 chromosome possibly linked to the regions from H-2D to Tla loci (*18*). Immunoglobulin systems started from cyclostomata (hag fish) (*38*), and situated in the left side in the same chromosome linked

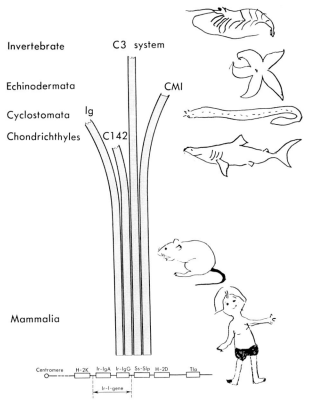

FIG. 6.   Phylogeny and gene location of C3 system, cell-mediated immunity (CMI), immuno-globulin system (Ig), and C142.

to the Ir-1 locus. C3 system is situated between these two systems in the center and is considered to be responsible for the central function of the immune system as revealed by its phylogeny and gene locations (Fig. 6). C142 started from chon-drichthyes (shark) (39) and the conjunction of the immunoglobulin system and the complement system is accomplished at this stage. If we consider these phylogeny and immunogenetical events, impaired cell-mediated immunity in a radiation- or disease-induced host, such as a lepromatous leprosy- (40), Wegener granuloma- (41) or tumor-bearing host (14), is considered to be a state of insufficiency in the pe-ripheral immune system and this is compensated for by the central immune system, that is, in these cases, increase of complement level. Therefore, our central function hypothesis of the complement system integrating the immunoglobulin system as well as the cell-mediated system in mammalian immune system is supported by (i) immunochemical flow analysis of the complement system in relation to im-munoglobulin and other cellular factors (Fig. 1), (ii) phylogeny of various immune systems, and (iii) genetic map observed in mouse H-2 gene analysis. Therefore based on these fundamental immunochemical and biological analyses of the im-mune system, potentiation of the complement system should be pursued as one of the most promising procedures to increase host defence against cancer.

REFERENCES

1. Nuttall, G. Experimente über die bakterienfeindlichen Einflusse des thierischen Körpers. Z. Hyg., *4*: 353–394, 1888.

2. Ritz, H. Über die Wirkung des Cobragiftes auf die Komplemente. Z. Immunol., *13*: 62–83, 1912.

3. Coca, A. F. A study of anticomplementary action of yeast of certain bacteria and of cobra venom. Z. Immunol., *21*: 604–622, 1914.

4. Ueno, S. Studien über die Komponenten des Komplementes. Japan. J. Med. Sci. VII, *2*: 201–225, 1938.

5. Mayer, M. M. Complement and complement fixation. *In;* E. A. Kabat and M. M. Mayer (eds.), Experimental Immunochemistry, ed. 2, pp. 133–240, Charles C. Thomas Publisher, Springfield, Ill., 1961.

6. Nelson, R. A., Jr. The immune adherence phenomenon. An immunological specific reaction between microorganism and erythrocytes leading to enhanced phagocytosis. Science, *118*: 733–737, 1953.

7. Nishioka, K. Measurements of complement by agglutination of human erythrocytes reacting in immune adherence. J. Immunol., *90*: 86–97, 1963.

8. Nishioka, K. and Linscott, W. D. Components of guinea pig complement. I. Separation of a serum fraction essential for immune hemolysis and immune adherence. J. Exp. Med., *118*: 767–793, 1963.

9. Linscott, W. D. and Nishioka, K. Components of guinea pig complement. II. Separation of serum fractions essential for immune hemolysis. J. Exp. Med., *118*: 795–815, 1963.

10. Inoue, K. and Nelson, R. A., Jr. The isolation and characterization of a new component of hemolytic complement, C3e. J. Immunol., *95*: 355–367, 1965.

11. Inoue, K. and Nelson, R. A., Jr. The isolation and characterization of a ninth component of hemolytic complement, C'3f. J. Immunol., *96*: 386–400, 1966.

12. WHO Immunology Unit. Nomenclature of complement. Bull. WHO, *39*: 935–938, 1968.

13. Müller-Eberhard, H. J. Patterns of complement activation. Prog. Immunol., *2*: 173–182, 1974.

14. Nishioka, K. Complement and tumor immunology. Adv. Cancer Res., *14*: 231–293, 1971.

15. Fu, S. M., Kunkel, H. G., Brusman, H. P., Allen, F. H., and Fotiuo, M. Evidence for linkage between HL-A histocompatibility genes and those involved in the synthesis of the second component of complement. J. Exp. Med., *140*: 1108–1111, 1974.

16. Démant, P., Capková, J., Hingová, E., and Voracová, B. The role of the histocompatibility-2-linked Ss-Slp region in the control of mouse complement. Proc. Natl. Acad. Sci. U.S., *70*; 863–864, 1973.

17. Ferreira, A. and Nussenzweig. V. Genetic linkage between serum levels of the third component of complement and the H-2 complex. J. Exp. Med., *141*: 513–517, 1975.

18. Gelfand, N. C., Sachs, D. H., Lieberman, R., and Paul, W. E. Ontogeny of B lymphocytes. III. H-2 linkage of a gene controlling the rate of appearance of complement receptor lymphocytes. J. Exp. Med., *139*: 1142–1153, 1974.

19. Henson, P. M. The immunologic release of constituents from neutrophil leucocytes. I. The role of antibody and complement on non-phagocytable surfaces or phagocytable particles. J. Immunol., *107*: 1535–1546, 1971.

20. Pepys, M. B. Role of complement in induction of antibody production *in vivo*. J. Exp. Med., *140*: 126–145, 1974.

21. Pepys, M. B. and Butterworth, A. E. Inhibition by C3 fragments of C3-dependent rosette formation and antigen-induced lymphocytes transformation. Clin. Exp. Immunol., *18*: 273–282, 1974.

22. Tamura, N. and Nelson, R. A., Jr. Three naturally occurring inhibitors of components of complement in guinea pig and rabbit serum. J. Immunol., *99*: 582–589.

23. Okada, H. and Nishioka, K. Complement receptors on cell membranes. I. Evidence for two complement receptors. J. Immunol., *111*: 1444–1449, 1973.

24. Okuda, T. and Tachibana, T. The third component of complement and complement receptors. Japan. J. Exp. Med., *44*: 531–538, 1974.

25. Lachmann, P. J. and Müller-Eberhard, H. J. The demonstration in human serum of conglutinogen-activating factor and its effect on the third component of complement. J. Immunol., *100*: 691–698, 1968.

26. Perlmann, P. and Hölm, G. Cytotoxic effects of lymphoid cells *in vitro*. Adv. Immunol., *11*: 117–193, 1969.

27. Thompson, R. A. and Lachmann. P. J. Reactive lysis: The complement-mediated lysis of unsensitized cells. J. Exp. Med., *131*: 629–641, 1970.

28. Brai, M. and Osler, A. Cobra venom-induced hemolysis. Activity levels in sera of patients with neoplastic and other diseases. J. Exp. Med., *136*: 950–955, 1972.

29. Sakamoto, M. and Nishioka, K. Studies on rat complement. II. Complement level in experimental tumor in rats. Japan. J. Exp. Med., 1975, in press.

30. Kawamura, I., Tsuji, T., Kumasaka, T., Ogawa, I., and Hayata, Y. Complement level in lung disorders. Clin. Immunol., *3*: 576–581, 1971 (in Japanese).

31. Ashikawa, K., Motoya, K., Sekiguchi, M., and Ishibashi, Y. Immune response in tumor-bearing patients and animals. II. Incidence of tuberculin anergy in cancer patients. Gann, *58*: 567–573, 1967.

32. Hornung, N. and Arquembourg, R. C. β1C globulin. An acute phase serum reactant of human serum. J. Immunol., *94*: 307–316, 1965.

33. Halpern, B. N., Biozzi, G, Stiffel, C., and Mouton, D. Inhibition of tumor growth by administration of killed *Corynebacterium parvum*. Nature, *212*: 853–854, 1966.

34. Okuda, T., Yoshioka, Y., Ikekawa, T., Chihara, G., and Nishioka, K. Anticomplementary activity of antitumor polysaccharides. Nature New Biol., *238*: 59–60, 1972.

35. Okada, H. and Baba, T. Rosette formation of human erythrocytes on cultured cells of tumor origin and activation of complement by cell membrane. Nature, *248*: 521–522, 1974.

36. Day, N. K. B., Gewurz, H., Johannsen, R., Finstad, J., and Good, R. A. Complement and complement-like activity in lower vertebrates and invertebrates. J. Exp. Med., *132*: 941–950, 1970.

37. Metchnikoff, E. Immunität, Gustav Fischer, Jena, 1897.

38. Lincithicum, D. S. and Hildemann, W. H. Immunologic responses of Pacific hagfish. III. Serum antibodies to cellular antigens. J. Immunol., *105*: 912–918, 1970.

39. Ross, G. D. and Jensen, J. A. The first component of the complement system of the nurse shark. Hemolytic characteristics of partially purified Cln. J. Immunol., *110*: 175–182, 1973.

40. Petchclai, B., Chutanondh, R., Prasongsom, S., Hiranras, S., and Ramasoota, T. Complement profile in leprosy. Am. J. Trop. Med. Hyg., *22*: 761–764, 1973.

41. Watabe, Y., Nagaki, K., and Fujita, T. Complement level in Wegener's granulomatosis. Proc. XIth Complement Symposium, 52–54, 1974 (in Japanese).

Discussion of Paper of Dr. Nishioka

DR. ALEXANDER: Do some malignant cells possess Fc or C3 receptors? Also, is there any alteration in the cell-mediated immune mechanisms you described in animals that are genetically deficient in one or more complement components?

DR. NISHIOKA: In Adv. Cancer Res., 1971, we reported finding C3b but not Fc receptors on nasopharyngeal carcinoma cells. We also demonstrated C3d as well as Fc receptors on Burkitt lymphoma tumors. The particular complement component one finds, if any, on a tumor cell may indicate something about its origin.

Secondly, there is only a limited amount of information related to tumorigenesis in complement deficient animals. Recently, patients lacking C3b inactivator, who were thus unable to block the positive feedback of C3b showing C3 deficiency, were reported to have decreased resistance to infection.

DR. HALPERN: Many species show a wide divergency in serum complement levels, the mouse having one of the lowest and the guinea pig probably the highest. Is there any correlation between the incidence of spontaneous tumors and the quantity of serum complement?

DR. NISHIOKA: It is generally accepted that experimental neoplasms are much more difficult to induce in the guinea pig than in the mouse and this will be in line with your suggestion. However, it appears that the values for serum complement levels one obtains depends greatly on the assay system employed. For example, in our laboratory Dr. Tamura has shown that it is very difficult to measure mouse complement activity using rabbit anti-sheep erythrocyte (SRBC) antibody, but rather easy when employing mouse anti-SRBC antiserum. One must therefore determine which type of antibody is most suitable for the complement system to be measured.

HOST DEFENSE AGAINST CANCER AND ITS POTENTIATION, D. MIZUNO ET AL. (EDS.),
UNIV. OF TOKYO PRESS, TOKYO / UNIV. PARK PRESS, BALTIMORE, PP. 97-111, 1975

Immunopotentiating Agents: Activity Profiles and Possible Mode of Action

P. Dukor, S. Vasella, E. Schläfli, B. Perren, R. H. Gisler, F. M. Dietrich, and D. Bitter-Suermann*

*Research Laboratories of the Pharmaceuticals Division, Ciba-Geigy Limited, Basel, Switzerland and Institut für Medizinische Mikrobiologie der Johannes-Gutenberg Universität, Mainz, Germany**

Abstract: In order to define the possible targets of systemically active immunopotentiating agents, numerous reference compounds were explored in different murine assay systems. Antibody responses to subimmunogenic doses of a thymus(T)-dependent antigen (bovine serum albumin (BSA)) were significantly enhanced by charged dextrans, carboxymethyl (CM)-cellulose, polyacrylic acid, poly A: U, concanavalin A (Con A), tetramisol, sphingosine derivatives, vitamins A and E, and other substances provided they were administered by the same route as the antigen (intraperitoneal). Poly I: C, pokeweed mitogen, lipopolysaccharide (LPS), Diribiotine, lysolecithin, and lentinan were active also when given by a different route (subcutaneous). Most of these agents failed to enhance the response to BSA in athymic mice or to the T-independent antigen DNP dextran, indicating that the cooperative cell system was required for the expression of the potentiating effect.

Some compounds (notably LPS) elicited antibody formation to BSA in non-immunized mice. There was an apparent correlation between this property, "T-cell substituting" ability *in vivo* and *in vitro*, C3-activating potency and intrinsic immunogenicity and mitogenicity for B cells. However, the effect of some of these substances was not restricted to B lymphocytes: LPS, levan, and SIII also potentiated the generation of alloantigen-specific cytotoxic T cells in one-way mixed lymphocyte cultures totally depleted of B cells. On the other hand, macrophages were required for the induction, though not the expression, of LPS-promoted cytotoxicity. The potentiating action of LPS (and of CM-pachymaran which neither enhanced antibody formation nor activated C3) was mimicked by some batches of serum, increased numbers of macrophages, and by 2-mercaptoethanol. In their presence, LPS and CM-pachymaran failed to enhance cytotoxic sensitization any further, while poly A: U and poly I: C still showed an additive effect.

In the pursuit of new approaches to the immunological control of neoplastic diseases, the development of systemically active immunoleptic agents capable of enhancing immune responses without concomitant injection of the target antigen (*1*) may represent an important step. Despite the rapidly growing knowledge of the surveillance mechanisms involved in host defences against cancer, it is still difficult to choose simple, sensitive, and predictive assay systems for the detection of clinically useful immunopotentiating compounds. We have therefore started to investigate a large number of reference substances in a variety of models. These included antibody formation to thymus (T)-dependent and T-independent antigens in the presence or absence of T cells both *in vivo* and *in vitro*, and the induction of cell-mediated cytotoxicity (CML) to allogeneic tumor cells *in vivo* and in unidirectional mixed lymphocyte cultures (MLC). In this communication we summarize some of our results and attempt to explore the possible link between bone marrow-derived (B) cell stimulation, activation of the alternative pathway of complement, and potentiation of T-mediated cytotoxicity, which may be relevant for the mode of action of tumor-inhibitory polysaccharides (*2–4*).

Effect of Immunopotentiating Agents on Antibody Formation in Mice

In a comparative investigation, activity profiles of known drugs were established in normal NMRI and in congenitally athymic nu/nu mice immunized with graded doses of T-dependent (bovine serum albumin (BSA)) and T-independent (DNP_{20}-aminoethyl dextran) antigens which were administered intraperitoneally (i.p.). Test substances were injected in different doses (up to the highest tolerated

TABLE 1. Effect of Various Immunopotentiating Agents on Antibody Formation to 10 μg BSA in NMRI Mice[a]

Agent[b]	mg/kg/day i.p.	Score values[c] in					
		Immunized mice			Non-immunized mice		
		Day : 0	0 to 4	−4 to 0	0	0 to 4	−4 to 0
Dextran sulfate	50	NS	4.6	—	—	4.3	—
DEAE-dextran	50	NS	13.5	—	—	0	—
CM-cellulose	500	NS	10.7	—	—	2.4	—
Polyacrylic acid	1	2.7	14.1	—	1.6	3.0	—
Poly I : C	5	4.9	14.6	NS	—	1.9	0.6
	0.5	16.2	7.8	11.6	0.6	0	0
Poly A : U	5	5.3	3.7	NS	—	0	1.25
Concanavalin A	0.1	4.3	NS	—	—	0.4	—
Pokeweed mitogen	20	12.3	NS	—	—	—	—
Lipopolysaccharide	5	14.8	19.3	20.8	—	15.1	21.2
	0.5	20.0	6.2		5.9	13.6	10.6

[a] BSA in buffered saline injected i.p. into groups of 10 mice on day 0. Serum sampling on day 9, 15, and 29. Antibody determination in individual sera by passive hemagglutination of glutaraldehyde-coupled BSA-SRBC (*5*) in microtiter plates. Titers expressed as $\log_2$ of reciprocal final agglutinating dilution (*6*). [b] Agents injected on day 0, 0 to 4, or −4 to 0. Injections on day 0 preceded antigen administration by 30 min. For details of compounds see Table 3. [c] Sums of differences between mean titers of drug-treated and -untreated mice on day 9, 15, and 29. Only differences >2 and statistically significant at $P<0.01$ (Wilcoxon rank test) are included (*6*). NS : not significant.

TABLE 2. Effect of Various Immunopotentiating Agents on Antibody Formation to 10 μg BSA in NMRI Mice[a]

Agent[b]	mg/kg/day i.p.	Score values[c] in					
		Immunized mice			Non-immunized mice		
		Day: 0	0 to 4	−4 to 0	0	0 to 4	−4 to 0
Lentinan	10	19.5	NS	17.8	2.9	2.3	—
	1	NS	NS	21.6	—	—	—
Diribiotine	(1 ml)	4.5	NS	5.4	1.1	—	0
Tetramisol	1	NS	3.3	—	—	1.1	—
Vitamin A	0.1	NS	6.4	NS	—	0	—
Lysolecithin	10	17.8	6.0	—	0	0	—
Norsphingosin	10	NS	10.6	—	—	0	—
Dehydrohomo- sphingosin	10	NS	17.6	—	—	0	—
L(+)-Cystein	30	NS	4.3	—	—	8.5	—
Vitamin E	30	5.9	NS	—	0	—	—
Al(OH)₃	50	10.7	—	—	3.6	—	—

[a],[b],[c] As in Table 1.

TABLE 3. Effect of Various Immunopotentiating Agents on Antibody Formation to 10 μg BSA in NMRI Mice[a]

Agent[b]	mg/kg/day s.c.	Score values[c] in					
		Immunized mice			Non-immunized mice		
		Day: 0	0 to 4	−4 to 0	0	0 to 4	−4 to 0
Poly I:C	5	NS	12.0	NS	—	0	—
Pokeweed mitogen	20	—	15.1	—	—	5.3	—
Lipopolysaccharide	5	NS	NS	18.4	—	—	23.6
	0.5	NS	NS	13.1	—	—	23.6
Lentinan	1	NS	NS	3.7	—	—	0
Diribiotine	(1 ml)	4.8	NS	NS	0.74	—	—
Lysolecithin	1	NS	4.4	NS	—	0	—
Al(OH)₃	50	4.9	—	—	0	—	—
Al(OH)₃-BSA[d]	(0.1 ml)	16.6	—	—	—	—	—
icFA-BSA[e]	(0.05 ml)	29.9	—	—	—	—	—

Compounds: dextran sulfate MW 5×10^5 (Serva), DEAE-dextran MW 2×10^6 (Pharmacia), CM-cellulose sodium salt and polyacrylic acid MW $0.5-1 \times 10^6$ (Fluka), poly I:C and poly A:U MW$>10^5$ (Miles), Con A (Calbiochem), pokeweed mitogen (Grand Island Biological), LPS *E. coli* 0111:B4 (Difco), lentinan (gift of Dr. G. Chihara), Diribiotine® (Saphal), tetramisol (synthesized by Dr. R. Bernasconi), vitamin E alcohol (Koch-Light), lysolecithin (Schwarz-Mann), norsphingosin and dehydrohomosphingosin (synthesized by Prof. E. Jenny), L(+)-cystein (Merck), vitamin E (Fluka), Alhydrogel® 2% Al₂O₃ (Superfos), incomplete Freund's adjuvant (icFA) (Difco).
[a],[b],[c] As in Table 2. [d] Mixed, 10 μg BSA and approx. 2 mg Al(OH)₃ in 0.1 ml. [e] Mixed, 10 μg BSA in saline and icFA 1:1 in 0.05 ml.

amount) either once 30 min before the antigen, or daily for 5 consecutive days ending or starting with the time of immunization. In each experiment, non-immunized but drug-treated animals were included as controls for the possible non-specific effect of the test agent on antibody formation. Sera were obtained at regular intervals and examined for anti-BSA or anti-DNP antibodies by passive hemagglutination using glutaraldehyde coupled BSA- and DNP-BSA-sheep red blood cells (SRBC). A synopsis of results derived from BSA-immunized NMRI mice is provided in Tables 1–3. Only data obtained with a subimmunogenic dose of 10 μg are reported, since the potentiating effect of most active compounds remained unchanged within a range of 1 to 10^4 μg of antigen. Moreover, only effective agents and in each case the optimal drug doses are shown.

It can be seen, that some typical patterns of drug-dependent potentiation of antibody formation emerged: the majority of the substances were far more effective if injected by the same route as the antigen (i.p.). A contribution of peritoneal irritation to the increased antigen-specific antibody response was made unlikely by the inability of gelatine, thioglycolate medium, and proteose-peptone broth to elicit more antibody in immunized than in non-immunized mice. Nevertheless, a merely local effect due to altered antigen handling in the peritoneal cavity cannot be safely discounted. Also, immunopotentiation by i.p. administered drugs in this model may rather correspond to phenomena occurring *in vitro*. However, several compounds were active even if given by a separate route (subcutaneous (s.c.)), thus reflecting a truly systemic effect. Poly I: C, pokeweed mitogen, lipopolysaccharide (LPS) and—to a lesser degree—lentinan, Diribiotine, lysolecithin, and $Al(OH)_3$ belong to this group.

There were also distinct differences with respect to the most effective drug timing. Lentinan was only active when administered prior to the antigen, poly I: C and LPS showed similar results before and after antigen, while vitamin E and poly A: U appeared to be rather more effective if given after the immunization.

The most striking feature was the increase in antibody titers of non-immunized mice elicited by LPS, pokeweed mitogen, dextran sulfate, and polyacrylic acid, reflecting probably polyclonal activation of B lymphocytes (7). Interestingly enough, a whole series of reducing agents which—with the minor exception of L(+)-cystein —all failed to promote antigen-dependent anti-BSA formation, greatly augmented the background titers. This was true for L(+)-cystein, 2-mercaptoethanol, S-(2-aminoethyl)-isothiouronium bromide-hydrobromide, L(+)-cysteinium chloride, and L(+)-ascorbic acid. Moreover, proteose peptone, gelatine, and thioglycolate medium had similar effects. Indeed, the latter three agents are commonly used for the induction of macrophage-rich peritoneal exudates, while thiols and disulfides are known to stimulate the replication of lymphoid cells *in vitro* (8, 9) and to substitute operationally for macrophages (10). It is tempting to interpret this in terms of increased macrophage activity and to speculate that the release of T- and B cell activating factors from phagocytic cells may constitute a common pathway for many immunopotentiating agents.

None of the substances mentioned in this section was capable of enhancing antigen-dependent antibody formation to DNP dextran, which itself of course possesses intrinsic B-cell stimulating properties (11). Furthermore, the inability of athymic nu/nu mice to respond to immunization with BSA could barely be overcome by the compounds included in this study. Nevertheless, a statistically significant but very small increase in anti-BSA antibody production by immunized nu/nu mice could be achieved by administration of dextran sulfate and polyacrylic acid. Similar T-cell substituting effects have been reported before (*12*) and were also observed in the case of LPS (*13*).

A detailed report of the results summarized in this section is going to be published elsewhere (*6*).

C3 Conversion and B-cell Activation by Immunopotentiating Agents

It has recently been established that many—if not all—T-independent antigens share the ability to activate B cells non-specifically, *i.e.*, that they possess intrinsic mitogenicity for B lymphocytes and trigger polyclonal antibody formation (*7*). Some of these antigens are also known to operationally substitute for T cells *in vitro* during otherwise T-dependent antibody responses (*7, 14, 15*). As is exemplified in Fig. 1, powerful B-cell mitogens such as LPS, cobra venom factor (*17*), and pokeweed mitogen, but not the T-cell specific mitogens concanavalin A (Con A) and phytohemagglutinin (PHA) (*18*) very efficiently promoted the induction

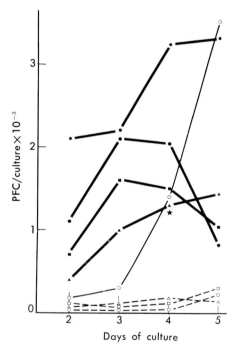

FIG. 1. "T-cell substituting" effect of cobra venom factor (VF), sepharose-coupled VF (SEPH-VF), DNP_{27}-dextran (DNP-DEX), pokeweed mitogen (PWM), LPS *E. coli* 0111: B4, but not of Con A and PHA on the 19S antibody response (direct plaque-forming cells) to SRBC in T-cell deficient cultures containing 7×10^6 nu/nu lymph node cells (B) and 3×10^5 nu/+ macrophages (M). B+M: control cultures. B+M+T: control cultures supplemented with 3×10^6 cortisone-resistant thymus cells (crT). Points represent means of triplicate cultures. For methods see Ref. *16*. ▲ VF; * SEPH-VF 40 μl; ★ DNP-DEX 10^{-2} μg; ■ PWM 16 μg; ● LPS 12 μg; □ Con A 4 μg; △ PHA 16 μg; —O— B+T+M; --O-- B+M.

of antibody formation to SRBC in T-cell deficient mosaic cultures (16). The same substituting effect was achieved by DNP dextran. A systemic investigation of T-independent antigens and B-cell mitogens has also revealed that a great majority of them activate C3 via the alternative pathway of the complement system (APC) (19). This has led us to propose that binding of activated C3 (C3b, C3d) to complement receptor bearing B lymphocytes could provide a second signal for B-cell triggering (20). However, the evidence linking C3 conversion to direct B-cell triggering has remained largely circumstantial and inconclusive (21).

Nevertheless, the fact that highly effective immunopotentiators such as dextran sulfate, polyacrylic acid, LPS, and pokeweed mitogen appear to activate B lymphocytes non-specifically, and to functionally replace T cells in some experimental situations, has prompted us to investigate the C3-converting ability of systemic adjuvants. The results are summarized in Tables 4 and 5. It can be seen that—as expected—there is an overall correlation between C3-conversion and B-cell activation by immunopotentiating agents: on the whole the specific potentiators such as DEAE-dextran, poly I: C, poly A: U, and lysolecithin were devoid of C3-activating properties while the non-specific potentiators were found to share the ability of converting C3. There were, however, some notable exceptions. As had been reported already by Okuda et al. (3) lentinan is a very active inducer of the alternative pathway, but its adjuvant activity is antigen-dependent and could not be dem-

TABLE 4. C3 Conversion and B-cell Activation by Immunopotentiating Agents

Agent[a]	C3 activation via APC[b]		T-independent immunogenicity and/or B-cell mitogenicity[c]	Non-specific potentiation of antibody formation		T-cell substitution	
	%C3 converted	at mg/ml		in vivo[d]	in vitro[c]	in vivo	in vitro[c]
Dextran sulfate	95	0.06	+	+	+	+(12)	
DNP$_{27}$-dextran	43	0.5	+(11)		+		+[e]
Polyacrylic acid	0	Up to 5		+		+(12)	
LPS E. coli 0111 : B4	33	0.5	+	‡‡‡	+	+(13)	+[e] (15)
Cobra venom factor	100	0.1	+(17)		+(17)		+[e] (17)
Pokeweed mitogen	28	0.16	+	+	+		+[e]
POL	21	1.5	+		+		+(14)
SIII	100	0.5	+		+		
Levan	62	0.5	+		+		
Lentinan	50	0.2		φ		φ[f]	
Pachymaran	30	1		φ			
HE-pachymaran	30	0.1		φ			
CM-pachymaran	0	Up to 5	φ[f]	φ			

[a] Agents not listed in Tables 1–3: dinitrophenylated amino-ethyl dextran MW 1.5×10^5 (synthesized by Dr. E. Rüde), cobra venom factor (purified chromatographically from Naja Naja venom (29)), polymerized flagellin (POL) (donated by Dr. J. Pye), type III pneumococcal polysaccharide MW 2×10^5 (SIII) and levan MW 2×10^7 (gifts of Dr. J. G. Howard), pachymaran, HE-pachymaran and CM-pachymaran (provided by Dr. J. Hamuro). [b] Loss of hemolytically active C3 (22) in C4-deficient guinea pig serum following 30 min 37°C incubation with test substance (19). Only optimum concentrations for C3 activation are shown. All compounds tested up to a concentration of 5 mg/ml. [c] Reviewed in Ref. 7. [d] Score values in non-immunized mice: $<3 = \phi$, $3-10 = +$, $11-20 = ‡‡$, $>20 = ‡‡‡$ (see Tables 1–3 and text). [e] See Fig. 1. [f] See text.

TABLE 5. C3 Conversion and B-cell Activation by Immunopotentiating Agents

Agent	C3 activation via APC[a]		T-independent immunogenicity and/or B-cell mitogenicity	Non-specific potentiation of antibody formation		T-cell substitution	
	% C3 converted at mg/ml			in vivo[b]	in vitro	in vivo[c]	in vitro
Dextran 500[a]	0	Up to 5	ϕ^{c}	ϕ	ϕ	ϕ	
DEAE-dextran	0[e]	Up to 5		ϕ		ϕ	
CM-cellulose	0	Up to 5		ϕ		ϕ	
Poly I : C	0	Up to 5		ϕ		ϕ	
Poly A : U	0	Up to 5		ϕ		ϕ	
Lysolecithin	0	Up to 5		ϕ			
Tetramisol	0	Up to 5		+			
Diribiotine	0	Up to 5 μl	ϕ^{c}	ϕ			
Concanavalin A	0[e]	Up to 5	ϕ (18)	ϕ		ϕ	ϕ^{f}

[a] As in Table 4. [b] Score values graded as in Table 4, data from Tables 1–3 and text. [c] See text.
[d] MW 3.7×10^5 (Pharmacia). [e] C3 consumption due to non-specific binding (19). [f] See Fig. 1.

onstrated in athymic mice. Indeed, the T-cell affinity of lentinan has been described in detail by Dresser some time ago (23). Pachymaran, hydroxyethyl (HE)-pachymaran and carboxymethyl (CM)-pachymaran failed to potentiate antigen-specific and non-specific anti-BSA formation in intact and athymic mice (6). In addition, CM-pachymaran was not mitogenic for B cells, but shared some other adjuvant properties with LPS, as will be shown in the next section. While pachymaran and HE-pachymaran were able to convert C3, CM-pachymaran appeared inactive in this assay. It would seem, therefore, that complement activation by these tumor inhibitory polysaccharides is not related to their immunologic qualities.

Potentiation of T-cell Functions by B-cell Activating Polysaccharides

The effect of B-cell activating polysaccharide antigens is by no means restricted

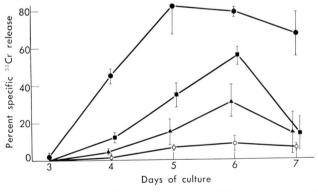

FIG. 2. Potentiating effect of LPS and of C57Bl/6 macrophages (M) on the development of cytotoxicity in one-way MLC set up with 1.9×10^6 C57Bl/6 crT and 5×10^5 700R-irradiated DBA$_2$ crT. Cytotoxicity assessed by specific isotope release from DBA$_2$ mastocytoma cells (killer: target ratio 15 : 1, 3-hr incubation). Points represent means of triplicate cultures $\pm$ standard deviation. For methods see Ref. 24. ○ control; ● LPS 4 μg/ml; ■ 2.5×10^4 M; ▲ 6×10^3 M.

to B cells. In fact, we have reported *(24)* that *E. coli* lipopolysaccharide 0111: B4, levan, and pneumococcal polysaccharide SIII were able to potentiate the generation of cytotoxic effector cells in MLC. As is shown in Fig. 2 LPS greatly enhanced cytotoxic sensitization in cultures containing exclusively cortisone-resistant thymus

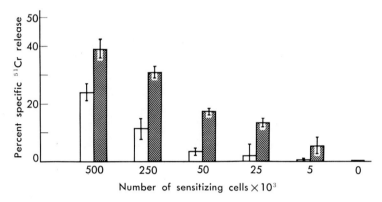

FIG. 3.   Alloantigen-dependence of LPS-mediated cytotoxic sensitization in MLC set up with 1.9×10^6 C57Bl/6 lymph node cells (LNC) and graded numbers of sensitizing 700 R-irradiated DBA$_2$ LNC in the presence (hatched bars) or absence (white bars) of 4 μg LPS/ml. Cytotoxicity assessed on day 5 as in Fig. 2. Bars represent means of triplicate cultures $\pm$ standard deviation.

TABLE 6.   Effect of Selective Removal of Macrophages, T Cells or B Cells on Development and Expression of LPS-mediated Cytotoxicity in One-way Mixed Cortisone-resistant Thymus Cell (crT)-cultures[a]

	Depletion procedure	Time of depletion	Type of antiserum	LPS 4 μg/ml present during culture period[b]	Cytotoxicity of 5 day cultures (% specific ^{51}Cr release from DBA$_2$ mastocytoma cells[c])
A	Incubation[d]	Prior to culturing	None (medium)	−	9.5 ± 2.8
			None (medium)	+	80.6 ± 2.7
			None (medium+C)[e]	+	84.2 ± 0.5
			Anti-mouse macrophage[f]+C	+	5.3 ± 3.1
B	Immuno-adsorption on Sephadex[g]	Prior to culturing	Anti-KLH (control)[g]	+	100.5 ± 4.5
			Anti-mouse light chain[g]	+	93.9 ± 7.3
C	Incubation[d]	After culturing, before cytotoxicity assay	None (medium)	+	58.9 ± 11.8
			None (medium+C)	+	64.9 ± 8.2
			None (NMS+C)[h]	+	49.0 ± 1.3
			Anti-θC3H[h]+C	+	2.5 ± 4.8
			Anti-mouse macrophage[f]+C	+	55.1 ± 13.0

[a] Method as in Ref. *24*. Responder cells 10^6 C57Bl/6 crT (A, C), 10^6 C3H crT (B), stimulator cells 10^6 750R-irradiated DBA$_2$ crT.   [b] LPS *E. coli* 0111 : B4 in A, B added *after* depletion procedure.   [c] Assay as in Ref. *24*.   Killer: target 15 : 1, 5-hr incubation.   [d] 30 min 37°C with antiserum (or medium), washing, 30 min 37°C with C (or medium), washing.   [e] Agarose-absorbed fresh rabbit serum 1 : 3.   [f] Raised in rabbits. Prepared and absorbed as in Ref. *27*.   [g] Column-passaged cells provided by Dr. L. Hudson *(28)*.   [h] Raised in AKR mice. Prepared and absorbed as in Ref. *16*.

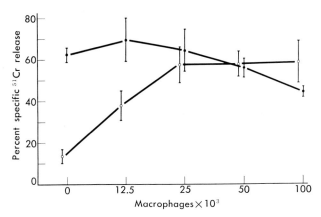

FIG. 4. Potentiation by LPS of cytotoxic sensitization in MLC supplemented with graded numbers of macrophages. Cultures set up with 1.9×10^6 C57Bl/6 crT, $5 \times 10\ 700^5$ R-irradiated DBA$_2$ LNC and different numbers of macrophages (as shown on the abscissa). Cytotoxicity assessed on day 5 as in Fig. 2. ○ cultures without LPS; ● cultures with LPS 4 μg/ml.

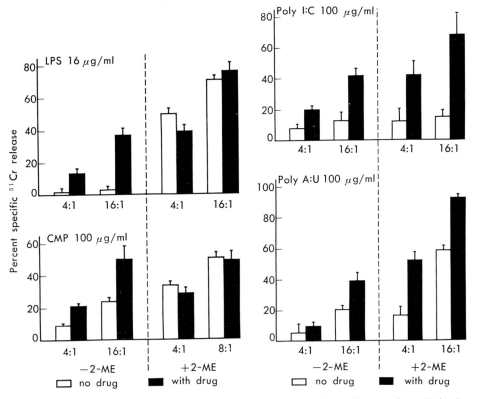

FIG. 5. Potentiating effect of LPS, CM-pachymaran, poly I : C and poly A : U *in vitro* on cytotoxic sensitization in one-way MLC (10^6 C3H LNC $+ 10^6$ 750 R-irradiated DBA$_2$ LNC). Dependence of drug effects on the presence of 5×10^{-5} M 2-mercaptoethanol (2-ME). Cytotoxicity after 5 days of culturing. Killer: target ratios as indicated on the abscissas, 5-hr incubation. Otherwise same legend as Figs. 2 and 3.

cells (crT) which constitute a relatively pure population of functional T cells (*16*). Macrophages or monocytes appear to be necessary both for T-cell proliferation and development of killer cells (*25, 26*). Indeed, as can be seen also in Fig. 2, addition of macrophages had a similar restoring effect on the poorly reactive crT cultures as had LPS.

Figure 3 demonstrates clearly that LPS-mediated cytotoxic sensitization in MLC occurred only in the presence of alloantigen, and other experiments proved that LPS-induced cytotoxicity is antigen-specific: C57B1/6 crT sensitized in the presence of LPS with DBA$_2$ cells gave rise to a killer cell population which could only lyse DBA$_2$, but not C3H cells. Moreover, as is shown in Table 6, LPS-mediated cytotoxicity is effected by a T-cell population, since cytotoxicity of the killer population could be abolished by treatment with highly specific anti-θ serum while a selective anti-macrophage serum proved ineffective.

The mechanism of LPS-mediated T-cell potentiation is not clear. The B-cell mitogenicity of LPS does not appear to be involved: total removal of the contaminating B cells from the crT-MLC prevented the development of Ig-staining cells during the culture period, but not of killer cells (Table 6). On the other hand, at least some macrophages were required for the action of LPS, because sensitization could be completely suppressed by incubating the seemingly pure crT population with anti-macrophage serum prior to culturing. Subsequent resupplementation with macrophages restored responsiveness to LPS.

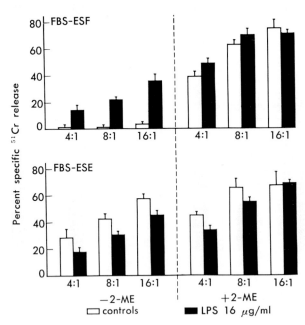

FIG. 6. Serum-dependence of potentiating LPS-effect on cytotoxic sensitization in MLC. Cultures set up with two different batches of fetal bovine serum (FBS=Rehatuin®, Reheis): ESF=Lot M 28505 and ESE=Lot M 28405. Otherwise identical culture and assay conditions as in Fig. 5.

As demonstratedi n Fig. 4, the potentiating action of LPS could be abolished by supplementing the crT cultures with a by-itself optimally stimulating number of macrophages. Moreover, enhancement of cytotoxicity by LPS could be mimicked by 2-mercaptoethanol (Fig. 5) and by an otherwise B-cell activating factor present in some batches of fetal calf serum (Fig. 6). In the presence of this factor or of 2-mercaptoethanol, LPS failed to enhance the generation of killer cells any further. The same was true for CM-pachymaran, while poly A: U and poly I: C still displayed an additive potentiating effect (Fig. 5). These results are compatible with the idea that poly A: U and poly I: C may directly interact with T cells, while LPS and CM-pachymaran may exert their action through macrophages. It remains to be shown whether macrophage activation, induction of exocytosis by split products of complements (21) and synergism with macrophage products may provide the common denominator for lymphocyte stimulation by complement active and inactive polysaccharides and by 2-mercaptoethanol.

REFERENCES

1. Mathé, G. Attempt at using systemic immunity adjuvants in experimental and human cancer therapy. *In ;* G. E. W. Wolstenholme and J. Knight (eds.), Immuno-potentiation (Ciba Foundation Symposium), vol. 18, pp. 305–326, Elsevier / Excerpta Medica / North Holland, Amsterdam / London / New York, 1973.

2. Chihara, G., Maeda, Y. Y., Hamuro, J., Sasaki, T., and Fukuoka, F. Inhibition of mouse sarcoma 180 by polysaccharides from *Lentinus edodes* (BERK.) SING. Nature, *222*: 687–688, 1969.

3. Okuda, T., Yoshioka, Y., Ikekawa, T., Chihara, G., and Nishioka, K. Anticomplementary activity of anti-tumour polysaccharides. Nature New Biol., *238*: 59–60, 1972.

4. Maeda, Y. Y., Hamuro, J., Yamada, Y. O., Ishimura, K., and Chihara, G. The nature of immunopotentiation by the anti-tumor polysaccharide lentinan and the significance of biogenic amines in its action. *In ;* G. E. W. Wolstenholme and J. Knight (eds.), Immunopotentiation (Ciba Foundation Symposium), vol. 18, pp. 259–281, Elsevier / Excerpta Medica / North Holland, Amsterdam / London / New York, 1973.

5. Avrameas, S., Taudou, B., and Chuilon, S. Glutaraldehyde, cyanuric chloride and tetraazotized *o*-dianisidine as coupling reagents in the passive hemagglutination test. Immunochemistry, *6*: 67–76, 1969.

6. Vasella, S. Zur Prüfung immunpotenzierender Stoffe. Ph.D. Thesis. University of Bern. Unpublished.

7. Coutinho, A. and Möller, G. Thymus-independent B cell induction and paralysis. Adv. Immunol., *21*: 113–236, 1975.

8. Heber-Katz, E. and Click, R. E. Immune responses *in vitro*. V. Role of mercaptoethanol in the mixed-leukocyte reaction. Cell. Immunol., *5*: 410–418, 1972.

9. Broome, J. D. and Jeng, M. W. Promotion of replication in lymphoid cells by specific thiols and disulfides *in vitro*. J. Exp. Med., *138*: 574–592, 1973.

10. Chen, C. and Hirsch, J. G. The effects of mercaptoethanol and of peritoneal macrophages on the antibody-forming capacity of nonadherent mouse spleen cells *in vitro*. J. Exp. Med., *136*: 604–617, 1972.

11. Gisler, R. H., Staber, F., Rüde, E., and Dukor, P. Soluble mediators of T-B interaction. Eur. J. Immunol., *3*: 650–652, 1973.

12. Diamantstein, T., Wagner, B., L'Age-Stehr, J., Beyse, I., Odenwald, M. V., and Schulz, G. Stimulation of humoral antibody formation by polyanions. III. Restoration of the immune response to sheep red blood cells by polyanions in thymectomized and lethally irradiated mice protected with bone marrow cells. Eur. J. Immunol., *1*: 302–304, 1971.

13. Andersson, B. and Blomgren, H. Evidence of thymus-independent humoral antibody production in mice against polyvinylpyrrolidone and *E. coli* lipopolysaccharide. Cell. Immunol., *2*: 411–424, 1971.

14. Schrader, J. W. Specific activation of the bone marrow-derived lymphocyte by antigen presented in a non-multivalent form. Evidence for a two-signal mechanism of triggering. J. Exp. Med., *137*: 844–849, 1973.

15. Watson, J., Trenkner, E., and Cohn, M. The use of bacterial lipopolysaccharides to show that two signals are required for the induction of antibody synthesis. J. Exp. Med., *138*: 699–714, 1973.

16. Gisler, R. H. and Dukor, P. A three-cell mosaic culture. *In vitro* immune response by a combination of pure B- and T-cells with peritoneal macrophages. Cell. Immunol., *4*: 341–350, 1972.

17. Dukor, P., Schumann, G., Gisler, R. H., Dierich, M., König, W., Hadding, U., and Bitter-Suermann, D. Complement-dependent B-cell activation by cobra venom factor and other mitogens? J. Exp. Med., *139*: 337–354, 1974.

18. Janossy, G. and Greaves, M. F. Lymphocyte activation. II. Discriminating stimulation of lymphocyte subpopulations by phytomitogens and heterologous anti-lymphocyte sera. Clin. Exp. Immunol., *10*: 525–536, 1972.

19. Bitter-Suermann, D., Hadding, U., Schorlemmer, H.-U., Limbert, M., Dierich, M., and Dukor, P. Activation by some T-independent antigens and B-cell mitogens of the alternative pathway of the complement system. J. Immunol., in press.

20. Dukor, P. and Hartmann, K. U. Bound C3 as the second signal for B cell activation. Cell. Immunol., *7*: 349–356, 1973.

21. Dukor, P., Dietrich, F. M., Gisler, R. H., Schumann, G., and Bitter-Suermann, D. Possible targets of complement action in B cell triggering. *In;* L. Brent and J. Holborow (eds.), Progress in Immunology II, vol. 3, pp. 99–109, North Holland, Amsterdam, 1974.

23. Dresser, D. W. and Phillips, J. M. The cellular targets for the action of adjuvants: T-adjuvants and B-adjuvants. *In;* G. E. W. Wolstenholme and J. Knight (eds.), Immunopotentiation (Ciba Foundation Symposium), vol. 18, pp. 3–18, Elsevier / Excerpta Medica / North Holland, Amsterdam / London / New York 1973.

24. Perren, B., Schläfli, E., Schumann, G., and Dukor, P. Cytotoxic sensitization in one-way mixed T cell cultures. *In;* D. Parker and J. L. Turk (eds.), Contact Hypersensitivity in Experimental Animals, Monogr. Allergy, vol. 8, pp. 125–135, Karger, Basel, 1974.

25. Gordon, J. Role of monocytes in the mixed leukocyte culture reaction. Proc. Soc. Exp. Biol. Med., *127*: 30–33, 1968.

26. Wagner, H., Feldmann, M., Boyle, W., and Schrader, J. W. Cell-mediated immune response *in vitro*. III. The requirement for macrophages in cytotoxic reactions against cell-bound and subcellular alloantigens. J. Exp. Med., *136*: 331–343, 1972.

27. Shortman, K. and Palmer, J. The requirement for macrophages in the *in vitro* immune response. Cell. Immunol., *2*: 399–410, 1971.

28. Schlossmann, S. F. and Hudson, L. Specific purification of lymphocyte populations on a digestible immunoadsorbent. J. Immunol., *110*: 313–315, 1973.

29. Bitter-Suermann, D., Dierich, M., König, W., and Hadding, U. Bypass-activation of the complement system starting with C3. I. Generation and function of an enzyme from a factor of guinea pig serum and cobra venom. Immunology, *23*, 267–281, 1972.

Discussion of Paper of Drs. Dukor et al.

DR. ALEXANDER: Why do you feel it is necessary to envoke a mechanism other than macrophage activation to explain the effects you note upon intraperitoneal injection of poly I: C or endotoxin followed by the antigen? We know that these materials can activate macrophages even at very low concentrations, and that the processes by which these cells handle antigens is different depending upon whether or not they are stimulated. Thus, it might be simple to hypothesize that the activated macrophages process the antigen so as to be able to present it in a more efficient way to the lymphocytes.

DR. DUKOR: I was only speculating that perhaps some mechanism apart from simple macrophage activation, such as the release of T- or B-cell stimulating products from these cells, might be operative, in some cases. A constant pattern of blocking of potentiation in the presence of stimulatory lots of fetal calf serum and 2-mercaptoethanol was observed with LPS and CM-pachymaran, but not with poly I: C or poly A: U. This may point to an essential difference in their mode of action. Whether it is a laboratory artifact or a meaningful result remains to be substantiated.

DR. HOBBS: Didn't you show that a tremendous stimulation in a unidirectional MLC obtained in the absence of macrophages?

DR. DUKOR: No, and I apologize for that apparently deceptive slide. Originally we believed this was true, as LPS invoked a good stimulatory response when adherent cells were removed by column absorption, so that there appeared to be no mononuclear phagocytic cells at the onset of our cultures. However, after 2 days of incubation, such cells were noted. Addition of anti-macrophage serum, that was not cytotoxic to lymphocytes, together with complement, at the beginning but not toward the end of the culture period, blocked this LPS-mediated cytotoxic sensitization. This, of course, does not prove that LPS acts through macrophages, but only that the final result is a macrophage-dependent event.

I must emphasize that one can resupplement such a culture with macrophages using as few as 5,000 cells. Also, one should be very careful not to employ induced cells; if they are thioglycolate induced, they're toxic.

DR. HOBBS: R. van Furth has stated that about 1.5% of the small round cells in the peripheral blood are macrophage precursors, and that may be the problem.

DR. NISHIOKA: I agree that the adjuvant action of the tumor-inhibitory polysaccharides you investigated may not be entirely based upon C3 activation. What concentration of these polysaccharides did you employ in your *in vitro* assay?

DR. DUKOR: All our test substances were used up to a maximum concentration of 5 mg/ml. The assay was performed using normal and C4-deficient guinea pig serum.

DR. NISHIOKA: In our experiments, doses of up to 10 mg/ml were used. We sometimes observed a critical dose dependence, sufficient to change a negative into a positive response within this range.

DR. DUKOR: I fully agree. Indeed, CM-pachymaran was much less potent than the other materials in this particular assay. It's extremely hazardous to extrapolate from such data to what is happening at the cellular level, however. We employed a fluid phase system without cells, while *in vivo* these tumor-inhibitory polysaccharides might become associated with cell membranes or other carriers and thereby acquire new properties with respect to complement activation, *etc*.

DR. MIZUNO: In agreement with your observations, we found a time-dependent decrease in the ability of LPS to stimulate macrophage cytotoxicity in the presence of allogeneic tumor cells. Such a decrease is not observed with lentinan. What is your interpretation of this difference?

DR. DUKOR: The LPS-mediated or -promoted cytotoxicity is identical to the normal alloantigen-induced cytotoxicity one obtains upon supplementation of cultures with the appropriate accessory cells or with stimulatory batches of fetal bovine serum or with 2-mercaptoethanol medium, so that they respond optimally. The kinetics are not changed by such additions.

DR. MIZUNO: I believe that, unlike lentinan, LPS may induce the formation of some inhibitory substance in the culture medium, capable of interfering with cytotoxicity.

DR. DUKOR: That's an attractive hypothesis, but I cannot offer any comparison between lentinan and LPS, as we have never examined lentinan in our culture system, in view of its insufficient solubility.

HOST DEFENSE AGAINST CANCER AND ITS POTENTIATION, D. MIZUNO ET AL. (EDS.),
UNIV. OF TOKYO PRESS, TOKYO / UNIV. PARK PRESS, BALTIMORE, PP. 113-130, 1975

The Role of Macrophages in the Host Defence against Cancer

Peter ALEXANDER

Chester Beatty Research Institute, Sutton, Surrey, U.K.

Abstract: Immunologically specific cytotoxic macrophages are found in tumour-bearing animals and their production requires the co-operation of thymus-dependent lymphocytes. There are at least two types of such macrophages on the basis of radiosensitivity and because some cause lysis of the tumour cells whereas others initially only inhibit DNA synthesis. In addition, there are immunologically non-specific cytotoxic macrophages which *in vitro* inhibit the growth of malignant cells but not of most normal dividing cells. Macrophages can be rendered non-specifically cytotoxic by certain polyanions such as dsRNA, endotoxin, and factors released by spleen cells. Immunologically specific cytotoxic macrophages acquire non-specific cytotoxicity to tumour cells following contact with the specific antigen.

In vivo both the specific and the non-specific cytotoxic macrophages contribute to resistance to tumour growth in certain, but probably not all, anatomical sites. The implications of these findings for immunotherapy and surveillance of spontaneously arising malignant cells will be discussed.

Tumours contain many more macrophages than is suggested by light-microscopic histology. There is a strong inverse correlation between the macrophage content of different tumours and their capacity to give rise to distant metastases. The macrophages in tumours are cytotoxic and reflect the immune reaction of the host to the tumour. These tumour macrophages are derived from host monocytes and a macrophage-rich tumour effectively competes for the monocytes of the host and as a result inflammatory reactions as well as delayed-hypersensitivity responses to unrelated antigens is greatly reduced in such animals. The so-called immunological anergy seen in advanced cancer is often not due to an impairment of lymphocyte function but is the result of a monocyte defect.

Macrophages exert several different functions in the complex interplay between malignant cells and the host. They contribute to the initiation of the immune response by processing antigens and presenting them in a suitable form to the lymphoid machinery. While no definitive experiments have been carried out to show that macrophages are essential if the host is to recognise tumour-specific transplantation type antigens (TSTA), it appears probable from studies with other antigens that they are. Whether phagocytosis by macrophages is involved in host resistance to tumours is also not clear. While suitably opsonised tumour cells are ingested by macrophages and destroyed, it is doubtful if this is a primary event under physiological conditions. From the point of view of tumour immunology the most important property of macrophages is their capacity to kill cells after a period of cell-to-cell contact. When cells have been killed in this way, they are then phagocytosed, but this is a late event and may be a "cleaning up" operation dependent on a primary cytotoxic reaction.

The term cytotoxic macrophages is used to describe cells which interfere with the normal growth of target cells with which they are in contact. This interference may be by lysis or by growth inhibition. In many of the experiments the end point measured has been the number of target cells which remain in contact with cyto-toxic macrophages after 24 or 48 hr of culture. Such a test will measure growth inhibition of target cells as well as lysis. In several experiments it has been shown that the initial event which occurs in the target cells is interference with DNA synthesis. However, the difference between growth inhibition and lysis is not absolute and macrophages which are principally growth inhibitory to one cell may be lytic when directed against another target. In any case after a period of growth inhibi-tion many target cells lyse. Operationally we distinguish between these two reac-tions by measuring release of isotope from prelabelled cells following 6 hr of contact with macrophages. Lytic macrophages are those which cause release, whereas growth inhibitory macrophages are those which interfere with DNA synthesis but do not cause release of isotopically labelled cell compounds within a relatively short time.

The Immunologically Specific Cytotoxic Macrophage

That macrophages obtained from the peritoneal cavity of suitably immunised mice are cytotoxic the allogeneic tumour cells and that this cytotoxic reaction shows an immunological specificity similar to that of complement-dependent antibodies has been known for 20 years from both *in vivo* and *in vitro* experiments (for a review, see Ref. *1*). However, convincing evidence that immunologically cytotoxic mac-rophages are involved in tumour immunity (*i.e.*, when the immunological reaction is directed against TSTA and not against allo-antigens) has only recently been obtained (*2, 3*). One reason why the role of macrophages in specific immunity is only now receiving detailed attention is that the bactericidal activity macrophages derived from animals immunised with a variety of micro-organisms is non-specific even though it is immunologically (*i.e.*, *via* lymphocytes) mediated (*4*). The paradox that the non-specific immunity exerted by macrophages against bacteria can be transferred with immunologically specific lymphocytes has in fact been resolved in experiments with tumour cells (*5*). There is now no conflict between the findings that immunity effected *in vivo* by macrophages against bacteria is immunologically non-specific yet macrophage-mediated immunity against tumours can be specific.

TABLE 1. Anti-tumor Macrophages

	X-ray dose needed to inhibit cytotoxicity	Produced by
Non-specifically cytotoxic		
a. Predominantly growth inhibitory		a. Polyanions
b. Preferentially attack malignant cells	>5,000R	b. Ag/Ab complexes
		c. Ag (acting on "immune macrophages
		d. Lymphokines
Specifically cytotoxic		
a. Growth inhibitory (lysis and phagocytosis occur subsequently)	<500R	a. From immune animal
		b. Direct contact with immune spleen cells
		c. "Armed" by SMAF
b. Rapidly lytic	>1,000R	From animals immunized with living cells

In vitro tests show that macrophages taken from the peritoneal cavity of mice immunised with either syngeneic or allogeneic tumour cells were cytotoxic to tumour cells in an immunologically specific way (2, 6). There is a quality difference in the macrophages derived from mice that have been immunised with living tumour cells and those which have been immunised with irradiated tumour cells as reflected in their mechanism of cytotoxicity and their sensitivity to X-rays (7) (Table 1). While both are growth inhibitory, lytic macrophages are produced predominantly following immunisation with living cells. The difference in the type of cytotoxicity is also reflected in their radiosensitivity; the lytic macrophages retain their cytotoxic action after 1,000 R of X-rays whereas the growth inhibitory macrophages lose their cytotoxic action following a dose of 500 R of X-rays.

Immunologically specific cytotoxic macrophages have also been produced by a process which we refer to as "arming." This can be achieved in two ways. (1) By incubating non-immune macrophages with immune lymphoid cells for more than 4 hr, after which they are specifically cytotoxic. This reaction is not mediated by a factor that can be found in the supernatant and appears to acquire direct cell-to-cell contact between the immune lymphoid cells and the macrophages. (2) By exposure to a soluble factor referred to as the specific macrophage "arming" factor (SMAF), which is released when the immune lymphoid cells are cultured with the specific antigen (8). The chemical nature of SMAF has not yet been elucidated but it is found in two distinct molecular sizes; in the order of 50,000 daltons and the other greater than 300,000 daltons (9). Both have an affinity for the macrophage surface and the specific antigens, and they may therefore be referred to operationally as cytophilic antibodies. Since the first discovery of SMAF evidence has accumulated that it is a product released by thymus-dependent lymphocytes (T lymphocytes) (9) and that macrophages are not armed by complement-dependent cytotoxic immunoglobulins. T lymphocytes are also necessary (12) for the formation following immunisation *in vivo* of immunologically specific cytotoxic macrophages (Table 2). The available data is consistent with the hypothesis that T lymphocytes are required both at the afferent and the efferent arm of the immune

TABLE 2. Role of T Cells in the Cytotoxic Action of Macrophages. Growth Inhibitory Effect of Immune Macrophages or Normal Macrophages Armed with Immune Spleen Cells to Allogeneic Lymphoma Cells (12)

Macrophages or spleen cells obtained from mice	Percent growth inhibition (48 hr)		
	Peritoneal macrophages	Non-immune macrophages armed with	
		Spleen cells	SMAF from spleen cell cultures
Not immunised	16	10	7
10 days after immunisation with lymphoma	96	82	65
Sham-thymectomised 10 days after immunisation	78	71	43
T-cell deprived 10 days after immunisation	22	5	0
Macrophages or spleen cells treated with anti-θ serum			
Treated not immunised	12	5	0
Not treated 21-day immune	87	97	66
Treated 21-day immune	85	11	10

response which leads to the appearance of immunologically specific cytotoxic macrophages.

The Non-specific Cytotoxic Macrophage (Previously Referred to as "Activated" Macrophage)

The recognition of the target cell and the subsequent expression of cytotoxicity by these macrophages is not determined by membrane antigens on the surface of the target cells such as histocompatibility, or tumour-specific antigens. Macrophages can be rendered non-specifically cytotoxic by procedures that do not involve the lymphoid apparatus of the host and in particular there appears to be no involvement of T cells. The fact that the cytotoxicity of these macrophages is not directed against specific surface antigens does not mean that their cytotoxic action is quite indiscriminate. When macrophages are rendered non-specifically cytotoxic in vitro they do not appear to attack normal types of host cells but they kill tumour cells (10). This observation appears to me to be one of the greatest interest since non-specifically cytotoxic macrophages may be more effective distinguishing between normal and transformed cells than any other in vitro test. The discrimination exerted by non-specifically cytotoxic macrophages may resemble the primitive protective mechanisms of invertebrates.

We used to refer to these non-specifically cytotoxic macrophages as being "activated" (11). While this terminology has the advantage of brevity it has led to confusion because the term "activation" has been used by others to describe changes induced in macrophages that are revealed by morphological, biochemical, and physiological criteria which do not necessarily correlate with the cytotoxic potentialities of the macrophage. For example, macrophages have been referred to as being "activated" if they have become larger than normal, show increased phagocytic capacity, show an increased rate of spreading on glass, have an increased metabolic activity or have more lysosomes. While non-specifically cytotoxic macrophages have many of these properties, there are many procedures which will cause "activation" according to these physiological criteria but which do not render macrophage non-specifically cytotoxic. It is not yet known whether treatments which increase the intracellular microbicidal activity of macrophages necessarily render them non-specifically cytotoxic.

The first procedure to be described, and still the simplest, for producing non-specifically cytotoxic macrophages is to expose them to minute quantities of endotoxin or dsRNA (whether derived from fungal viruses or made synthetically like poly I/poly CI (11)). After such treatments macrophages which do not normally inhibit the growth of lymphoma and sarcoma cells do so and this effect is not due to a direct toxic action of these agents on the target cells. The active principle of endotoxin is lipid A and not the polysaccharides moiety. Johnson (13) has found that poly A/poly U is also an efficient agent for this purpose. Perhaps the most interesting substance which has been found to render macrophages cytotoxic is the simple

pepto-disaccharides shown above and isolated from bacterial cell walls. Recently we found that immune complexes and aggregated IgG's will also convert non-cytotoxic into cytotoxic macrophages. It would also appear that in addition to the release of the SMAF immune lymphoid cells when they are cultured with the specific antigen will, under certain conditions, produce lymphokine which renders macrophages non-specifically cytotoxic. The nature of this factor is not known.

An entirely different method of producing non-specific macrophages is to incubate specific cytotoxic macrophages with the antigen to which they have been sensitised (5). This phenomenon is shown diagrammatically in Fig. 1 and probably explains why non-specifically macrophages can be found in the peritoneal cavity of mice carrying a persistent infection. This phenomenon was first described by Remington et al. (14) in mice infected with toxoplasmodia but is now known to apply to other types of persisting infection. Those strains of BCG which give rise

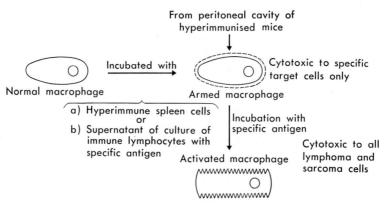

Fig. 1.   Mechanism of macrophage cytotoxicity.

to persistent infection in mice cause the appearance of non-specific cytotoxic macrophages, whereas other forms of BCG (like that produced by Glaxo) which are rapidly erradicated in mice produce immune macrophages which can be rendered non-specifically cytotoxic by contact with antigen. Without adding antigen macrophages from mice inoculated with Glaxo BCG are not non-specifically cytotoxic.

The mechanism by which non-specifically cytotoxic macrophages exert their activity which in most cases is that of cytostasis (*i.e.*, inhibition of DNA synthesis) lysis being a late event, although there are some target cells which are lysed quite rapidly by non-specifically toxic macrophages. It is not yet clear whether to achieve this effect the target cells have to be in intimate contact with the macrophage or whether the toxic action is caused by a factor released from the non-specifically cytotoxic macrophages. There is some evidence that macrophages following treatments which render them non-specifically cytotoxic release into the supernatant macromolecules which are capable of stopping DNA synthesis but the activity of this factor is low. It must be emphasised that macrophages release very many biologically active macromolecules into the surrounding fluid and that the rate of release of some of these materials—in particular enzymes capable of hydolysing macromolecules—is greatly increased by treatments which also render macrophages cytotoxic. It is therefore an attractive hypothesis that the mechanism of non-specific cytotoxicity is mediated by humoral factors perhaps and that the need for close proximity between the target cell and the macrophage is that the action of the humoral factor is antagonised by components in the medium.

Evidence for an In Vivo Role of Cytotoxic Macrophages

Evans (*15*), using various criteria, such as adhesion to glass or plastic in the presence of trypsin, lysis by specific antimacrophage serum, and phagocytic ability, showed that the number of macrophages in tumours is often much greater than conventional histopathological methods indicate. In a series of primary transplanted tumours in the rats the macrophage contents range from 4–60% of the cell population of the tumour. Since tumour cells which have been freed of macrophages and then transplanted into syngeneic recipients gave rise to tumours with typical macrophage contents, it is clear that reversal of the macrophages in the tumours are the monocytes from the blood. The macrophages in tumours are in general non-specifically cytotoxic although in some experiments immunologically specific cytotoxicity has been detected.

Tumours which are grown in animals deprived of T lymphocytes but have a normal bone marrow function (and therefore are able to provide monocytes in normal numbers), do not contain nearly as many macrophages as grow in normal rats (Fig. 2). This shows that the macrophages enter into the tumour as part of an immune response required in T lymphocytes and that the difference in the macrophage contents of tumours is not due to difference in blood supply (*16*). That there is a relation in the immune reaction invoked by the tumour and the macrophage content was shown (*16*) by the fact that the macrophage content of tumours is directly related to their immunogenicity (Table 3). It is of particulari nterest that

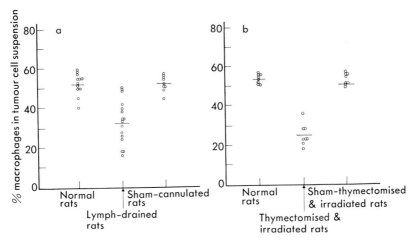

FIG. 2.   Effect of immunosuppression on % macrophages in tumours grown in deprived rats. a, controls; b, rats with thoracic duct lymph drainage; c, sham-cannulated rats; d, thymectomised and irradiated rats; e, sham-thymectomised rats. The thoracic ducts of rats were cannulated and tumours implanted 1 day later. Drainage was terminated after 8–10 days when the number of lymphocytes collected over 24 hr had fallen to 0.1% of the first day's yield. Sham-cannulated rats underwent anaesthesia and laparotomy, but the duct was left intact. Other rats were thymectomized at 4 weeks and then received 3×300 rad whole-body irradiation (X-rays) at 2-week intervals. To ensure recovery of the bone marrow, an interval of 4 weeks was allowed between the last dose of irradiation and implantation of the tumour. At this time, treated rats were able to develop normal inflammatory macrophage exudates in response to intraperitoneal oyster glycogen stimulation, indicating normal monocyte production. Thymuses of sham-thymectomised rats were exposed but not removed and received no irradiation. The tumour used was a benzpyrene-induced fibrosarcoma (HSBPA) which had been passage 20–25 times in syngeneic Hooded rats. All tumours were grown i.m. in hind limbs, excised 14 days later when they were approximately 2 cm in diameter, and their macrophage contents assessed by Evans' methods. Each point represents one rat, and the horizontal bar is the mean of the group. (a) Effect of thoracic duct lymph drainage of host on % macrophages in HSBPA tumour. (b) Effect of previous thymectomy and irradiation of host on % macrophages in HSBPA tumour.

TABLE 3. Macrophage Content, Incidence Metastases, and Immunogenicity of Chemically Induced Rat Fibrosarcomata Transplanted into Syngeneic Recipients

Tumour	Mean % macrophages (and range)	Incidence of metastases (%)	Immunogenicity
MC-3	8 (2–12)	100	$< 10^3$
HSH	12 (10–15)	100	10^3–2×10^4
ASBPI	22 (18–26)	50–55	10^5
MCI-M	38 (36–42)	20–30	10^6
HSN	40 (34–44)	30–35	5×10^6–10^7
HSBPA	54 (42–63)	10–12	10^7–5×10^7

The incidence of metastases was measured after excision of tumours which had been growing intramuscularly (i.m.) in hind limbs for 14 days. Immunogenicity was assessed as the number of cells required for tumour growth in rats which were immunised by excision of i.m. tumour 14 days previously.

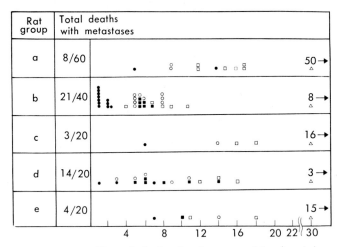

Time of death after tumour excision (weeks)

FIG. 3. Effect of immunosuppression on incidence of metastases after excision of HSBPA tumour. HSBPA tumours were grown i.m. in hind limbs of various groups of immunosuppressed rats (lymph drained, b, and thymectomised and irradiated, d) and appropriate controls (a, c, e) untreated rats a, and sham-cannulated c, or sham-thymectomised c, for 14 days. The tumour-bearing limbs were then amputated, and the animals kept for observation on the development of metastases for up to 30 weeks. ● deaths with no evidence of metastases; ○ deaths with lymph node metastases; □ deaths with lung metastases; ■ deaths with lymph node and lung metastases; △ survivals.

there is a direct correlation between the tendency of tumours to give rise to distant metastases and their macrophage content (Table 3). Those tumours which have high macrophage contents have a low incidence of spontaneous metastases. Following removal of T cells the macrophage content of the tumour is lowered (Fig. 2) and at the same time the metastatic potential of such tumours is greatly increased (Fig. 3).

More direct evidence for the *in vivo* relevance of immunologically specific cytotoxic macrophages came from studies in which mice were immunised with irradiated syngeneic lymphoma cells, a procedure which renders them resistant to a subsequent challenge with the cells. The lymphocytes from such immune mice were not found to be cytotoxic to the tumour cells *in vitro* but transferred immunity *in vivo* (*17*). In other syngeneic tumour systems lymphocytes from immune donors can be shown to have some cytotoxic activity *in vitro* but in general such cytotoxicity is weak and is much less than the cytotoxicity produced when the same lymphoid cells are tested *in vivo* by the so-called Winn test, in which the lymphoid cells of the host are mixed with tumour cells and then injected into normal animals. Under these conditions lymphocytes from immune animals which were not cytotoxic at all or only very feebly cytotoxic *in vitro* inhibited most efficiently tumour growth *in vivo* in an immunologically specific manner. Moreover it can be shown that the Winn test works only if the recipients of the mixture of immune lymphoid cells and tumour cells have a normally functioning bone marrow. If the recipient is exposed to whole body radiation or to injection of silica, then the mixture of immune lymphoid cells and tumour cells grows. This data is consistent with the view that a "macrophage or monocyte" present in the recipient are "armed" by the immune lymphoid cells and that it is this "armed" cell that destroy the tumour cells. Specifically immune macrophages can also under rather restricted conditions be used for immunotherapy but they do not act systemically because injected macrophages do not distribute themselves throughout the body but tend to be trapped in liver and spleen (*18*). Immunologically specific monocytes are likely to be more useful than macrophages for immunotherapy since monocytes would be expected to produce a systemic rather than only a local effect.

The *in vivo* significance of non-specific and cytotoxic macrophages in tumour control is open to conjecture. Remington *et al.* (*14*) found that the incidence of virally induced leukaemia was delayed in mice that had been infected with toxoplasmodia but the effect was small and in general there have been few reports which indicate that the induction of tumours is either significantly reduced or delayed in animals carrying a persistent infection (and therefore having non-specific and cytotoxic macrophages). The well-known anti-tumour action of endotoxin and double-stranderd dsRNA cannot be wholly attributed to the fact that the reagents induce non-specific cytotoxicity of macrophages *in vitro* as well as *in vivo*. An essential component of this anti-tumour action, which is unquestionably multifactorial, is that they induce haemorrhagic necrosis within established tumours. There are however some indications that macrophages rendered non-specifically cytotoxic by these agents play a contributory role in the *in vivo* anti-tumour effects (*19*).

Experiments from our laboratory show quite clearly that macrophages from immune animals are rendered non-specifically cytotoxic on meeting the specific antigen not only *in vitro* but also when the contact with antigen occurs *in vivo* (*5*). This is of course the situation under which a delayed hypersensitivity reaction is induced in the skin. Both in man and in experimental animals skin tumours can be made to regress if a delayed hypersensitivity reaction to an unrelated antigen is induced in the area of skin involved with tumour. These delayed hypersensitivity reactions are usually induced by sensitising the donor to dinitrochlorobenzene or to BCG and then producing a delayed hypersensitivity reaction by injecting the sensitizing antigen of purified protein derivative (PPD). We were able to show (*20*) by studies of tumours growing in the peritoneal cavity that the rejection of tumours during the course of a delayed hypersensitivity reaction correlates directly with the appearance of non-specifically cytotoxic macrophages. The fact that the non-specifically macrophages are selectively active against malignant cells makes them a most valuable tool for eliminating tumours.

The relation of adjuvant activity and the induction of changes in macrophages which render them non-specifically cytotoxic is very close. Thus dsRNA, endotoxin and in particular the peptoglycans isolated from bacterial cell wall are all most potent adjuvants. This suggests the possibility that when tumour cells meet non-specifically cytotoxic macrophages they are not only destroyed but that as a result of their interaction with the cytotoxic macrophages they give rise to a higher degree of immunity than if they had met normal (*i.e.*, non-cytotoxic) macrophages.

A speculative but very attractive hypothesis is that non-specific cytotoxic macrophages may exert a surveillance mechanism in the body against spontaneously arising malignant cells. There are several lines of evidence which suggest that malignant transformations occur much more frequently than do tumours and that the reason for this is that the body eliminates the vast majority of malignantly transformed cells before they can give rise to a tumour. However, the hypothesis that the *in vivo* control of malignantly transformed cells occurs *via* T lymphocyte-mediated immunity has run into problems. There are several clear and decisive animal experiments which show that after removal of T cells mice do not become more susceptible to spontaneous tumours or to tumours induced by chemical carcinogens. The only carcinogenic process to which they are more vulnerable is the induction of tumours by viruses that normally are only oncogenic in new-born animals. We are therefore faced with the possibility of either abandoning the concept of surveillance altogether or of postulating a surveillance mechanism which is not based on the conventional immune system but on a non-specifically cytotoxic macrophage.

REFERENCES

1. Pearsall, N. N. and Weiser, R. S. The Macrophage, Lea and Febiger, Philadelphia, 1970.
2. Evans, R. and Alexander, P. Cooperation of immune lymphoid cells with macrophages in tumour immunity. Nature, *228*: 620–622, 1970.
3. Takeda, K. Immunology of Cancer, Hokkaido Univ. School of Med., Japan, 1969.
4. Mackaness, G. B. The influence of immunologically committed lymphoid cells on macrophage activity *in vivo*. J. Exp. Med., *129*: 973–992, 1969.
5. Evans, R. and Alexander, P. Mechanism of immunologically specific killing of tumour cells by macrophages. Nature, *236*: 168–170, 1972.
6. Otter, W. den, Evans, R., and Alexander, P. Cytotoxicity of murine peritoneal macrophages in tumour allograft immunity. Transplantation, *14*: 220–226, 1972.
7. Otter, W. den, Evans, R., and Alexander, P. Recognition of two types of cytotoxic macrophages on the basis of difference in radiosensitivity. Transplantation, *18*: 421–428, 1974.

8. Evans, R. and Alexander, P. Rendering macrophages specifically cytotoxic by a factor released from immune lymphoid cells. Transplantation, *12*: 227–229, 1971.

9. Evans, R., Grant, C. K., Cox, H., Steele, K., and Alexander, P. Thymus-derived lymphocytes produce an immunologically specific macrophage-arming factor. J. Exp. Med., *136*: 1318–1322, 1972.

10. Hibbs, J. B., Jr., Lambert, L. H., Jr., and Remington, J. S. Possible role of macrophage mediated non-specific cytotoxicity in tumour resistance. Nature New Biol., *235*: 48–50, 1972.

11. Alexander, P. and Evans, R. Endotoxin and double stranded RNA render macrophages cytotoxic. Nature New Biol., *232*: 76–78, 1971.

12. Grant, C. K., Evans, R., and Alexander, P. Multiple effector roles of lymphocyte in allograft immunity. Cell. Immunol., *8*: 365–376, 1973.

13. Johnson, A. Personal communication.

14. Hibbs, J. B., Jr., Lambert, L. H., Jr., and Remington, J. S. Resistance to murine tumours conferred by chronic infection with intracellular Protozoa, Toxoplasma gondii and Besnoitia jellisoni. J. Infect. Dis., *124*: 587–592, 1971.

15. Evans, R. Macrophages in syngeneic animal tumours. Transplantation, *14*, 468–473, 1972.

16. Eccles, S. A. and Alexander, P. Macrophage content of tumours in relation to metastatic spread and host immune reaction. Nature, *250*: 667–669, 1974.

17. Alexander, P., Connel, D. I., and Mikulska, Z. B. Treatment of murine leukaemia with spleen cells or sera from allogeneic mice immunised against the tumour. Cancer Res., *26*: 1508–1519, 1966.

18. Alexander, P., Evans, R., and Mikulska, Z. B. Relationship between concomitant immunity and metastasis—The role of macrophages in concomitant immunity involving the peritoneal cavity. *In ;* S. Garattini and G. Franchi (eds.), Chemotherapy of Cancer Dissemination and Metastasis, pp. 177–185, Raven Press, New York, 1973.

19. Parr, I., Wheeler, E., and Alexander, P. Similarities of the anti-tumour actions of endotoxin, lipid A and double-stranded RNA. Brit. J. Cancer, *27*: 370–389, 1973.

20. Alexander, P. Activated macrophages and the anti-tumour action of BCG. Natl. Cancer Inst. Monogr., *39*: 127–133, 1973.

Discussion of Paper of Dr. Alexander

DR. HALPERN: It has recently been shown that the reticuloendothelial system hyperplasia which follows injection of *Corynebacterium parvum* into mice can be completely abolished by sublethal total body X-irradiation, while local radiation is without effect. I think this lends support to the idea that cells responsible for this hyperplastic phenomenon in the liver and spleen bone marrow-derived monocytes. If the macrophages found in the tumors you examined are also bone marrow-derived, similar total body irradiation would probably abate this infiltration, and might markedly after the evolution of the macrophage-rich tumors.

Secondly, after surgical excision of certain tumors, such as the Lewis fibrosarcoma, the rate of metastases is increased. It would be interesting to see the pattern of macrophage infiltration of such neoplasms.

DR. ALEXANDER: The experiment you suggested has been done (see Eccles and Alexander, Nature, *250:* 667, 1974), and your prediction is entirely correct. The infiltration of macrophages or monocytes into tumors is dependent on T cell-mediated reactions, T-cell depletion of an animal in the absence of bone marrow damage leads to a greatly diminished macrophage infiltrate. One should be cautious in interpreting results based upon total body irradiation or anti-lymphocyte serum treatment, as along with the immunodepression the bone marrow is greatly damaged.

DR. KOBAYASHI: Did you obtain morphological evidence that the macrophages you observed were indeed macrophages, as they are sometimes very similar to lymphocytes?

DR. ALEXANDER: Morphology is of little value, and I was pleased when Dr. Dukor emphasized this. There is a whole population of cells which are pre- or early monocytes, that do not immediately adhere to glass or infest carbon particles, but which manifest glass adherence or phagocytosis after a day of culture. If one takes a culture of spleen or buffy coat cells and incubates them, many will adhere to glass within 2 hr. But removal of the culture supernatant after 24 hr yields another population of macrophages. Thus, there are host mononuclear cells which have the potential of differentiating into monocytes or macrophages. The only definitive way of removing them is with a specific anti-macrophage serum, one which is not cytotoxic to thoracic duct lymph cells. By such treatment one will not obtain a second adherent population after 24- hr incubation.

DR. KOBAYASHI: Where were the macrophages located with respect to the tumor tissue?

DR. ALEXANDER: A small ring of macrophages surrounded the tumors, but the majority were uniformly distributed throughout the neoplasms. The problem is that ordinary histological sections prepared for the light microscope will not specifically reveal a macrophage. One may be misled if the electron microscope or a whole battery of histologic stains are not employed.

DR. KOBAYASHI: You mentioned that the macrophage content of the various tumors you examined paralleled the grade of its antigenicity. Is this perhaps because the macrophages themselves affected the grade of tumor antigenicity?

DR. ALEXANDER: I spoke of "immunogenicity," which is a complex parameter involving 1) the magnitude of the host's immune reaction which the tumor evokes, and 2) the effectiveness with which the tumor escapes or responds to it. All six of the tumors here described evoke a host reaction of approximately equal magnitude, and examination of cells from the draining lymph nodes reveals an equal immunologically specific cytotoxicity. The reason why only some are immunogenic, *i.e.*, a tumor challenge is rejected by immune animals, is that in some cases the tumor cells are able to avoid destruction. Thus, as I have here defined it, it is "escape" which determines how immunogenic the tumors are, but there may be other systems in which inherent tumor antigenicity plays a role also. One could argue that macrophages infiltrate tumors merely as passengers or by-products of the immune response, as in T cell-deprived animals there are many fewer macrophages in the tumor. It is very difficult to assay the cytotoxicity of macrophages within a tumor.

DR. JERNE: I assume that when you refer to a "specific macrophage," you mean a cell that has been armed by some lymphocyte factor. Is it known whether this is an antibody or T-cell product?

DR. ALEXANDER: There is evidence for both points of view. My own prejudice is that it is an immunologically specific macromolecule. It has been conclusively shown that a T-cell factor of unknown chemical nature can render macrophages specific, and I suspect a B-cell product can as well. The active substance may be analogous to IgE, which is very cytophilic for macrophages.

DR. AMOS: In attempting isolation of pure macrophage populations from animals that have rejected a tumor, we discovered a peculiar affinity between macrophages and lymphocytes. Many of these sticky lymphocytes themselves adhering to iron particles. Therefore, might not some of the effects you've presented be due to lymphocytes transferred along with macrophages, or to the generation of new cells in the reconstituted host, especially in an allogeneic combination?

    Secondly, Dr. Jerne previously referred to the work of Fauve in Jacob's laboratory, who found that a small molecule which causes macrophage immobility

is powerfully anti-inflammatory. The failure of macrophages to appear in the peritoneal cavities of some of your tumor-bearing animals could be explained on the
basis of such a molecule. Did you do differential leukocyte counts to see whether
there actually was a depletion of macrophages or monocytes from the circulation
in the tumor-bearing rats, as you've implied?

DR. ALEXANDER: We were very conscious of the need to deal with pure macrophage preparations, and we obtained populations consisting of more than 99%
macrophages, with virtually every cell phagocytizing several opsonized sheep erythrocytes, by a technique developed by Dr. Evans, in which monolayers were prepared from peritoneal exudate cells and allowed to adhere to glass in the presence
of trypsin and extensive washings. In addition, these cells were all destroyed by
our anti-macrophage serum not by ALS, both sera being defined in terms of their
action on thoracic duct lymphocytes. With such cells, from which all sticky lymphocytes should have been eliminated, we were able to transfer a local immunity
to the peritoneal cavity.

We considered the possibility that a humoral factor was responsible for the
macrophage depletion of these animals, but we were unable to produce monocyte
exhaustion by serum transfer. PPD-induced delayed hypersensitivity occurred in
BCG-sensitized rats given 5 ml of serum from a rat bearing a high macrophage
content tumor. The number of monocytes consumed in such a tumor is enormous,
on the order of 10^9 cells. Indeed, we now use macrophage rich tumors rather than
peritoneal exudates for the isolation of macrophages in large quantities.

DR. AMOS: How do you know that the macrophages are actually consumed by
the tumor, and not just non-specifically sticking there?

DR. ALEXANDER: Perhaps I should say they home there, for they are not destroyed.
The tumor macrophages are of host origin, and not a product of tumor cell dedifferentiation as the macrophages infiltrating parental tumors growing in F_1 hybrids
are of F_1 phenotype.

DR. NAUTS: Have you similarly examined the macrophage content of various
tissues surrounding human neoplasms, as this might be of value in planning immunotherapy?

DR. ALEXANDER: Valid results in our system can be obtained only with complete
tumor cell suspensions. By means of trypsin and collagenase treatment of rat sarcomas it is possible to salvage virtually all the cells in such tumors. With most
human neoplasms, use of sufficient enzymatic treatment to totally disperse all cells
results in much cell death, whereas mild enzymatic exposure leaves a residue of aggregated cells. Either method results in cell selection. It is a purely technical problem.
Malignant melanoma behaves more like rat sarcomas in this regard, and I was thus
able to present the macrophage contents of nine patients with melanoma.

DR. NISHIOKA: What is the nature of the cytotoxic factor in macrophages? Have you measured the release of lysosomal enzymes from these cells? Also, do your target cells possess C3b, as Dr. Pearlman described C3b on the surface of his target cells involved in macrophage and lymphocyte-mediated cytotoxicity?

Dr. Alexander: The active principle of the immunologically specific macrophage is unknown. With reference to the non-specific cells, your suggestion that it is due to the release of enzymes is probably correct, albeit perhaps not lysosomal enzymes, as the macrophage is an enzyme exporter whereas lysozyme is likely to be released only during a cell's death. It is difficult to determine whether supernatants of macrophage cultures can abolish target cell DNA synthesis or whether cell contact is indeed required, and there have been discordant results even in our own laboratory. I suspect this is because serum factors can compete with macrophage enzymes, so that when a macrophage and target cell are in intimate contact these hydrolytic enzymes can act immediately on the target. A group at the Rockefeller University has recently shown that activated macrophages (defined as having certain biochemical characteristics, but not all of which are cytotoxic) release certain hydrolytic enzymes in greater quantities than do normal macrophages.

We have not looked for C3b on our target cells, and would not expect the pure lymphocyte populations in thoracic duct lymph or nodes to have C3b bound to their surface. The complement effect you described is predominantly important in non-specific cytotoxicity, whereas ours is specific.

Dr. Janković: Do you consider foot pad thickness a better measurement of delayed hypersensitivity to PPD than the skin reaction?

Dr. Alexander: We've had great difficulty reading skin flank reactions in the rat. Foot pad swelling is a moderately reliable criterion when combined with histologic examination to insure that one is dealing with a mononuclear cell infiltrate.

Dr. Janković: Do you have quantitative data concerning macrophages in lymphoid and other tissues of tumor-bearing rats?

Dr. Alexander: The macrophage content of draining lymph nodes increases dramatically. At 7 days after tumor transplantation one can find directly cytotoxic T-cells there, but by 14 days after tumor transplantation the macrophage content is high, and it is now the predominant cytotoxic cell.

Dr. Janković: In order to be sure that there is an infiltration of the tumor by host macrophages one should expect a macrophage depletion in other tissues or a higher proliferative rate of macrophages.

Dr. Alexander: The macrophage is a fixed cell, and I don't believe that once a monocyte has differentiated into a macrophage in either the peritoneal cavity or a lymphoid organ, that it migrates. It is the competition for circulating monocytes that is important, while macrophages themselves may never migrate out of the lymphoid tissues into tumors.

DR. JANKOVIĆ: Are you sure that macrophages don't proliferate in the tumor-bearing animal?

DR. ALEXANDER: No, but macrophage proliferation doesn't occur during graft rejection. Mackaness and others have shown that differentiated macrophages can divide, but while many ³H-thymidine labelled macrophages appear during the course of an infection such as with BCG, we have never observed similarly labelled macrophages in tumors.

DR. DRESSER: What is the function of the SMAF? Is it to agglutinate the target material onto the surface of macrophages so that they simply have to phagocytize it, or does it stimulate the macrophage to become more active, in a way analogous to some of the other factors you've described?

DR. ALEXANDER: SMAF probably does have the dual functions you outlined, as it causes agglutination of the target cells to macrophages as well as macrophage activation, similar to the manner in which IgE and antigen act on mast cells. Non-specifically activated macrophages are most likely relatively ineffective, as several hours are required before irreversible cell damage is accomplished and, in the absence of specific agglutination, the macrophage and target will not remain in close proximity for a sufficient length of time. *In vitro,* gravity insures that the target cell makes contact with the macrophage.

DR. DRESSER: In your answer to Dr. Jerne's question, you raised the possibility that SMAF might be both an antibody and of T-cell origin. Despite the original claims of Marchalonis and Cohn that immunoglobulin was present on the T-cell surface, recent evidence collected by R.M.E. Parkhouse and others indicates that immunoglobulin is neither synthesized by nor present on the surface of T cells. Parkhouse and a New York group have now reported finding, in mice, an immunoglobulin molecule very similar to human IgD, which is synthesized by B cells and it is a candidate for an immunoglobulin which gets onto the T-cell surface by a cytophilic process. (Now shown by Parkhouse and Abney not to occur on T cells —April 1975). Is your proposed SMAF "antibody" perhaps similar to this IgD-like molecule?

DR. ALEXANDER: This is possible.

DR. DRESSER: The work I mentioned was performed using disc acrylamide gels. The "IgD" is characterized by circumstantial evidence concerning molecular size, and not directly by means of an anti-IgD class specific anti-serum.

Is it implicit in your description of SMAF that if one were to prepare a hybrid antibody molecule between an anti-macrophage antibody and anti-target cell antibody, and then added a non-specific factor, one could create a situation as efficient as SMAF?

DR. ALEXANDER: Yes, and a failure using such a system could always be rationalized on the basis of steric problems.

DR. KENNEDY: Did you attempt to correlate the ability of an animal to resist a tumor challenge while its primary was *in situ* with your ordering of immunogenicity based upon resistance to a tumor cell challenge following removal of the primary? For you assumed that patients with malignant melanoma and metastases had less resistance than those without secondaries.

DR. ALEXANDER: A study of concomitant immunity is complex, because it depends upon what site one challenges. Even with the most immunogenic of these rat tumors, very little concomitant immunity is detectable with a subcutaneous tumor challenge, but a strong reaction occurs following intravenous administration. There was little difference in the intravenous concomitant immunity among the various tumors utilized.

DR. KENNEDY: It appears that the most immunogenic of the tumors you investigated had the highest content of macrophages and were associated with the lowest levels of peripheral blood monocytes. Can one draw the conclusion that survival is more likely in the face of a dearth of circulating monocytes, and that a normal level of monocytes in the blood is a bad prognostic sign?

DR. ALEXANDER: No, although it is true that those rats bearing large tumors and exhibiting a good delayed hypersensitivity to PPD could not be cured surgically, whereas those animals showing poor delayed hypersensitivity responses could be so cured. But this was only noted with very large tumors, on the order of 20 g in a 200 g rat, and such an extreme situation is rarely approached clinically.

DR. KENNEDY: Our clinicians will be interested to hear that, as many depend upon skin tests to predict a patient's ability to reject his tumor.

DR. ALEXANDER: However, this was only one of the six parameters I mentioned which may contribute to the anergy of a tumor-bearing individual. Clinically, one does not often approach the ideal situation of being able to identify cases where one factor in a multi-factorial process predominates.

DR. KENNEDY: Did any of your rats, especially those with macrophage rich tumors, develop anemia? For, the usual anemia of neoplasia is indistinguishable from the anemia found in situations of chronic antigenic stimulation, as in autoimmune diseases and chronic low grade infections. Any depletion of peripheral blood monocytes observed might thus represent a failure of production as the result of an immune response leading to chronic antigenic stimulation, rather than to the sequestration of monocytes in the tumors.

DR. ALEXANDER: There is some bone marrow abnormality in these animals, as they present unusual peripheral blood smears. They are full of erythrocyte precursor elements, resembling the blood picture of a folic acid depleted animal. With large tumors animals may indeed become folate deficient, but these primitive cells remained in the absence of such a deficiency.

DR. HOBBS: We have been attempting to raise the monocyte counts in cancer patients based on the idea that it might aid in rejection of their tumors. As a result we have performed many careful peripheral monocyte counts in individuals with stage II and III malignant melanoma, and have not found a monocytopenia. Invariably, however, there is K cell depletion. Does your anti-macrophage serum delete K cells?

DR. ALEXANDER: One must realize that the K cell is actually a spectron of mononuclear cells capable of killing antibody coated targets. This activity is greatly reduced upon the addition of our anti-macrophage serum to buffy coat or peritoneal exudate cells. Macrophages, of course, can also lyse antibody coated cells.

Your monocyte counts may not include cells not easily recognizable on morphologic grounds as classical monocytes. At least this is the case in rats. Also, your patients don't share the enormous tumor load these animals bore.

DR. HOBBS: In our cancer patients, the difference between the total leukocyte count and the sum of lymphocytes with markers and the easily recognizable white blood cells is only 1–2%. In normals it is 6–10%, the difference being due to small round cells (lymphoid in appearance), presumably K cells. These seem to have been abrogated in cancer patients.

DR. HOBBS: As there are so many macrophages in some of the tumors you examined, and as the macrophage is a very long-lived phagocyte, why don't they keep accumulating and eventually overcome the tumor? Are macrophages short-lived in tumors, perhaps due to some toxic factor?

DR. ALEXANDER: These macrophages form typically long-lived granulomas, as defined by Speetor and Willoughby. It is possible that in the process of killing a tumor cell, mutual suicide results, as suggested by Granger and Wiser. There are problems with their data, and I don't think the macrophage actually dies in the process, but it may become disarmed. There are, of course, many other possible explanations such as that net tumor growth is the product of tumor cell division and tumor cell destruction by macrophage.

HOST DEFENSE AGAINST CANCER AND ITS POTENTIATION, D. MIZUNO ET AL. (EDS.),
UNIV. OF TOKYO PRESS, TOKYO / UNIV. PARK PRESS, BALTIMORE, PP. 131–141, 1975

The Effect of Tumor Ascitic Fluid on Lymphocyte Trapping and Its Relationship to Immune Function

Philip FROST

Department of Immunology and Microbiology, Wayne State University School of Medicine, Detroit, Michigan, U.S.A.

Abstract: Lymphocyte trapping is an early response of the immune system to the presence of antigen. The interaction of macrophages with antigen triggers a sequestration of recirculating lymphocytes within the stimulated lymphoid organ.

The demonstration of trapping is dependent on a number of variables including the dose, route, timing, and nature of the stimulating antigen. The trapping response is non-specific and can be induced by inert particulate materials. A specific selection phase follows the trap and accounts for the recruitment of antigen-sensitive cells from the recirculating pool.

Trapping is impaired by the growth of ascitic tumors and by the injection of ascitic tumor fluids (TAF) into normal mice. The failure of trapping is, however, probably due to a host rather than tumor factor, for non-tumor peritoneal exudate fluids (PEF) also inhibit trapping. The failure of trapping results in a depressed cellular and humoral immune response, though the precise relationships of these two events is complicated by the marked mitogenic effect of TAF and PEF.

The recirculation of lymphocytes represents one of the most dynamic aspects of immune function. The daily flow of lymphoid cells between the blood, lymphatic tissue, thoracic duct, and back to the blood again, has few counterparts in biologic systems. It was an early hypothesis that this dramatic lymphocyte movement could provide a mechanism for optimizing contact between antigen and its specific reactive cells. It is this concept that forms the basis for the studies described herein.

An original observation of Hall and Morris (*1*) demonstrated that antigen has a dramatic effect on the flow of cells out of a lymph node. These observations have been expanded by many investigators (*2–8*) to the extent that the effect of antigen on lymphocyte recirculation has come to be accepted as one of the earliest steps in the immune response.

This report will attempt to discuss the mechanism of these effects, circumstances whereupon these effects can be inhibited, the possible mechanism of the inhibition, and the subsequent effects of the inhibition on the immune response.

Background

1. *Lymphocyte trapping is a term which describes the sequestration of recirculating lympho-cytes within antigen-stimulated lymphoid organs (7, 8)*

Trapping is demonstrated by the intravenous injection of ^{51}Cr-labelled syn-geneic lymphoid cells into mice which had received antigen either intraveneously one hour earlier or subcutaneously 24 hr earlier, or received no antigen. Twenty-four hours later the animals are sacrificed and the percent localization of label within varied tissues is determined in a gamma spectrometer. Table 1 describes a typical experiment of this kind. While a variety of factors such as the dose, route, timing, and type of antigen injected influence the ultimate trapping response, the phenomenon is remarkably reproducible and very difficult to inhibit (8, 10).

A large number of agents have been tested for their ability to induce trapping. These materials have been divided into five groups as listed in Table 2. Group I antigens will induce trapping in virgin animals. These agents are similar in their

TABLE 1. Antigen-induced Lymphocyte Trapping in C3H Mice

| | Percent localization of labelled cells | | | Percent trapping |
	Left peripheral lymph nodes	Right peripheral lymph nodes	Spleen	
Control	2.1 ± 0.2	2.0 ± 0.08	14.6 ± 0.9	
SRBC-SC	3.2 ± 0.4	1.8 ± 0.3	15.1 ± 1.1	43
SRBC-IV	2.0 ± 0.5	1.9 ± 0.2	22.6 ± 1.3	55

Groups of mice are injected with 5×10^8 sheep erythrocyte (SRBC)-IV or -SC followed by the IV in-jection of 5×10^6 ^{51}Cr-labelled syngeneic lymph node cells.

TABLE 2. Agents Tested for Trapping Potential

Group I	Group III
Sheep erythrocytes	Complete and incomplete Freund's adjuvants
Keyhole limpet hemocyanin	Vitamin A alcohol and palmitate
Salmonella " H " antigen	Pertussis
Pneumococcal polysaccharide	*Corynebacterium parvum*
Xenogeneic sera	Endotoxin
Skin allografts and xenografts	
Syngeneic and allogeneic tumors	Group IV
Ethyl stearate, methyl palmitate	Silica
	Latex
Group II	Carbon
Bovine gamma globulin	Carrageenan
Bovine serum albumin	
Tetanus toxoid	Group V
DNP-polylysine	Syngeneic and allogeneic sera
	Syngeneic erythrocytes and lymphocytes
	Skin isografts
	Mineral oil

large molecular size or particulate nature. Their precise chemical nature is unimportant, for lipid, protein, and polysaccharides all induce trapping. Group II antigens are totally ineffective in eliciting trapping in non-immunized animals, but are effective trappers in specifically sensitized recipients.

All adjuvants tested (Group III) have been found to be potent trappers, though they differ from antigens in two ways. Firstly, they need not be immunogens, e.g., vitamin A alcohol. Secondly, while antigens induce trapping for 48–72 hr, adjuvants produce a persistent trap for as long as 45 days. This information coupled with a large series of other experiments has led us to postulate that one way in which adjuvants enhance the immune response is by creating a persistent "trap" which increases the potential selection of antigen-sensitive cells (9).

Group IV are inert particles (inert in the sense that they are not immunogenic) which share a common clearance by macrophages. These are all good trappers.

Finally, some agents (Group V) do not induce trapping under any circumstances.

2. The cellular origin of trapping

Though our original belief was that lymphoid cells were central to the trap mechanism considerable circumstantial and direct evidence now supports the thesis that macrophages are the control cells in the initiation of lymphocyte trapping (8, 11). The evidence in favor of this thesis can be summarized as follows:

1) Procedures which severely deplete lymphocytes in vivo, e.g., treatment of mice with irradiation, cyclophosphamide, hydrocortisone, acetate or anti-lymphocyte serum; do not hinder the trap mechanism.

2) Thymectomized, irradiated, and bone marrow-reconstituted animals still "trap" even if exposed to an additional 1,000 R irradiation.

3) Particulate materials are potent initiators of trapping whether they be immunogenic or not.

4) Conditions which encourage phagocytosis (passive or active immunization, cytophilic antibody) enhance the trapping potential of Group II antigens.

5) Animals tolerant to bovine gamma globulin (BGG) trap effectively when challenged with aggregated BGG or when passively immunized and challenged with soluble BGG.

6) Cell populations rich in macrophages are better at adoptively transferring trapping potential to irradiated hosts.

These observations form a cohesive body of evidence favoring the role of macrophages in the initiation of trapping.

3. The anatomic location of lymphocyte trapping and the cell trapped

The demonstration of trapping is independent of the cell type labelled. Any lymphoid cell which recirculates can be "trapped." Thus, the injection of labelled lymph node, spleen, bone marrow, thymus, or even lymphoid cells from donors tolerant to the challenge antigen, may all act as indicators of the presence of trapping (12).

The location of trapped cells is dependent on the inherent homing properties of the cell utilized. Lymph node cells are trapped in the thymus (T)-dependent areas of the spleen while spleen cells localize in both the T-dependent and T-independent areas of the splenic white pulp. Autoradiographic studies have revealed no discrete labelled cell localizations within trapping lymphoid organs, but rather a diffuse accumulation of cells in a pattern difficult to distinguish from normals. No labelled cells were seen in the red pulp.

4. The mechanism of trapping

So far we have reviewed the non-specific aspects of trapping. We prefer to call this the initiation phase, the phase related to macrophage functions. A subsequent series of specific events then occur; the selection phase, during which specific antigen reactive cells are retained within the stimulated lymphoid organ. These events have been described by several investigators (2, 3, 5) and will not be reviewed here.

We believe the initiation phase probably result from a mechanical obstruction of outflow from the hilum of the lymph node or from the white to the red pulp of the spleen. The obstruction is probably mediated by an activation of macrophages lining the hilar sinusoids of lymph nodes. A similar clear exit channel from the spleen has not as yet been defined, but the recent work of Mitchell (13), describing bridging channels between the white and red pulp, may well resolve this problem.

5. The relationship of lymphocyte trapping to tumor growth

The intraperitoneal injection of a variety of syngeneic tumors results in lymphocyte trapping in the spleen which is evanescent and disappears within a few days (depending on the initital tumor dose) despite continued tumor growth (14). This failure of trapping is non-specific, for animals bearing ascitic tumors will not demonstrate trapping upon challenge with a variety of antigens and adjuvants (Table 3). Contrary to these findings solid tumors continue to induce trapping for as long as the animals survive and do not interfere with trapping initiated by unrelated antigens (14–16).

TABLE 3. The Failure of Lymphocyte Trapping in Ascitic Tumor-bearing Mice (Day 4)

	% localization of labelled cells in the spleen		% trapping (control only)
	Control	Tumor bearers	
No antigen	14.4 ± 0.4	16.9 ± 0.5	
SRBC-IV	23.4 ± 1.2	17.3 ± 0.8	63
C. parvum-IV	25.3 ± 1.4	16.4 ± 0.9	75

Mice bearing Meth/A ascitic tumor (10^7 tumor cells injected intraperitoneally on day 0) and controls were challenged with 5×10^8 SRBC or 0.2 ml of *Corynebacterium parvum* given intravenously one hour prior to 10^7 ^{51}Cr-labelled syngeneic lymph node cells.

Since the failure of trapping occurs only in ascitic tumor bearers and is systemic in nature, we considered that the effect could be mediated by some tumor product or host factor liberated into the ascitic fluid. This proved to be true, for the injections of cell free tumor ascitic fluid into normal mice abrogated their ability to trap when challenged with a variety of antigens and adjuvants (Table 3).

6. The nature of the anti-trapping factor (ATF)

Our original belief that ATF is of tumor origin has been seriously weakened by the finding that peritoneal exudate fluid (PEF) induced by protease pepteone or Fuller's Earth (FE) also ablate lymphocyte trapping in normal animals. The intravenous injection of 0.5 ml of PEF ablates trapping in a manner similar to tumor ascitic fluid (TAF).

These findings negate the possibility of the ATF being of a purely tumor source. It seems instead that a host factor produced in the peritoneum in response to the tumor is responsible for the observed effects.

7. The mechanism of action of ATF

Several possible explanations for ATF action have been investigated. One possibility was that the trap failed because the lymphoid organs were already maximally trapping in response to the ATF. This could then result in "congestion" and a diminished inflow of cells into lymph nodes and spleen. To test this hypothesis groups of ATF-treated animals were injected with either 5×10^6 or 100×10^6 ^{51}Cr-labelled spleen cells, and the number of cells localizing in the spleen and lymph nodes was calculated as a percentage of the number injected. The number of cells localizing in lymph nodes and spleen after the injection of 5×10^6 spleen cells was 2.2×10^5 and 1.1×10^6, respectively. Comparable localizations after the injection of 100×10^6 spleen cells was 45×10^5 in lymph nodes and 26×10^6 in the spleen. It is evident from these results that the lymphoid organs of ATF-treated animals can sustain marked increases in cell traffic and that lymphoid organ congestion is unlikely to be responsible for the failure of the trap.

Since we believe the macrophage to be the central cell in the initiation of trapping, the effect of ATF on macrophage endocytic activity *in vivo* was evaluated. We found that the clearance of ^{125}I-labelled aggregated BGG, a measure of phagocytosis and radio-labelled colloidal gold a measure of pinocytosis, were identical in control and ATF-treated animals (12). These findings imply that macrophage endocytic activity is unaffected by ATF, but do not indicate if subsequent macrophage activities are impaired.

A third possible explanation for the ablation of trapping is that ATF alters the normal pattern of lymphocyte recirculation. To test this hypothesis lymph node and spleen cells from normal and ATF-treated animals were labelled and injected into normal or ATF-treated animals. While some alterations in the distribution of cells was found, the differences were minor when compared to the total number of cells involved. Thus, lymph node cells from ATF-treated animals have a greater number of spleen seeking cells, while spleen cells from these animals have a decreased number of lymph node seeking cells (12).

During the course of these studies we noted that mice treated with ATF developed a peripheral lymphadenopathy and splenomegaly. Because of the dramatic nature of these changes attempts were made to correlate these findings with the failure of trapping (17).

The nature of the organomegaly noted has been found to result from a marked mitogenic effect of syngeneic tumor ascitic fluid. Simple weight measurements re-

TABLE 4.   The Mitogenic Effect of Syngeneic Peritoneal Fluids

	Weight (mg)			^{125}IUdR uptake (cpm $\times 10^3$)		
	Normal	TAF-treated	PEF-treated	Normal	TAF-treated	PEF-treated
Peripheral lymph nodes	21.8±0.3	32.8±5.6	28.4±2.6	13.9±0.97	27.1±5.2	26.9±3.1
% change		↑50% $P=0.01$	↑30% $P=0.01$		↑94%	↑93%
Mesenteric lymph nodes	69.7±0.8	63.3±6.2	58.3±2.9	35.1±2.6	38.2±4.2	27.0±3.9
% change		NS	↓16.4% $P=0.001$		NS	NS
Spleen	122±5.2	211±26	185±16	82.5±10.6	387.7±41.1	184.3±2.1
% change		↑73%	↑52%		↑369%	↑94%
Thymus	41.3±6	38± 3	40.3±2.9	15.9±2.1	19.3±0.65	20.8±4.9
% change		NS	NS		NS	NS

Groups of six animals were injected with phosphate-buffered saline (PBS) or peritoneal fluid on day 0. Three days later all groups received a single intraperitoneal pulse of 15 μCi ^{125}IUdR and were sacrificed one hour later. The weights and ^{125}IUdR uptake were then assessed. ↑: increase. ↓: decrease. NS: not significant ($P>0.05$).

vealed an increase of peripheral lymph node weight (axillary, brachial, and inquinal) from 21.8±1.4 to 32.8±2.5 mg (an increase of 50%) within three days of a single intravenous injection of 0.5 ml TAF. Spleen weights increased even more dramatically from a mean of 110±6 to 270±32 mg in 3 days (an increase of 145%). Mesenteric nodes appeared not to be effected while thymic weight decreased. These changes were accompanied by a dramatic increase in ^{125}IUdR (iododeoxyuridine) uptake in the organs effected. These changes are summarized in Table 4.

Histologic studies revealed a large number of blast forms and mitotic figures in the cortex of the lymph nodes and in the T-dependent and-independent areas of the spleen. No such changes were seen in the thymus or mesenteric nodes.

These observations led us to postulate that lymphoid tissues in such a dramatic state of change could well be incapable of responding to antigen by the induction of trapping. Unfortunately, this explanation for the effect of TAF of trapping was weakened by the finding that low molecular weight fractions of TAF (prepared by passing TAF through a series of Amicon filters) which were capable of inducing mitogenesis were incapable of blocking trapping. This finding trends to argue against the presence of mitogenesis being responsible for the failure of trapping. However, we should note that we have never seen the ablation of trapping without some evidence of mitogenesis.

8.   Evidence for the host origin of ATF

One of the original questions regarding the anti-trapping effects of TAF was whether it was of host or tumor origin. Since tumors injected subcutaneously did not effect trapping in any way, some doubt as to the tumor origin of the active agent arose. We therefore conducted a series of experiments utilizing PEF derived from animals injected intraperitoneally with FE. To our surprise these peritoneal fluids both ablated trapping and induced mitogenesis in syngeneic mice. These findings have held true despite repeated attempts at attributing the effects of PEF to foreign contaminants of the peritoneal fluid. It therefore appears that the irritation of the peritoneum of normal animals by tumors or other agents stimulates the production by the host of factors which effect lymphocyte trapping and which stimulate mitogenesis within the host.

9.   The effect of TAF on cellular and humoral immune responses

A large number of observations have shown that TAF derived from a variety of tumors can suppress both cellular and humoral immune responses (*18–22*). In our hands this has generally held true, though we have occasionally observed an enhanced response to sheep erythrocytes in animals undergoing considerable splenic mitogenesis. Allograft rejection, both first and second set, have however consistently been prolonged for four and three days respectively, despite evidence of a mitogenic response. Similarly, tumor growth has been enhanced in animals treated with TAF prior to and after tumor challenge (*10*).

The relationship between the ablation of trapping and impaired immune responsiveness seems clear, but is complicated by the mitogenic effect of TAF. We presently are in the midst of examining fractions of TAF which induce mitogenesis but do not impair trapping in an effort to separate these two events.

REFERENCES

1.   Hall, J. G. and Morris, B. The immediate effect of antigen on the cell output of a lymph node. Brit. J. Exp. Pathol., *46*: 450–454, 1965.
2.   Ford, W. L. and Gowans, J. L. The role of lymphocytes in antibody formation. II. The influence of lymphocyte migration on the initiation of antibody formation in the isolated perfused spleen. Proc. Roy. Soc., Ser. B., *168*: 244–262, 1967.
3.   Rowley, D. A., Gowans, J. I., Atkins, R. C., Ford, W. L., and Smith, M. E. The specific selection of recirculating lymphocytes by antigen in normal and preimmunized rats. J. Exp. Med., *136*: 499–513, 1972.
4.   Dresser, D. W., Taub, R. N., and Krantz, A. R. The effect of localized injection of adjuvant material on the draining lymph node. II. Circulating lymphocytes. Immunology, *18*: 663–670, 1970.
5.   Sprent, J., Miller, J. F. A. P., and Mitchell, G. F. Antigen induced selective recruitment of circulating lymphocytes. Cell. Immunol., *2*: 171–181, 1971.
6.   Emerson, E. E. and Thursh, D. R. Immunologically specific retention of long lived lymphoid cells in antigenically stimulated lymph nodes. J. Immunol., *106*: 635–643, 1971.
7.   Zatz, M. M. and Lance, E. M. The distribution of ^{51}Cr labelled lymphocytes into antigen-stimulated mice. J. Exp. Med., *134*: 224–241, 1971.
8.   Frost, P. and Lance, E. M. The cellular origin of the lymphocyte trap. Immunology, *26*: 175–186, 1974.
9.   Frost, P. and Lance, E. M. The relation of lymphocyte trapping to the mode of action of adjuvants. *In;* G. E. W. Wolstenholme and J. Knight (eds.), Immunopotentiation (Ciba Foundation Symposium), vol. 18, pp. 29–45, Elsevier / Excerpta Medica / North Holland, Amsterdam / London / New York, 1973.

10. Lance, E. M. and Frost, P. The role of lymphocyte dynamics in the regulation of the immune response. Second International Congress of Immunology, 1974, in press.
11. Frost, P. Further evidence for the role of macrophages in the initiation of lymphocyte trapping. Immunology, *27*: 609–616, 1974.
12. Frost, P. Thesis: The mechanism and function of lymphocyte trapping. Council of National Academic Awards, London, 1974.
13. Mitchell, J. Lymphocyte circulation in the spleen: Marginal zone bridging channels and their possible role in cell traffic. Immunology, *24*: 93–107, 1973.
14. Frost, P. and Lance, E. M. Abrogation of lymphocyte trapping by ascitic tumors. Nature, *246*: 101–103, 1973.
15. Gillette, S. and Bellanti, J. A. Kinetics of lymphoid cells in tumor-bearing mice. Cell. Immunol., *8*: 311–320, 1973.
16. Zatz, M. M., White, A., and Goldstein, A. L. Alterations in lymphocyte populations in tumorigenesis. I. Lymphocyte trapping. J. Immunol., *111*: 706–711, 1973.
17. Frost, P. The mitogenic effect of syngeneic peritoneal fluids and its relation to the ablation of lymphocyte trapping. Unpublished.
18. Grohsman, J. and Nowotny, A. The immune recognition of TA3 tumors, its facilitation by endotoxin and abrogation by ascites fluid. J. Immunol., *109*: 1090–1095, 1972.
19. Hrśak, I and Marotti, T. Immunosuppression mediated by Ehrlichs ascites fluid. Eur. J. Cancer, *9*: 717–724, 1973.
20. McCarthy, R. E., Coffin, J. M., and Gates, S. L. Selective inhibition of the secondary immune response to mouse skin allografts by cell-free Ehrlich ascites carcinoma fluid. Transplantation, *6*: 737–743, 1968.
21. Robinson, E., Galakai, V. K., and Schlesinger, M. Studies on the mechanism of prolonged survival of allografts from tumor-bearing donors. Cancer Res., *281*: 462–464, 1968.
22. Yamazaki, H., Nitta, K., and Umezawa, H. Immunosuppression induced with cell-free fluid of Ehrlich carcinoma ascites and its fractions. Gann, *64*: 83–92, 1973.

Discussion of Paper of Dr. Frost

DR. ALEXANDER: I believe it would be less confusing if you referred to your ascites tumor fluid as ATF rather than TAF, as the latter is also the abbreviation for tumor angiogenic factor.

DR. FROST: Thank you. I'll follow your suggestion.

DR. M. HOZUMI: Have you characterized the anti-trapping factor in your ascites fluid, and have you ideas on its mechanism of production?

DR. FROST: It contains protein, has a molecular weight greater than 50,000 daltons, and can be centrifuged at 105,000 g for 4 hr without loss of potency. We're presently analyzing it in more detail. I have no information bearing on its mechanism of production.

DR. DRESSER: You noted that solid tumors, in contrast to ascitic ones, do not exhibit a systemic blocking of the trapping phenomenon. If you inject antigen ipsilaterally to the tumor, will you get an additional trapping effect?

DR. FROST: No, and I've performed that experiment a number of times. Animals with solid tumors were followed for their entire survival time, up to 60 days after tumor implantation, and trapping in the draining nodes invariably persists, even in the face of massive tumors.

DR. DRESSER: When you described the effect of ATF on the plaque-forming cell (PFC), which class of PFC were you noting? In certain circumstances the IgG PFC response can be as much as 100-fold more dependent on T-cell help than the IgM PFC. Delineation of both indirect and direct PFC's might thus provide valuable information concerning a possible differential effect of ATF.

DR. FROST: In the presentation we recorded only the IgM responses, but we have examined IgG PFC's, which are depressed but not as greatly as that of IgM. The memory response is also depressed in these animals.

DR. JERNE: Does trapping imply an increased passage of lymphocytes through the lymph node capillary walls?

DR. FROST: I don't know. Ford and J. Hall have attempted to define what happens at the post-capillary venules during trapping. There appears to be an increase in the percentage of cells entering a node after antigen administration, and thereafter a slowing of flow occurs, although there are still a large number of emigrating cells. This idea was confirmed by Ford's experiments in the isolated, perfused rat spleen. It is not clear whether there is an increased number of cells entering these nodes from the blood.

DR. JERNE: Isn't that the only way cells can come in?

DR. FROST: Yes, but cells are also leaving so that, by a simplistic analysis, if there are the same number of cells entering a node but an obstruction then occurs at the outlet, an increased number of cells remain sequestered.

DR. JERNE: Trapping appears to be a very mysterious process, as it is selective.

DR. FROST: Trapping, as we define it, is a non-specific phenomenon, as initially it is not selective. The selection phase, as demonstrated by others in thoracic duct depletion experiments, is a secondary mechanism which probably occurs about 24 hr after the original trap, for it's not until 3–4 days later that blasts appear in the afferent lymph and thoracic duct.

DR. HALPERN: With reference to the reticuloendothelial (RE) hyperplasia you observed, did you determine whether it was due to a proliferation of phagocytic cells by, for example, clearance measurement studies? I don't believe that RE cells are responsible for this phenomenon, as such cells do not easily multiply, and the hyperplasia produced by stimulation with materials such as *Corynebacterium parvum* is rather due to an influx of bone marrow monocytic cells.
   Secondly, is that ATF phenomenon similar using allogeneic and syngeneic tumors? Also, is trapping radiosensitive?

DR. FROST: The clearance mechanisms, *i.e.*, clearance of aggregated radio-labelled BCG, are similar in normal, tumor-bearing, and ATF-treated animals. This, of course, doesn't relate to whether there are other changes in macrophage activity. I believe that lymphocytes rather than macrophages are probably involved in the hyperplastic response.
   Both allogeneic and syngeneic tumors respond similarly in our assays. The trapping phenomenon is extremely radio-resistant.

DR. T. TOKUNAGA (National Institute of Health, Tokyo):   In complementation of your results, we noted that the 24-hr foot pad swelling delayed hypersensitivity reaction to SRBC was entirely abrogated in highly SRBC-sensitized mice if they were given intraperitoneal injections of Ehrlich ascites tumor fluid just before assay. Here, TAF appears to suppress expression of delayed hypersensitivity. Spleen cells from these animals responded to phytohemagglutinin (PHA) and concanavalin A (Con A), while spleen cells from Ehrlich ascites tumor-bearing mice did not.

DR. FROST: In collaboration with Dr. W. H. Adler, we have also shown that the normal lymphocyte response to PHA, Con A, endotoxin or in an mixed lymphocyte culture (MLC) can be markedly inhibited by the addition of ATF or peritoneal exudate fluid.

DR. DUKOR: Are the effects of ATF linked to enzymic activity, so that they could be mimicked by proteases or suppressed by the addition of a protease inhibitor?

DR. FROST: I don't know.

DR. KITAGAWA: You noted that all adjuvants are good trappers. Is the trapping or migration of effector cells, i.e., sensitized lymphocytes, in the antigen injection site also augmented by adjuvants?

DR. FROST: There is great controversy surrounding the concept of specific homing sensitized cells to an antigen depot. Ford and Tilney recently reported an increase in the localization of specific cells following injection of histo-incompatible cells into grafted animals but this increase was very small.

HOST DEFENSE AGAINST CANCER AND ITS POTENTIATION, D. MIZUNO ET AL. (EDS.),
UNIV. OF TOKYO PRESS, TOKYO / UNIV. PARK PRESS, BALTIMORE, PP. 143-155, 1975

Factors in the Immune Response to Tumors and Potential Methods for Increasing Their Effectiveness*

D. Bernard AMOS

Division of Immunology, Duke University Medical Center, Durham, North Carolina, U.S.A.

Abstract: Ascites tumors are produced by transplanting lymphocytes or sarcomas in the peritoneal cavity. After several transfers many free floating cells are produced. Transferred to a new host these cells divide exponentially for eight to ten days. In the compatible (syngeneic) host growth continues but at a slower rate. In the incompatible (allogeneic) host there is an abrupt fall in the number of tumor cells and none are found after the eleventh day. Lymphocytes from the peritoneal cavity of mice that have rejected an allogeneic tumor are extremely powerful killers of tumor cells *in vitro*. Killing is in two stages. The first is the binding stage and is very dependent upon: (1) the presence of Mg^{2+} and Ca^{2+} ions; (2) the metabolic stage of the target cell. Binding is not highly temperature dependent. Cytolysis or the actual killing stage is very dependent upon: (1) successful binding; (2) a serum lipoprotein, and (3) temperature. The peritoneal lymphocytes are capable of transferring immunity to another animal. Optimum results are observed when these lymphocytes are mixed with tumor cells. Under these conditions the recipient develops his own immunity and his own killer cells, even when the second animal is compatible with the tumor.

One of the most enduring attributes of the tumor immunologist is optimism, since continued optimism and perseverance are necessary to offset the repeated difficulties encountered. One wonders how Gaylord, Clowes, and Baeslack would have phrased their report to the Commissioner of Health of the State of New York in 1905 had they been given foreknowledge of the path ahead (*1*). They wrote "It gives us great pleasure to report to you an unusually prosperous year in the researches which we are conducting. We are enabled at this time to present to you the completed reports covering the most interesting and significant subject of the spontaneous cure of cancer in animals, a number of preliminary communications on

* Supported by USPHS Grants AI-18399 and CA-14049.

143

the evidence of immunity to cancer and several interesting papers relating to the growth of cancer in animals, considered from a biological chemical standpoint. Our researches for this year, as recorded in the articles above enumerated, have been rewarded by the demonstration of the fact that *cancer is in principle a curable malady.*" Now nearly 50 years later, I am priviledged to report that again very rapid progress has been made in the last few years and we are beginning to have an insight into the processes that can be harnessed for the destruction of tumor cells. I also realize that Gaylord *et al.* were as successful as we in the destruction of a spontaneous tumor and that we too may have far to go. In this presentation I wish to review some of the findings from our laboratory on lymphocyte-mediated cytotoxicity against tumors, to discuss the inherent potential of synergistic interactions between antibody and lymphocytes in cytolysis and to draw your attention to a potential therapeutics procedure that I believe to have widespread applicability and that appears to be presently overlooked, that of the action of antibody to a hapten adsorbed to a tumor.

Lymphocyte-mediated Cytotoxicity

The system we have studied is one in which the ascites form of C57B1 lymphoma EL4 is injected into the peritoneal cavity of BALB/c mice. Since BALB/c and C57B1 differ at the H-2 and at many minor histocompatibility loci, incompatibility between the strains is strong and rejection is rapid. Tumor cells usually multiply exponentially for 7–8 days after their introduction but then vanish from the peritoneal cavity by the 10th day leaving an accumulation of several million host cells within the peritoneal cavity. Immune peritoneal exudate cells harvested on the 11th day are thus of host origin and composed of lymphocytes and macrophages in about equal proportions (*2*). Most macrophages (and some lymphocytes) are removed by passage through nylon wool columns. The small-to-medium-sized lymphocytes (IPEL) that pass the column have many ribosomes and a very active Golgi apparatus. The nucleus frequently has a deep cleft tightly packed with ribosomes. The nuclear cleft often appears to open into the Golgi region (*3*). Only occasional mitotic cells are seen and it is believed that the population contains a high proportion of fully differentiated cytotoxic effector cells.

By injecting IPEL into rats, we were able to induce an antibody which, after absorption with mouse red cells and thymus, would react with about 80% IPEL (*4*). This serum would not react with thymus, bone marrow, or normal PEL (NPEL), but would react against IPEL from mice of several strains immune to EL4 or to a different tumor. Thus there appeared to be specificity for a class of cell involved in homograft rejection, but no specificity for strain distribution or for a particular tumor. We therefore, regard the IPEL as having a differentiation antigen, "Ka," which is expressed on lymphocytes but not thymocytes (*4*). Ka is not a receptor antigen in the sense that Kimura has reported (*5*); antibody-treated IPEL were still fully cytotoxic for EL4. All activity was, however, lost when complement was added, demonstrating that the Ka-positive population did indeed include the cytotoxic effector cells. The marker was also present in a small proportion of spleen and lymph node cells (4), the number of positive cells varying from animal to animal, but averaging about 20% for normal peripheral lymph node cells and 30% for lymph node cells from immune donors. Normal spleen appeared to include about 10% Ka-positive cells and immune spleen about 15–20%. Although NPEL failed to react, the exudate induced by thioglycolate include some 40% Ka-positive cells (6).

Cells carrying the Ka marker are interesting in that many of them also appear to carry other antigens. Whereas 80–90% of IPEL are Ka-positive, 80% also carry the Thy-1 marker and appear to carry bone marrow-derived (B)-cell markers in addition (4). It is difficult to be dogmatic about the coincidence of 3 markers on a single cell because of the usual problems of specificity of anti-B-cell sera, but absorption with thymus left reactivity against IPEL in rabbit anti-B-cell serum prepared against spleen cells from X-irradiated bone marrow-reconstituted donors (6). The data suggest that some IPEL carry 3 class markers; this could be as high as 80%, but it cannot be below 40%, and in this case, 60% would carry 2 of the markers.

We know little of the origin of these interesting cells. Cytotoxic effector cells can be demonstrated as early as the 7th day after tumor rejection, but we do not know if they are formed in the peritoneal cavity, or if they migrate from other lymphoid organs.

Because of the high proportion of specific effector cells we were able to investigate the phases of cytolysis. These studies were facilitated by the use of a new monolayer technique (7). Target cells added to tissue culture dishes that have been coated with poly-L-lysine (PLL) adhere to the dish. Any free PLL residues are quenched with serum. The monolayer is resistant to EDTA treatment. A proportion of IPEL added to monolayers formed with PLL adhere to the target cells. The non-adherent cells can be removed with barbital buffer and the adherent cells can then be eluted with EDTA and examined separately. Most of the killing is by adherent cells. Since there is a low level of killing with the non-adherent cells, it is possible that the effectors pass through phases, at times being active and at others being unable to bind.

Adherence, or binding, precedes lysis. Binding occurs at 25°C but not readily at 7°C, although transient binding has been reported at 4°C (8). It does not occur in the absence of divalent cations, and the degree of binding is governed by the concentration of Mg^{2+} and, to a lesser degree, of Ca^{2+} added to the medium (7). Serum is not required for this phase. Binding takes place quite rapidly, and in the assay system generally used, that of Canty and Wunderlich (9), it is facilitated by rocking the tissue culture dish. Rocking is believed to act by increasing the number of contacts between target and effector cells.

In contrast to binding, lysis is highly temperature dependent and takes place very slowly at 25°C. It is thus possible to rock plates at 25°C to allow binding and then to raise the temperature to 37°C to allow killing (10, 11). Under these conditions, the actual killing step does not require the continuation of rocking. We take this as evidence that binding is necessary for killing and that a bound cell can proceed to kill when environmental conditions (temperature, and the presence of serum) are appropriate. Serum can facilitate lysis. The effect of serum is most noticeable at low concentrations, thus the addition of 2% fetal calf serum (FCS) to a serum-free system gives a marked elevation in cytotoxicity (12). The molecule responsible is resistant to boiling.

Serum also contains inhibitory factors which do not however exert their effect until the glucose concentration falls below 2 mg/ml (12). The inhibitor is not toxic. Target cells placed in glucose-free serum medium and then transferred to glucose-containing medium are fully viable, and can now be killed by IPEL.

We have also studied the effects of a number of drugs and alterations in physical conditions on cytolysis. This can be done by inducing specific changes in either the killer or the target when the effect of the agent is irreversible, or by imposing the change on both killer and target where the agent is reversible. For example, the killer cell can be treated with proteolytic enzymes, then washed, and its ability to bind or to kill determined (13). Trypsin at 1 μg/ml can potentiate both binding and killing (13), while higher concentrations produce increasing degrees of inhibition of both. These changes are reversible with time. Papain and pronase are also inhibitory at high concentrations but augment killing to a small but reproducible extent when present in low concentration, while neuraminidase at a variety of concentrations potentiates killing. These findings may be an indication that enzymes which remove sialic acid (neuraminidase directly and proteolytic enzymes indirectly through their action on a glycoprotein), reduce surface charge thus facilitating the approach of the killer to the target.

The identity of the effector cell receptor remains elusive. While there are many reports of the importance of immunoglobulins in T-cell binding, this remains a controversial subject. In our laboratory we have been unable to demonstrate such an immunoglobulin, nor can we release by enzyme or detergent or even by simple disruption any cell membrane component able to bind to target cells (14).

While there is no good agreement about the nature of the effector cell receptor, the nature of the site recognized on the target cell is also not completely resolved. Studies by Brondz (15) and independently by many others showed the relevance of H-2 targets to cytolysis by allogeneic effectors. Cerrotini and Brunner report that blocking is specific for single haplotypes of an F_1 hybrid (16). However, the H-2 haplotype is a multicomponent genetic system which controls the production of at least four, and probably more, components, two of which are defined by the usual anti-H-2 sera and which are chemically distinctive. Other components, e.g., those designated Ia can be distinguished by their presence on some, but not all, lymphocytes (17), some probably being expressed on B lymphocytes and other on T lymphocytes. The literature on this point is not conclusive and many critical studies, e.g., by absorption and with highly purified sera, have not yet been done. The extent to which the Ia specificities are recognized by effector cells is not known.

Edidin and Henney have removed H-2 antigens by repeated capping with antibody and found the treated cells can still be killed by lymphocytes (18). This result would argue against H-2 participation. Nabholz, in contrast, has found that antibody to H-2.33 can block killing of cytotoxic lymphocytes directed against the K region of H-2b (19). This finding is difficult to reconcile with the Edidin and Henney's result, unless the Nabholz antibody also contained other antibodies —*e.g.*, to Ia.

In our own experiments we find that antibody against normal C57B1 tissues can block binding and cytolysis as can antibody raised against EL4 in BALB or antisera raised in congenic mice against H-2b antigens, again suggesting a relationship to the H-2 complex (*20, 21*). Some of the antisera used give only a single peak in precipitation of detergent-solubilized iodine-labeled membranes corresponding to H-2, together with a smaller peak corresponding to β_2 microglobulin (*22*). However, many treatments that do not destroy H-2 activity on the cell abolish binding. These include partial dehydration, treatment with cytochalasin, sodium azide or alcohol and with heat or osmotic shock (*23*). Thus, from antibody inhibition studies it is clear that H-2 must lie close to the target site, and the possibility exists that a portion of the molecule other than the site for antibody binding and which is held in a particular conformation is important. Alternatively, the target site may be a macromolecular complex of which H-2 is a part, or H-2 may lie in close proximity to such a complex (*22*).

The dynamic state of the target cell surface appears to be very important in lymphocyte-mediated cytotoxicity, although it seems to be much less important in antibody-mediated cytotoxicity in the presence of complement. What the situation will be with respect to cytolysis of tumor antigens is unsure. Data on antibody-combining sites are relatively easy to obtain whereas data on the target for cell-mediated reactions are always more difficult to interpret.

In considering tumor cell destruction by a host it is necessary to bear in mind that the host has many potential immune response processes, any or all of which may be mobilized to make varying contributions. Thus while lymphocyte-mediated cytotoxicity may be a very potent weapon for *in vitro* cytolysis against certain tumors, it may be considerably less effective in others and, as will be discussed below, antibody can also make a major contribution. We also have to show how *in vitro* cytotoxicity relates to *in vivo* tumor destruction. The usual type of adoptive transfer of immune lymph node or spleen cells does not answer the question of *in vivo* relevance of single processes, since the cell suspension includes cytotoxic effector cells, antibody-producing cells and macrophages and while an elusive entity in animal systems, cells transferred could also elaborate transfer factor and thus, rapidly sensitize the recipient. Adoptive transfer with IPEL provides a cleaner system since the population transferred is more homogeneous, 80% or more of such cells carrying the Thy-1 marker. Transfer of IPEL immune to EL4 or to neuroblastoma A from A strain mice in a Winn-type assay shows that IPEL are indeed capable of protecting the recipients. In a series of experiments, 10^6 IPEL from BALB/c donors were mixed with 2.5×10^5 EL4 tumor cells and injected subcutaneously (s.c.) into BALB/c, C57B1/6, (C57B1/6×A) F_1 hybrids, or into the C57B1/G0 subline obtained from Dr. Grunenberg's laboratory. This last subline was used by Gorer for the production of the EL4 tumor. In control animals receiving tumor alone, transient growth was observed in BALB/c mice. All C57B1 and the hybrid with A showed progressive tumor growth, the hybrids surviving for about 6 days longer than C57B1. In mice receiving IPEL, all BALB/c mice, and F_1 hybrids survived, as did 89.4% of C57B1/6 and 95% of C57B1/G0 (*24*). This shows that IPEL can give quite good protection in compatible hosts in which the BALB IPEL would have been quickly eliminated. This finding led to the supposition that the recipients of the IPEL and tumor might have developed an active immunity. Indeed, when challenged 3 weeks later with EL4 cells s.c., 64% of F_1, 37% of B1/6, and 68% of B1/G0 survived (*24*). When later challenged intraperitoneally (i.p.), their peritoneal exudate cells were cytotoxic for EL4 *in vitro*. That the new effector cells could actually be generated in the C57B1 hosts was shown by the sensitivity of cells from protected C57B1 mice to lysis by antibody produced in BALB against C57 and resistance to C57 anti-BALB antibody (*25*).

This leads us to consider the peculiar interaction that occurs when allogeneic effector cells are mixed with live tumor cells and how this may be used in the treatment of tumors, and to the presently insoluble problem of how to destroy an established tumor. The protective effect we see is initially restricted to the local site. Tumor cells do not grow when mixed with IPEL and injected on one side of the thorax. Tumor cells injected on the opposite side of the animal grow unchecked allogeneic IPEL alone do not induce immunity. Therefore, the procedure is unlikely to be effective in the presence of a growing tumor. Transfer of cells immune to a tumor together with attenuated tumor cells might, however, be considered after surgery of an apparently non-metastasizing tumor to control recurrence or late metastasis. Generation of effector cells would have to be by *in vitro* cultivation with tumor. Our data indicate that fractions from stable tissue culture cell lines are effective in this respect (*26*). The Ginsburg or Häyry maneuver of two cycle stimulation could be a useful means of augmenting the number of effector cells generated (*27, 28*). However, the recent paper by Fauve *et al.* (*29*) on the production of a small molecule with anti inflammatory and macrophage immobility properties can mean that no immunotherapeutic attack can reach the tumor unless means are found to overcome the anti-kinin effects of the molecule. Active inflammation at the tumor site would favor the delivery of immunocytes or antibodies to the tumor.

Lymphocyte-mediated cytotoxicity is just one means of tumor cell cytolysis. Emphasis is now growing on the potential of antibody in combination with lymphocytes, and as mentioned in the introduction, I should like to discuss two distinct possibilities for therapy with antibody. The first of these is lymphocyte-antibody-lymphocyte interaction (LALI) or lymphocyte-dependent antibody-mediated cytotoxicity (LDA). The second involves treatment with hapten and anti-hapten produced in animals.

Interaction between Lymphocyte and Antibody

In LALI, antibody combines with a ^{51}Cr-labeled target cell, normal lymphocytes are then added, and the mixture is incubated for 3 hr or longer. Lysis is determined by the amount of chromium released. The target can be a tumor cell, a stable tissue culture cell line, a mitogen-stimulated or even a normal lymphocyte (*30*). Under these conditions, in our hands high levels of killing results, provided that the attacking lymphocyte: target cell ratio is 100: 1 or higher and the antibody concentration is high (*31*). With lesser antibody concentration, ^{51}Cr release falls rapidly to a low level but then remains significantly above background levels despite progressively falling antibody. Titers of 100,000 or more are reported in the literature but usually the specific release of chromium is rather low. Our own experience in humans is limited to antibodies against antigens of the HL-1 system which includes HL-A (*32*), and to antibodies against the H-2b lymphoma EL4 in the mouse. Results in both systems appear to be closely comparable. We also have inferential information suggesting LALI may be operative *in vivo*. In man, the specificity is directed against components of the HL-1 system but does not appear to be mediated by conventional HL-A antibodies and the reactivity is greatly affected by this genotype of the attacking cell (*33*).

The results of two family studies can be outlined, details will be presented elsewhere (*31*). Family A included father, mother, and 5 sibs. The HL-A haplotypes of the father were: 2-5 (A), 1-7 (B). The haplotypes of the mother were: 10-W16 (C), W30/31-12 (D). The resultant sib genotypes were: Sib Su, AC; Sib Ma, AC; Sib Chi, AD; Sib Ir, AD; and Sib Ni, BD. The mother's serum contained an anti-5-W5 broadly reactive antibody, cytotoxic for the father and Sibs Su, Ma, Chi, and Ni. In LALI, Ni, who differed at both haplotypes, provided the best attack cell from within the family when Ma provided the target, Ma being the least effective attack cell for his own target. HL-A identical Sib Su, also gave a low level of killing against Ma, Chi, and Ir, who shared the 2-5 haplotype, were intermediate. Almost identical results were obtained when Su cells were the target. Similarly, Ni provided the best attack cell for Chi target cells; other reactions are still being examined. In this family the reactivity agreed with the distribution of the 2-5 haplotype.

In the B family, the father's haplotype were A, 1-8 and B, W25-X, the mother's were C, 1-W21 and D, W25-5. The children had haplotypes Ka BD, Ch AD, and Sa BC. The father and Ch provided sensitive targets for the mother's serum. Ka and Sa did not, using the mother or two unrelated donors as attack cells. As with the previous family, there was good reproducibility between experiments, and the reactivity appeared to be directed against the 1-8 haplotype. Serum from the mother contained no cytotoxic antibodies when tested in cytotoxicity tests of varying sensitivity. Of considerable interest is the finding that the serum is unreactive when tested against cells from 3 unrelated individuals with the 1-8 haplotype. We hope to determine the relevance of this reactivity to the distribution of the MLR-S factors in the population.

In the mouse, excellent killing of mouse tumor cells *in vitro* is observed using lymph node cells from non-immune donors and hyper-immune anti-H-2 sera. We also believe that LALI provides an explanation for an *in vivo* observation that we were long unable to interpret adequately. Batchelor and Silverman had described a model system for the study of enhancement that allows the enhancing activity of serum to be titrated against the lytic action of lymphoid cells. Lymph node cells from C57Bl mice immune to C3H ascites sarcoma BP8 harvested 14 days after immunization have relatively little cytotoxic potential in adoptive transfer tests. These cells, when mixed with an enhancing dose (1 μl) of immune serum, produced a dramatic cytotoxic effect. This synergistic effect was not seen if the lymphoid cells were harvested 5 days after immunization. When the results were published (*34*) we suggested that a small amount of antibody produced by the lymphoid cells was additive with the hyper-immune serum. While this remains a possibility, it now seems more likely that the antibody was being used in LALI by the injected lymphocytes, the immunization possibly having enriched the complement of attack cells in the population.

Immunotherapy by Hapten-anti-hapten Interaction

Turning to the final approach to tumor immunity, I wish to discuss how pharmacologists could collaborate with immunologists to devise a more effective approach. L-Phenylalanine mustard (PAM) is a compound used as a chemotherapeutic agent in cancer therapy and known to be concentrated in the tumor or in tissues close to the tumor (*35, 36*). Coupled to a carrier such as serum protein it also acts as an effective hapten. If a protein from a different species is used as a carrier it is necessary to absorb out antibodies to the carrier protein: if the protein is homologous, this is not necessary. A heterologous protein might, however, give a more protent antibody in some hapten-carrier-host combinations, so both sources of carrier should be tried. In the experiments reported by Burke, PAM was complexed to human gamma globulin (HGG) and injected, with adjuvant, into rabbits (*37*). The antiserum produced was absorbed with HGG to leave anti-PAM. Mice bearing an ependynoma were inoculated intravenously (i.v.) with sub-cytotoxic doses of PAM and allowed to equilibrate for 30 min. Anti-PAM was then injected i.v. Tumor growth was markedly inhibited and the tumors showed marked histological changes (*37*). The effect of the PAM-anti-PAM combination was less when used against a poorly vascularized carcinoma, and was minimal against a leukemia.

The importance of this procedure is its versatility and lack of inherent toxicity. The hapten need not be a chemotherapeutic agent, the only qualifications are that it must localize to the surface of the tumor cells, that it must be capable of acting as a hapten and it should not be toxic. Agents such as actinomycin might be eminently suitable. The PAM-anti-PAM type of procedure could also be tried in combination therapy with LALI or lymphocyte-mediated cytotoxicity (LMC). In this approach, a predetermined dose of the hapten would be administered. As soon as the hapten had cleared the bloodstream and danger of anaphylaxis had passed, anti-hapten would be given the resultant reaction would be cytotoxic for the tumor and would also produce a violent inflammatory reaction. This could probably occur depites anti-inflammatory influences of some tumors. The anti-PAM would be followed after a suitable time period and when inflammation was maximal (probably 6–24 hr), by an injection of antibody to the tumor togetherwith, if indicated, immune or normal lymphocytes. The number of variables that could be tried is great, and the system has limitless potential. Obviously, close cooperation between a pharmacologist who could select drugs for their ability to reach and to localize on the tumor cell surface, and the immunologist would be highly advantageous.

REFERENCES

1. Gaylord, H. R., Clowes, G. H. A., and Baeslack, F. W. Preliminary report on the presence of an immune body in the blood of mice spontaneously recovered from cancer (Adenocarcinoma, Jensen) and the effect of this immune serum upon growing tumors in mice affected with the same material. *In;* Contributions to the Subject of Immunity in Cancer, from the Annual Reports of the New York State Cancer Laboratory, pp. 5-8, J. B. Lyon Company, Albany, New York, 1910. Reprinted from Medical News, Jan. 14, 1905.

2. Berke, G., Sullivan, K. A., and Amos, D. B. Rejection of ascites tumor allografts. I. Isolation, characterization, and *in vitro* reactivity of peritoneal lymphoid effector cells from BALB/c mice immune to EL4 leukosis. J. Exp. Med., *135*: 1334-1350, 1972.

3. Sullivan, K. A. and Amos, D. B. Unpublished.

4. Sullivan, K. A., Berke, G., and Amos, D. B. An antigenic determinant of cytotoxic lympocytes. Transplantation, *16*: 388-891, 1973.

5. Kimura, A. Inhibition of specific cell-mediated cytotoxicity by anti-T-cell receptor antibody. J. Exp. Med., *139*: 888-901, 1974.

6. Sullivan, K. A., Ph.D. Dissertation, Division of Immunology, Duke University Medical Center, Durham, NC, 1973.

7. Stulting, R. D. and Berke, G. Nature of lymphocyte-tumor interaction. A general method for cellular immunoabsorption. J. Exp. Med., *137*: 932-942, 1973.

8. Wagner, H. and Rollinghoff, M. T cell-mediated cytotoxicity: discrimination between antigen recognition, lethal hit and cytolysis phase. Eur. J. Immunol., *4*: 745-750, 1974.

9. Canty, T. G. and Wunderlich, J. R. Quantitative *in vitro* assay of cytotoxic cellular immunity. J. Natl. Cancer Inst., *45*: 761-772, 1970.

10. Berke, G., Sullivan, K. A., and Amos, D. B. Rejection of ascites tumor allografts. II. A pathway for cell-mediated tumor destruction *in vitro* by peritoneal exudate lymphoid cells. J. Exp. Med., *136*: 1594-1604, 1973.

11. Berke, G. and Sullivan, K. A. Temperature control of lymphocyte-mediated cytotoxicity *in vitro*. Transplant. Proc., *5*: 421-423, 1973.

12. Kemp, A. S., Berke, G., Dawson, J. R., and Amos, D. B. The influence of normal serum components on lymphocyte-mediated cytolysis *in vitro*. Transplantation, *17*: 447-452, 1973.

13. Todd, R. F. Functional characterization of membrane components of cytotoxic peritoneal exudate lymphocytes. II. Trypsin sensitivity of the killer cell receptor. Transplantation, in press.

14. Todd, R. F. and Berke, G. Functional characterization of membrane components of cytotoxic peritoneal exudate T lymphocytes. Immunochemistry, *11*: 313-320, 1974.

15. Brondz, B. D. and Snegirova, A. E. Interaction of immune lymphocytes with the mixtures of target cells possessing selected specificities of the H-2 immunizing allele. Immunology, *20*: 457-468, 1971.

16. Cerottini, J.-C. and Brunner, K. T. Cell-mediated cytotoxicity, allograft rejection and tumor immunity. Adv. Immunol., *18*: 67-132, 1974.

17. Shreffler, D. C. and David, C. S. The H-2 major histocompatibility complex and

the I immune response region: Genetic variation, function, and organization. Adv. Immunol., *20*: 125–195, 1975.

18. Edidin, M. and Henney, C. S. The effect of capping H-2 antigens on the susceptibility of target cells to humoral and T cell-mediated lysis. Nature New Biol., *246*: 47–49, 1973.

19. Nabholz, M., Vives, J., Young, H. M., Meo, T., Miggiano, V., Rijnbeek, A., and Shreffler, D. C. Cell-mediated cell lysis *in vitro*: Genetic control of killer cell production and target specificities in the mouse. Eur. J. Immunol., *4*: 378–387, 1974.

20. Todd, R. F., Stulting, R. D., and Berke, G. Mechanism of blocking by hyperimmune serum of lymphocyte-mediated cytolysis of allogeneic tumor cells. Cancer Res., *33*: 3203–3208, 1973.

21. Todd, R. F., Stulting, R. D., and Gooding, L. Unpublished.

22. Todd, R. F., Stulting, R. D., and Amos, D. B. Lymphocyte-mediated cytolysis of allogeneic tumor cells *in vitro*. I. Search for target antigens in subcellular fractions. Cell. Immunol., *18*: 304–323, 1975.

23. Stulting, R. D., Todd, R. F., and Amos, D. B. Lymphocyte-mediated cytolysis of allogeneic tumor cells *in vitro*. II. Binding of cytotoxic lymphocytes to formaldehyde-fixed target cells. Cell. Immunol., in press.

24. Crowell, J. and Amos, D. B. Unpublished.

25. Kemp, A., Berke, G., Crowell, J., and Amos, B. Induction of cell-mediated immunity against leukemia EL4 in C57Bl mice. J. Natl. Cancer Inst., *51*: 1877–1882, 1973.

26. Corley, R., Dawson, J. R., and Amos, D. B. Lymphocyte stimulation *in vitro*: Generation of cytotoxic effector lymphocytes using subcellular fractions of a lymphoid cell line. Cell. Immunol., *16*: 92–105, 1975.

27. Ginsberg, H. Cycles of transformation and differentiation of lymphocytes *in vitro*. Transplant. Proc., *3*: 883–887, 1971.

28. Häyry, P. and Andersson, L. C. T " memory " cells in allograft response *in vitro*. Transplant. Proc., *7*: 243–245, 1975.

29. Fauve, R. M., Herin, B., Jacob, H., Gaillard, J. A., and Jacob, F. Antiinflammatory effects of murine malignant cells. PNAS, *71*: 4052–4056, 1974.

30. Perlmann, P., Perlmann, H., and Wigzell, H. Lymphocyte mediated cytotoxicity *in vitro*. Induction and inhibition by humoral antibody and nature of effector cells. Transplant. Rev., *13*: 91–114, 1972.

31. Ferreira, E. and Amos, D. B. Unpublished.

32. Yunis, E. J., Krivit, W., Reinsmoen, N., and Amos, D. B. Inheritance of a recombinant HL-A haplotype and genetics of the HL-1 region in man. Nature, 248: 517–519, 1974.

33. Corley, R., Chung, S., and Amos, D. B. Unpublished.

34. Hutchin, P., Amos, D. B., and Prioleau, W. H. Interactions of humoral antibodies and immune lymphocytes. Transplantation, *5*: 68–75, 1967.

35. Brown, W. S. *In;* Nitrogen Mustards and Related Alkylating Agents, vol. 2, pp. 243–295, Academic Press, New York, 1963.

36. Soloway, A. H., Nilas, E., Kjelberg, R. N., and Mark, V. H. Penetration of brain and brain tumor by intravenous injections of alkylating agents. IV. J. Med. Pharm. Chem., *5*: 1371–1376, 1962.

37. Burke, J. F. Induced immunological response to tumors. Cancer Res., 29: 2363–2367, 1969.

Discussion of Paper of Dr. Amos

DR. ALEXANDER: Do cytotoxic small lymphocytes bearing the Ka marker possess a θ marker as well?

DR. AMOS: A certain proportion of these cells certainly do, for exposure of immune peritoneal exudate cells to anti-Ka serum results in 80% cytotoxicity, while treatment of this same population with anti-θ serum also kills about 80%. We have not as yet performed double fluorescence labeling studies.

DR. HOBBS: Does your anti-Ka serum destroy macrophages or K cells? For, our estimation of the K-cell population in humans is about 8% of the small round cells of the peripheral blood, a figure too large to be equivalent to van Furth's estimation of approximately 1.5% of such peripheral cells being macrophage precursors. In Northwick Park, England, they have found a child having a complete K-cell deficiency in the presence of normal monocytes and T and B cells. This condition appears to be hereditary, suggesting that K cells may be a special subclass of lymphoid cell, subject to defined genetic control.

DR. AMOS: We haven't tested the activity of this antiserum against macrophages or K cells. With regard to your comment, a recent paper described two effector populations in lymphocyte-mediated killing. One is the peritoneal exudate macrophage, which is responsible for an EDTA-independent cytotoxicity, and the other is a peripheral lymphocyte, involved in an EDTA-dependent scheme (J. Immunol., *113*: 1527–1532, 1974).

DR. ALEXANDER: In Dr. Burke's experiments, as the tumor-bearing animals were initially primed by i.v. or intra-lesional administration of nitrogen mustard and then only later treated with anti-hapten antibody, am I correct in assuming that part of the tumor load was first deleted by the mustard?

DR. AMOS: No, for in some experiments the nitrogen mustard was given in a very low dose which, by itself, was non-toxic, and was followed by antibody within 2 hr.

DR. SIMMONS: How was localization of the mustard exclusively to the tumor achieved?

DR. AMOS: Presumably it is attaching to other tissues as well, although one might postulate that it adheres longer to the tumor. There may also be preferential uptake, as, for example, some of the newly isolated antibiotics appear to non-specifically concentrate on tumor cell surfaces.

DR. STOCK: Were other tissues beside the tumor examined histologically following administration of the anti-hapten antiserum? For, some of the more rapidly proliferating cells might be expected to localize part of a systemically administered nitrogen mustard.

DR. AMOS: I'm not sure, but I don't want to emphasize this single example. A completely non-toxic agent could have been utilized, provided it could serve as a hapten and bind selectively to tumors. Indeed, I here mentioned these studies to bring them to the attention of pharmacologists, who could be equipped to better define the abilities of various agents to localize in different types of neoplasm.

DR. KENNEDY: There are certain substances which demonstrate such properties. For example, hematoporphyrin concentrates mainly in neoplastic tissue, but also to some extent in the liver. Here regional instillation might be of value.

DR. AMOS: A typical test system could be malignant melanoma, where there is great precedent for administration of various materials.

DR. KENNEDY: Might the effects observed in Dr. Burke's system be similar to the synergistic relationships noted by Schreffler and others between a small dose of a chemotherapeutic agent and a specific anti-tumor antibody?

DR. AMOS: In this study an anti-hapten rather than an anti-tumor antibody was employed. Both will ideally eventually localize to the tumor cell, but the advantage of the former agent is that it evokes a strong inflammatory response which can facilitate the penetration of an antibody. Perhaps treatment with a hapten followed by an anti-hapten antiserum could also precede anti-tumor antibody administration with a favorable result.

DR. KOBAYASHI: The immunizing effect you demonstrated with allogeneic tumors seems very strong. Is it possible to thus cure an already proliferating tumor?

DR. AMOS: No. However, I should like to try increasing the vascular permeability of these tumors utilizing the hapten/anti-hapten antibody system, and then test the effect of immune killer cells on a growing neoplasm.

DR. HOBBS: By the addition of K cells or macrophages, Fakhri and I have been able to rescue an animal up to 5 days after the establishment of a peritoneal tumor. Here the K cells function independently of complement, while the macrophages are encouraged by it.

DR. AMOS: This would appear to be a type of mass action phenomenon. Can you also protect these animals by intraperitoneal administration of antibody?

DR. HOBBS: By itself, specific antibody will rescue an animal only 1 day following tumor   inoculation.

DR. NISHIOKA: Are both Mg^{2+} and Ca^{2+} ion required for the binding stage of lymphocytes to target cells?

DR. AMOS: No. Either Mg^{2+} or Ca^{2+} alone can suffice. Binding is more dependent on Mg^{2+}, and higher concentrations of Ca^{2+} are required to provide the same effects. This phase is serum independent whereas in the killing phase serum potentiates cytotoxicity. A great augmentation of cytotoxicity is obtained by the addition of a highly heat stable serum factor (resistant to heating at 100°C for 5 min) in the presence of glucose.

DR. NISHIOKA: You noted binding inhibition in the presence of EDTA. Was this system reconstituted upon the addition of Ca^{2+} or Mg^{2+}?

DR. AMOS: We washed the cells and then put them into fresh medium and binding occurred. We also looked at the binding phase during addition of increasing concentrations of Ca^{2+} or Mg^{2+} to medium lacking these ions.

DR. H. OKADA (National Cancer Center Research Institute, Tokyo):   Is it possible that one of the reasons for the high specific cytotoxicity you obtained is a stimulation of precursor cells by their reaction with target cells during the binding phase of your scheme?

DR. AMOS: We conducted our experiments under relatively short-range conditions, so that binding proceeded for only 30–60 min. We have also noted that our peritoneal exudate lymphocytes show a very rapid and active proliferative response to allogeneic cells. I don't know whether the population responding in a mixed lymphocyte culture is the same pouplation that binds, however.

HOST DEFENSE AGAINST CANCER AND ITS POTENTIATION, D. MIZUNO ET AL. (EDS.),
UNIV. OF TOKYO PRESS, TOKYO / UNIV. PARK PRESS, BALTIMORE, PP. 157-179, 1975

Different Approaches to Stimulation of Host Defence

J. E. Castro

Royal Postgraduate Medical School, London, and Hammersmith Hospital, London, U.K.

Abstract: Most autochthonous tumours are antigenic, so the central problem of
immunotherapy is to make immunity more effective in control of tumour growth.
Stimulation or depression of different components of the immune response to different degrees and at will is the goal for immunological destruction of tumours. At
present, however, it is not possible to implicate any one mechanism in the immune
elimination of tumours, and four methods of immunological potentiation are possible: (1) increased cytotoxic antibodies, or better localisation of them; (2) suppression
of serum or cellular inhibitory factors; (3) increased or more effective macrophage
function; (4) in creased or more effective cell-mediated immunity.

Preferential production or physical separation of cytotoxic antibody is not always possible but potentially cytotoxic sera can be assessed "*in vitro*" before use "*in
vivo*." Localisation of cytotoxic antibodies might be improved by combination with
other chemicals, by selective perfusion of tumours, or by combination with other
immunological manipulations. Alternatively, antibodies might act as a vehicle for
concentrating therapeutic agents on tumour cells.

The exact nature of serum factors which stimulate tumour growth is still a matter for debate. Selective suppression of antibody-forming cells might be achieved by
chemotherapy or alloantisera, whilst circulating inhibitory factors may be removed
by immunoadsorption. Antigen-antibody complexes, if they are important, could
be dissociated with the added benefit that cytotoxic antibodies are released. Alteration of normal homeostatic control of immune responses might be achieved by interference with regulatory cells once this subpopulation of lymphocytes has been more
clearly defined.

Resistance to tumours parallels reticuloendothelial phagocytic activity. *Corynebacterium parvum* is an example of a substance that stimulates phagocytosis (whilst
depressing cell-mediated immunity) and in defined circumstances it has powerful
effects against primary tumours and their metastases. The mechanism of these antitumour effects is not clear; antigen processing for lymphocytes, macrophage cyto-

toxicity or maintenance of the balance between cellular immunity and enhancement by removal of inhibitory factors are possible explanations.

Several methods are available for stimulation of cell-mediated immunity. Adoptive transfer of immunised allogeneic lymphocytes has only limited application because of their rapid rejection. The use of transfer factor overcomes this problem but suitable donors are rarely available, assay is difficult, and populations of cells that will respond may not be present in the recipient. Cell-mediated immunity may be stimulated by altering the antigenicity of tumour cells either by acetoacetylation, gluteraldehyde treatment, enzyme degeneration of the cell membrane, or by incorporation of viruses into the cells. Conjugation of tumor cells with hapten could increase antigenicity by more helper cell effects or by providing new targets for immunological attack. Most immunological adjuvants stimulate cellular and humoral immunity but lentinan and orchidectomy may have selective effects upon cell-mediated immunity.

Elimination of tumours may result from alteration of several different and opposing components of the immune response and a unifying hypothesis of immune stimulation is not possible at present. However, encouraging results have been obtained for treatment of experimental and clinical tumours using these approaches.

With the demonstration by Foley (1) and others (2, 3) that experimental tumours exhibit specific antigenicity, the possibility of changing the course of human cancer by manipulation of this host response is attractive. It has been shown by a variety of techniques that most, if not all, autochthonous human tumours are antigenic. Antibodies or cytotoxic lymphocytes have been demonstrated against malignant melanoma (4), osteosarcoma (5), Burkitt's lymphoma (6), neuroblastoma (7), and carcinomas of the colon, lung, larynx, lip, and breast (8). Because these tumours are antigenic, the central problem of immunotherapy is to make such existing immunity more effective in the control of tumour growth. The stimulation of host resistance could be specific and designed to cope with a particular neo-antigen expressed by a particular tumour, but as we have little knowledge of the nature and relative importance of such tumour neo-antigens, it is necessary to protect against all of them and, therefore, non-specific stimulation of defences is a more reasonable approach at the present time.

The goal of non-specific immunological control of tumours should be the potentiation or depression of different components of the immune response to different degrees and at will. However, a prerequisite of such manoeuvres is an understanding of those components of the immunological mechanisms that are advantageous to tumour destruction. At present, the immunological mechanisms of tumour destruction are not known and there is disagreement as to the relative roles of the separate components of the immunological apparatus in this process. It has not been possible to implicate any one cytotoxic mechanism in immune elimination of tumours and different mechanisms seem to dominate in different circumstances.

Recent investigations show at least two cellular cytotoxic mechanisms: one involves thymus-processed cytotoxic cells (T cells) which recognise target cell antigens (9) and the other is effected by a thymus-independent effector cell which has no direct affinity for target cell antigen (10); these cells are triggered to kill by antibody bound to the target cells. On other occasions, antibodies (11) or macrophages (12) may be important in tumour cell destruction. Most attempts at the immunological control of tumours have been dominated by the concept that stimulation of cellular mechanisms is beneficial whilst humoral immunity should be depressed since it is likely to produce antibodies which promote tumour growth. This simplistic view, however, takes no account of the role of cytotoxic antibodies and of macrophages in tumour destruction.

It would seem that with present knowledge, four methods of stimulation of host responses are available which might retard tumour growth: (1) increased or improved localisation of cytotoxic antibody; (2) suppression of blocking factors; (3) more effective macrophage activity; (4) more effective cell-mediated immunity.

Cytotoxic Antibody

Physical separation of cytotoxic from enhancing immunoglobulins (13) is, as yet, an unsolved problem which is important both to tumour and transplantation biologists. Several features are important in the preferential stimulation of antibodies having a particular biological function, for example, the dose of antigen used to raise antibody, its route of administration to the animal in which antibody is being raised, and the time interval between priming and harvesting. In the recipient, the dosage of antibody and its route of administration are also important in obtaining a particular biological reaction.

Despite these difficulties, cytotoxic antibodies may be of use in the treatment of tumours. Carefully timed serum samples could be taken from a patient at intervals after surgical removal of a tumour and the cytotoxicity of the serum could be determined *in vitro*. Those samples showing cytotoxicity might be used *in vivo* to treat residual or recurrent tumours (14). Alternatively, allogeneic serum from patients with histologically similar or cross-reacting tumours could be used and even xenogeneic sera specifically absorbed might be useful.

Some of the antigens on virus-induced tumours are cross-reacting, showing virus specificity. Antibodies raised against the virus genome might therefore be useful in tumours of different histological types but induced by the same oncogenic virus. There is, however, increasing evidence that chemically induced tumours express cross-reacting antigens and at least some of these are phase-specific or foetal antigens (15). Despite the frequent observations that pretreatment with foetal tissues will alter the growth of subsequent tumour challenge (16, 17), we have, as yet, been unable to influence the growth of tumour by administration of xenogeneic antifoetal antibody but this could reflect the weak immunogenicity of foetal antigens.

In contrast, xenogeneic sera against tumour-specific transplantation antigen may have an effect upon tumour growth. We have used a rabbit anti-mouse Meth/A tumour serum which was shown to have cytotoxic activity against Meth/A cells *in vitro*. When intravenous antiserum was given and the ascitic Meth/A tumour was

TABLE 1. The Effect of Intravenous Rabbit Anti-Meth/A Mouse Tumour Serum on the Growth of Meth/A Tumour *In Vivo*

Interval between serum and tumour cells (days)	Degree of protection	
	Ascitic tumour	Solid subcutaneous tumour
0	++	++
14	++	0

given intraperitoneally, so that it grew in ascitic form, there was a good protective effect. This protection decreased with prolongation of the interval between tumour and antibody administration. There was, however, still good protection when the interval was two weeks between intraperitoneal tumour and intravenous antibody. When intravenous antiserum was given and the ascitic tumour was injected subcutaneously, so that it grew in solid form, different results were obtained. If antiserum and tumour were given subcutaneously good protection was obtained, but with prolongation of the tumour-antibody interval protective effects of antiserum were less, and when the interval was two weeks the antiserum had no antitumour action (Table 1).

The failure of antiserum to destroy or inhibit established solid tumours could be a problem of antibody distribution so that the antibody and tumour cells do not make contact. Such contact could be facilitated by combining cytotoxic antibodies with pharmaceutical agents which would improve their penetration or, alternatively, by infusion or regional perfusion of the tumour. The combination of antibody administration with other immunological manipulations might facilitate tumour inhibition or destruction.

An alternative use for antitumour antibodies is to use them as vehicles for transporting anti-tumour agents to the tumour surface so that high concentration of such agents is obtained at the tumour site whilst the generalised systemic side effects of the antitumour agents are minimised (*18*).

Blocking Factors

Serum blocking factors which interfere with the normal interaction of cytotoxic cells and tumour cells have been described both in laboratory animals and in humans. Their occurrence and disappearance after conventional treatments seem to correlate with the clinical course of tumours (*19*) but their exact nature is not clear. Antibody, antigen excess (*20*) and antibody-antigen complexes (*21*) have been invoked and these different agents may be important either at different points in the immune response or in different circumstances.

Despite these defects of knowledge, there are theoretically more approaches to the removal of blocking factors than to stimulation of antibody formation of a particular biological class. With removal of blocking factors, then the normal antitumour mechanisms may be able to eliminate tumour cells. Selective suppression of these cells, which are responsible for antibody production, has been claimed after the use of cyclophosphamide (*22*) and in animals antisera have been raised against antibody-producing cells (23). In practice, however, use of these antisera is disappointing. Once blocking factors are present, they might be removed by immuno-absorption or by plasmaphoresis. Antigen-antibody complexes, if they are important, could be dissociated with the added benefit that the liberated antibody might itself be cytotoxic.

Macrophages

During growth of transplanted syngeneic tumours, there is increased production (24) and function of macrophages (25) and this increased function results from changes of cellular factors rather than opsonins (26). Furthermore, the resistance of laboratory animals to tumours parallels reticuloendothelial activity (27). The ways in which macrophages are involved in tumour destruction are not clear. There is morphological evidence from electron-microscopic studies of interaction between macrophages and lymphocytes at the onset of immune responses (28) and it is well accepted that macrophages process some antigens, including tumour antigens, for lymphocytes (29).

However, there are other functions of macrophages that may be important for the control of tumours. It has been shown that macrophages recovered from suitably immunised hosts are activated by contact with the tumour cells used for immunisation but after this they will also kill unrelated tumour cells that grow in their presence (30). The relationship of in vitro macrophage cytotoxicity to the protection observed in vivo is difficult to interpret because of the interaction of macrophages with other cell types.

Macrophages are important in other immunological reactions. For example, small numbers of macrophages are essential if lymphocytes are to respond to phytohaemagglutinin (31). Furthermore, they may play an important part in maintaining a balance between cellular immunity and enhancement of tumour growth, by removing excess antigens or antigen-antibody complexes from the circulation (32).

Corynebacterium parvum is a powerful stimulant of reticuloendothelial activity (33) which we have studied. When given intravenously or intraperitoneally, it increased spleen and liver size (34) (Table 2) and histological examination of these organs showed enlargement was due to increased macrophages. There was also evidence of increased function of macrophages, for particulate carbon was cleared more rapidly from treated mice (35). Concomitant with these changes, resistance to tu-

TABLE 2. Effects of Two Doses of 0.2 ml C. parvum on the Thymus, Spleen, and Liver Weights Two Weeks after Injection with the Vaccine

Animals	Organ weights (mg)		
	Thymus	Spleen	Liver
Control mice	38.2 ± 10.6	79 ± 7.0	$1,278 \pm 116$
Mice given C. parvum	10.9 ± 1.9	524 ± 84	$2,037 \pm 228$

Values are mean±standard deviation (SD).

TABLE 3. Percentage of Controls and *C. parvum*-treated Mice to Show the Effect of ALS on the Anti-tumour Activity of *C. parvum*

Treatment	Percentage survival after treatment at		
	30 days	40 days	50 days
Control+tumour	92	55	45
Control, ALS+tumour	66	8	0
C. parvum, ALS+tumour	83	83	75
C. parvum+tumour	100	100	100
C. parvum+ALS	92	75	50

C. parvum was given intraperitoneally (i.p.) on days 1 and 2, and ALS on days 3, 4, 5, and then weekly. Tumour cells were given i.p. on day 0.

mours develops (*36, 37*) and we have shown that pretreatment with *C. parvum* decreased death rate of BALB/c mice inoculated intraperitoneally with Meth/A ascitic tumour (Table 3), CBA mice given S37 ascitic tumour and C3H/He mice given Ehrlich's ascitic tumour (*38*). It is interesting that intravenous *C. parvum* did not affect the death rate from solid Meth/A tumour but in a study of the effects of *C. parvum* on the growth of the primary Lewis lung tumour (*39*) it was shown that some inhibition of tumour growth was obtained after intravenous or intraperitoneal *C. parvum* but that subcutaneous inoculation of the vaccine had no effect. These data would suggest that *C. parvum* is more effective when tumour cells are dissociated rather than when they are growing as a solid vascularised tumour.

The interaction of macrophages with other cell types makes it difficult to establish their importance in tumour therapy. It could be that the anti-tumour effects of *C. parvum* were mediated directly through increased macrophages themselves or by increase of macrophages with associated changes in lymphocytes responsible for humoral or cell-mediated immunity. It seems unlikely that increased cell-mediated immunity was implicated in the anti-tumour effects of *C. parvum*, for it prolonged survival of murine skin allografts both in H2 identical and non-identical strain combinations. It also caused atrophy of the thymus (Table 2). Furthermore, the anti-tumour effects of *C. parvum* were maintained despite adult thymectomy or treatment with antilymphocyte serum (ALS) (Table 3), manoeuvres which inhibit cell-mediated immunity. These observations agree with those of Woodruff (*40*), who has shown an antitumour effect of *C. parvum* in mice made deficient in cell-mediated immunity by thymectomy, irradiation, and reconstitution with syngeneic bone marrow. Whilst not excluding the necessity of a small limiting number of cells responsible for cell-mediated immunity, these data suggest that the increased antitumour activity of *C. parvum*-treated mice is not related to an increase of T cells and they lend indirect support to the hypothesis of Howard (*41*), which suggests a negative regulatory effect of macrophages on T cells.

Interaction of macrophages with antibody-producing cells was evidenced by the observation of increased direct response to sheep erythrocytes (SRBC) in mice given *C. parvum* but whether this reflects more efficient antigen handling by macrophages or changes in the numbers of antibody-producing cells was not clear. However, the observation that there was no increase of cytotoxicity to H2 antigens after

C. parvum makes it unlikely that increased cytotoxic bone marrow-derived cell (B-cell) function is the mechanism of antitumor activity of *C. parvum*.

In other experiments we have shown that the protective effects of intraperitoneal *C. parvum* on ascitic Meth/A tumour was maximal with low tumour dose and the duration of its effect was between 25 and 50 days. Splenectomy did not affect the anti-tumour activity and, despite the recent studies that suggest large doses of BDG given orally retains some of the anti-tumour effects seen after injection, we were unable to observe any immunological effects of oral *C. parvum* despite massive doses of the vaccine. Particularly, oral *C. parvum* did not significantly increase spleen weight, increase antibodies against *C. parvum* itself, and it had no effect upon the growth of tumours which are inhibited by intravenous administration of the vaccine (*42*).

C. parvum and Tumour Metastases

Because of the superior effects of *C. parvum* on dissociated rather than solid tumours, we have observed the effects of *C. parvum* treatment on the primary Lewis lung carcinoma and its metastases in female C57/BL mice. When intravenous or intraperitoneal *C. parvum* was given at the same time as subcutaneous inoculation of the tumour, there was significant reduction in the primary tumour mass and the number of pulmonary metastases detected by the methods described by Wexler (*43*) (Table 4). In contrast, contralateral subcutaneous *C. parvum* had no effect on either the primary tumour or its metastases.

When the Lewis lung tumour was inoculated subcutaneously in normal mice,

TABLE 4.   The Effect of *C. parvum* on Pulmonary Metastases from the Lewis Lung Tumour When Given at the Same Time as Subcutaneous Tumour Inoculation

Treatment	Number of mice	Average number of metastases	Range of metastases
Controls (untreated)	9	24	10–37
0.1 ml *C. parvum* i.v.	9	4[a]	0–11
0.1 ml *C. parvum* i.p.	9	4[a]	0–8
0.1 ml *C. parvum* s.c.	9	18	7–36

i.v.: intravenously.   s.c.: subcutaneously.   [a] $P > 0.01$.

TABLE 5.   The Effect of Combined *C. parvum* and Surgery on the Number of Pulmonary Metastases of the Lewis Lung Tumour

Day on which *C. parvum* was given :	Number of metastases as percentage of those in the untreated control group		
	i.v. *C. parvum*	i.p. *C. parvum*	s.c. *C. parvum*
7	10.5[a]	29	66
8	33[b]	33[b]	94
9	59	41	93
10	65	74	90

The tumour was excised on day 10.   [a] $P > 0.001$.   [b] $P > 0.01$.

pulmonary metastases were not observed 10 days after tumour inoculation but, despite excision of the primary tumour at this same time (10 days), pulmonary metastases develop consistently 21 days after inoculation.

In order to simulate a clinical situation, the combined effects of surgical excision of the primary tumour at day 10 and intravenous injection of *C. parvum* on pulmonary metastases were studied. It was found that when surgery and *C. parvum* administration were on the same day there was only minimal protection but if *C. parvum* was given one or more days before tumour excision, there was significant protection and the earlier before surgery it was given the greater the protective effects. Indeed, some mice were permanently cured of tumour both at the primary site by surgery and of their metastases by treatment with *C. parvum* (Table 5). Such results suggest that in defined conditions *C. parvum* can prevent pulmonary metastases from the Lewis tumour and it may be a useful adjuvant for tumours that have poor prognosis after surgery alone.

Cell-mediated Immunity

Despite the demonstration of antitumour activity without increase of cell-mediated immunity after *C. parvum*, there is no doubt of the importance of cell-mediated immunity in some tumour situations. For example, we have shown that orchidectomy increased cell-mediated immunity, as evidenced by an increase of thymus size (Table 6) both in pre- and postpuberal (44) animals and increase of immunological reactions which manifest cell-mediated immunity. It was shown that orchidectomy caused accelerated rejection of murine skin allografts, an increase in the early (cell-mediated) response to oxazolone and stimulation of the direct response to SRBC (45). Such findings agree with the observation of Graff (46), who also observed accelerated rejection of murine skin allografts, and Kaplan and Rosston (47), who found protection against wasting disease in mice after orchidectomy. The accelerated rejection of skin allografts after orchidectomy as due to immunological causes, rather than metabolic or vascular ones, as suggested by abrogation of this effect by adult thymectomy or administration of ALS (Fig. 1), both of which deplete cell-mediated immunity. The response to SRBC depends upon T cells and B cells and increased response to this antigen may result from changes in either cell-mediated or humoral immunity. However, recent work by Campbell (48) suggests that T cells are in fact the limiting factor in this response and it would suggest that orchidectomy potentiates the response by an effect upon

TABLE 6. Percentage of BALB/c Mice with Subcutaneous Sarcomas after Injection with 0.05 μg Methylcholanthrene per Mouse

	Days after methylcholanthrene				
	50	100	150	200	250
Controls	0	25	67	88	88
Orchidectomised	0	16	35	65	65

Forty mice in each group.

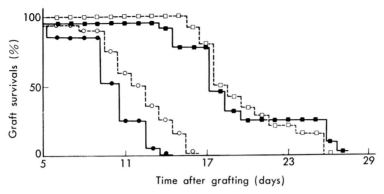

FIG. 1. Accelerated rejection of skin allografts produced by orchidectomy and the result of ALS on this effect. ○ control; □ control+ALS; ● orchidectomised; ■ orchidectomised+ALS.

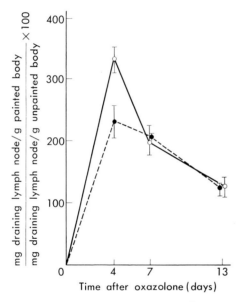

FIG. 2. Increased early (cell-mediated) response of orchidectomised mice to *in vivo* stimulation with oxazolone but no difference in the late (humoral) response (mean values±SD). ● control; ○ orchidectomised.

this population of cells. The investigations of Davies (*49*) have shown that application of oxazolone to the skin of mice causes stimulation of cell-mediated immunity in the regional lymph nodes 4 days after antigen, but by 8 days the response was due to increased antibody production. In our experiments the response of control and orchidectomised mice to *in vivo* oxazolone was compared and it was found that the response at 4 days (the time of maximal cell-mediated immunity) was significantly greater in the orchidectomised mice but at 8 or 13 days (the times when antibody responses predominate) there was no difference between the two groups of mice (Fig. 2).

These findings suggest that orchidectomy caused non-specific active immuno-

TABLE 7. The Effect of Orchidectomy and Synchronous Orchidectomy and Thymectomy on the Thymus, Spleen, and Lymph Node Weights One Week after Surgery

	Organ weights (mg)		
	Thymus	Spleen	Lymph node
Sham-operated controls	35.6± 6.6	106±21	1.8±0.3
Orchidectomised	67.1±12.3	123±16	2.5±0.4
Orchidectomised and thymectomised	—	121±14	1.7±0.3

Values are mean±SD.

potentiation and particularly those responses that depend upon cell-mediated immunity for expression. The effect of orchidectomy on tumour induction and transplantation in mice were studied. The effect of orchidectomy on the induction of subcutaneous sarcomas by methylcholanthrene was to delay the rate of tumour appearance and also to decrease the number of mice that developed tumours (Table 7), a finding that agrees with the observations of Hopewell (50) who induced brain tumours in rats using carcinogenic chemicals and Bertram and Craig (51) on the induction of leukaemia. However, once tumour growth was established, the rate of growth was similar in both control and orchidectomised mice so that survival curves paralleled graphs of tumour induction.

In tumour transplantation experiments, the Meth/A tumour which originated in the laboratory of Old (52) was used. We confirmed that it is an antigenic tumour, it is syngeneic with BALB/c mice, exhibits a good dose response curve and on electron microscopy it does not contain viral particles. It is not obviously endocrine-dependent, for the tumour can be grown in tissue culture with addition of hormonal supplements, and it grows almost equally well in males and females (the slightly superior growth in males probably reflects their decreased immunological reactivity (53, 54). On histological examination it has the appearances of a soft-tissue sarcoma, a tumour not normally thought of as being endocrine dependent. When the Meth/A tumour was grown intraperitoneally, orchidectomy had only a slight but significant protective effect against death from the tumour. When the same cells grew as a solid, subcutaneous tumour, protection was considerably increased (Fig. 3).

Two pieces of evidence suggested that the protective effects of orchidectomy on tumours was an immunological one. Firstly, abrogation of the protective effect of orchidectomy by administration of ALS and secondly, partial abrogation by synchronous thymectomy with orchidectomy (55).

The superior effect of orchidectomy (which stimulated cell-mediated immunity) on growth of the solid form of tumour contrasts with the observations after C. parvum administration, which stimulates macrophage function, and had most effect upon dissociated tumours.

The effect of orchidectomy on the occurrence of leukaemia in AKR mice was also studied. Normally 50–90% of these mice develop leukaemia by 7–10 months (56) and the incidence is higher in females than males (57). Histologically, tumours are lymphoblastic or lymphocytic and an intact thymus is essential for their develop-

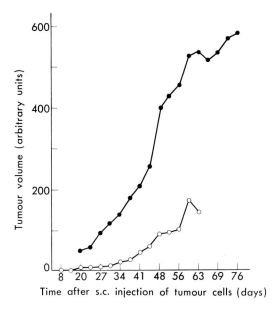

Time after s.c. injection of tumour cells (days)

FIG. 3.   Mean tumour volumes of control and orchidectomised mice after subcutaneous injection of viable Meth/A tumour cells. ● control; ○ orchidectomised.

ment. In contradistinction to the findings with other tumours, the effect of orchidectomy on AKR leukaemia was to accelerate appearance of tumours and death from it and this finding is in agreement with those of others (*58*). The explanation is probably that orchidectomy by causing thymic hypertrophy increased the number of cells at risk of malignant transformation.

Other methods for stimulation of cell-mediated immunity are possible. Adoptive transfer of allogeneic lymphocytes from subjects immunised against tumours or from subjects that have undergone spontaneous or surgical cure of tumours have been used (*59, 60*) but with only limited success because of the short life span of transferred allogeneic lymphocytes (*61*). Transfer factor (*62*) which is a dialysable, non-antigenic non-immunoglobulin of 10,000 molecular weight resident in circulating leucocytes, obviates these problems. Administration of transfer factor *in vivo* converts non-sensitive recipient circulating lymphocytes to a responsive state to specific antigens, including tumour antigens. However, suitable donor sources are not readily available, it is difficult to assay, and populations of cells which respond to transfer factor may not be present in the recipient. So far, reports of the use of transfer factor for treating tumours have been limited to anecdotal case reports, particularly of patients with malignant melanoma and, although some success has been claimed (*63*), the specificity of transfer factor has recently been questioned. It has been suggested that it is acting as a non-specific potentiator of immune responses.

Most immunological adjuvants act on several components of the immune system but selective stimulation of cell-mediated immunity has been claimed for lentinan (*64*), a polysaccharide extracted from the edible Japanese mushroom (*Lentinus edodes*). The effects of lentinan on normal mice seem to be variable, for we have found that it does not affect skin allograft survival and has no effect on thymus or lymph node weight. We have been unable to demonstrate a protective effect in BALB/c mice given Meth/A tumour either intraperitoneally or subcutaneously, CBA mice given S37 ascites sarcoma or C3H/He mice given Ehrlich's ascites tumour. It would seem that the previously reported antitumour effects of lentinan are limited to specific tumours in particular strains of mice.

Because of these difficulties of stimulating intrinsic cell-mediated responses, attempts have been made to cause stimulation by altering antigenicity of tumour cells, for example by acetoacetylation (65), enzymatic changes in the cell surface (66), or by gluteraldehyde treatment. Sanderson and Frost (67) have demonstrated the use of gluteraldehyde-treated cells for the induction of immunity to Meth/A tumour in syngeneic murine hosts. Gluteraldehyde solution contains polymeric α- and β-saturated aldehydes. These react rapidly with protein amino groups in mild conditions and cross-link the protein molecules. The modification is irreversible and does not disorder the crystalline structure, and for these reasons gluteraldehyde is used as a fixative for electron microscopy and X-ray diffraction. Non-immunised control mice challenged with 10^5 tumour cells survived for approximately 20 days whereas mice immunised with gluteraldehyde-treated cells were completely protected against this challenge but not against 10^6 tumour cells. In contrast, mice immunised with the same number of irradiated cells showed less protection. These results applied when the interval between gluteraldehyde-treated cells and tumour challenge was 2 weeks but when mice were left for 27 days between immunisation and challenge, only partial protection was obtained indicating that immunity decreased at that time. Two factors might operate in producing this immunity: firstly, gluteraldehyde may be preserving the tumour antigenicity and secondly, the chemical modification of the proteins may produce an enhanced cellular immunity at the expense of humoral response.

The incorporation of virus into tumour cells (68, 69) is another approach to increasing tumour immunogenicity. It has been observed that mice that recover from transplantation of tumours after viral oncolysis were immune when challenged with uninfected tumour cells. It is possible that the virus used in oncolysis might act as a carrier for haptenic determinants of tumour cells, and evidence for this explanation has been provided by the observation that antiviral antibody added in excess to a virus oncolysate inhibited the antitumour response. The possibility that antigens become incorporated into the virus envelope is the most easily testable explanation for adjuvanticity of viruses but it is not the only possible mechanism, for it could result from increased immunogenicity of host cell debris. Host antigens become attached to the viral proteins and the resulting molecules could carry antigenic determinants which are characteristic of the host cell in addition to the possible carrier-hapten type (70). Other less specific interactions are possible: effects of neurominidase in uncovering new antigenic sites after the removal of sialic acid are well established (71) and nucleic acids have adjuvant effects (72). Local immunostimulation, perhaps by attraction of specialised cells to critical sites, is also possible; some bacteria have been shown to act in this way and it is probably also true for most viruses. Certainly, the conjugation of tumour cells with hapten could theoretically increase antigenicity either by increasing helper cell effect or providing new targets for immunological attack.

Stimulation of Tumour Growth by the Immune Response

Recently, Prehn (73) has suggested that stimulation of the immune response may stimulate tumours to development. He suggested that although specific immune reactivity may sometimes be adequate to control a neoplasm, lesser degrees of immune reactivity may promote the growth of latent tumours. According to this hypothesis, immune reaction may at times produce better tumour growth than would occur in the complete absence of immune reactivity. If the immunological response to antigenic tumours is biphasic, a similar situation should exist in connection with other immunological rejections. A possible example has been reported with respect to the parasite *Plasmodium berghei* infection in mice (74). It has been found that ALS decreased the number of parasites and prolonged the life of infected hosts, but only in situations when there was little natural resistance. In mouse strains with more immunity, ALS shortens life from this same infection. These data are similar to the situation with the mouse mammary tumour (75); C3H mouse tumour produced by milk agent is quite immunogenic when grown in C3H mice which lack the virus, but when grown in a subline which contains virus, it has very little immunogenicity. Attempts at immunisation against the tumour implants in virus-containing mice sometimes lead to enhanced tumour growth and X-irradiation of neonatal thymectomy may decrease the growth of transplants of this tumour. In the C3H mice in which the tumours are more immunogenic, reduction of immune capacity by thymectomy or irradiation increased tumour growth. The results could, however, be explained by alteration in the balance between blocking factors and cellular immunity.

There are other data which support the immune stimulation theory. When thymectomised, X-irradiated mice were injected with various numbers of spleen cells from specifically immunised mice but mixed with a constant number of target tumour cells, different results were obtained dependent on the proportions of the cell populations. Small numbers of immune spleen cells caused acceleration of tumour growth when compared with controls of either non-immune spleen cells or spleen cells from animals immunised against different non-cross-reacting tumours. Large numbers of specifically immune spleen cells, however, produced inhibition of tumour growth (76). Such data suggests that early in the course of disease, or in situations where the immune reaction to tumour is weak, stimulation of tumour growth may occur, whereas inhibition of tumour growth occurs at other times.

The *in vitro* experiments of Jeejeebhoy (77) also support the theory. At an early stage of tumour development when tumours were not palpable, the cellular antitumour immune responses of mice were found to be capable of specifically stimulating tumour growth. However, when the tumours enlarged and were palpable, it was found that the stimulatory pattern seen early in tumour development had changed to an inhibitory one.

These observations on tumour stimulation may also offer an explanation for some of our own experiments which involved the use of foetal tissue to influence the growth of subsequent tumour challenge. These experiments were based on the suggestion that at least some of the neo-antigens expressed by tumours were similar to those of foetal tissues (*78*). The evidence for occurrence of such foetal antigens is now considerable for in addition to the classical observation by Gold and Freedman (*79*), which showed that colon carcinomas express antigens similar to those occurring in foetal gut, liver, and pancreas during the first trimester. Baldwin (*80*) has shown by immunofluorescence that chemically induced experimental tumours have foetal antigens on their surfaces. We have shown that adult syngeneic animals are capable of constantly restricting the growth of syngeneic foetal tissue implants (*81*). The evidence suggests that this is in fact an immunological mechanism, for pretreatment with foetal tissues modifies the growth of a second foetal pretreatment with foetal tissues modifies the growth of a second foetal tissue implant. Furthermore, the occurrence of lymphocyte infiltrate into syngeneic foetal tissue implants in non-immunologically suppressed animals is evidence of an immune mechanism and the observation that foetal tissue implants grow preferentially in immunologically deprived animals when compared to normal immunologically competent mice is again suggestive that the moderation of foetal tissue growth is effected by immunological mechanisms.

In view of the suggestion that tumour antigens are re-awakened foetal antigens (*82, 83*), we investigated the effects of initial exposure to foetal antigens on transplantation of tumours. We found that pretreatment with irradiated foetal tissues from 11 day foetuses given 10 days before inoculation with intraperitoneal Meth/A tumour cells confirmed protection against this tumour but pretreatment with non-irradiated tissues caused enhancement of tumour growth (*84*) (Fig. 4). Irradiation of foetal inocula was found to be essential by Coggin (*85, 86*) for pro-

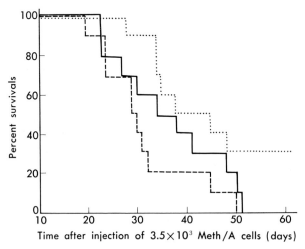

FIG. 4.   Comparison of survival in mice pretreated with irradiated or non-irradiated syngeneic foetal tissues (FT) and given Meth/A tumour cells intraperitoneally. —— control; ······ irradiated FT; - - - - non-irradiated FT.

tection against subsequent tumour challenge. It may be that irradiation, by preventing the maturation of foetal tissues, effectively increased the dose of immunity against foetal antigens but in the non-irradiated foetal tissue implants the mild degree of immunity engendered by maturating foetal tissues which lose their characteristic antigens is an example of tumour stimulation related to a mild degree of immunity.

CONCLUSIONS

The data presented suggests that antitumour activity can result from separate components of the immune response. For example, both *C. parvum* and orchidectomy have antitumour effects but *C. parvum* appears to stimulate macrophages whilst depressing cell-mediated immunity, whereas orchidectomy stimulates cell-mediated immunity with small effects upon macrophages. In some circumstances, stimulation of the immune response actually enhances tumour growth. It is therefore not possible at present to fit the mechanisms of immunopotentiation into a unifying hypothesis. It is this defect that led Burnet (*87*) to say "I expect in 20 years' time three major areas to be written off as blind alleys—anaphylaxis, *the use of complex adjuvants*, and experiments on intercellular transfer of immunological elimination. They are blind alleys in the sense that the findings within the corresponding field of experiment study cannot be transferred without the greatest circumspection into a general context." It is at present not possible to fit the mechanisms of immunopotentiation into a unifying hypothesis and in this sense it is correct to consider study of adjuvants of this type as a blind alley, but the encouraging results obtained in treating laboratory tumour models and now being reported in clinical practice make it worthy of further study.

ACKNOWLEDGMENTS

Sir Peter Medawar, Dr. Eugene Lance, and Dr. Tessa Sadler were scientific collaborators in some of the work reported; Miss Wendy Cass and Mrs. R. Hunt gave technical assistance and it is a pleasure to acknowledge them all. The Cancer Research Campaign has supported studies with *Corynebacterium parvum*.

REFERENCES

1. Foley, E. J. Antigenic properties of methylcholanthrene induced tumours in mice of the strain of origin. Cancer Res., *13*: 835–837, 1953.
2. Prehn, R. T. and Main, J. M. Immunity to methylcholanthrene induced sarcomas. J. Natl. Cancer Inst., *18*: 769–778, 1957.
3. Rapp, F. The role of the viral genome in oncogenesis. Cancer Res., *28*: 1832–1834, 1968.
4. Lewis, M. G., Ikonopisov, R. L., Nairn, R. C., Phillips, T. M., Fairley, G. H., Bodenham, D. C., and Alexander, P. Tumour specific antibodies in human malignant melanoma and their relationship to the extent of the disease. Brit. Med. J., *3*: 547–552, 1969.

5. Morton, D. L., Malmgren, R. A., Holmes, E. C., Ketcham, A. S. Demonstration of antibodies against human malignant melanoma by immunofluorescence. Surgery, *64*: 233–240, 1968.

6. Klein, E., Klein, G., Adkarni, J. S., Adkarni, J. J., Wigzell, H., and Clifford, P. Surface 1Gm-kappa specificity on a Burkitt lymphoma cell *in vitro* and in derived culture lines. Cancer Res., *28*: 1300–1309, 1968.

7. Hellstrom, I. E., Hellstrom, K. E., Pierce, G. D., and Bill, A. H. Demonstration of cell bound and humoral immunity against neuroblastoma cells. Proc. Natl. Acad. Sci. U.S., *60*: 1231–1238, 1968.

8. Hellstrom, I. E., Hellstrom, K. E., Pierce, G. E., and Yang, J. P. Cellular and humoral immunity to different types of human neoplasms. Nature, *220*: 1352–1354, 1968.

9. Blomgren, H., Tagasugi, M., and Friberg, S. Specific cytotoxicity by sensitised mouse thymus cells on tissue culture target cells. Cell. Immunol., *1*: 619–631, 1970.

10. Hersey, P., Cullen, P., and MacLennon, I. C. Lymphocyte dependent cytotoxic antibody activity against human transplantation antigens. Transplantation, *16*: 9–16, 1973.

11. Evans, C. A., Gorman, L. R., Ito, Y., and Weiser, R. S. Anti-tumour immunity in the Shope papilloma-carcinoma complex of rabbits. J. Natl. Cancer Inst., *29*: 277–285, 1962.

12. Evans, R. and Alexander, P. Co-operation of immune lymphoid cells with macrophages in tumour immunity. Nature, *228*: 620–622, 1970.

13. Fuller, T. C. and Winn, H. J. Immunochemical and biological characterisation of alloantibody active in immunological enhancement. Abstr. Papers, 4th Int. Congr. Transplant. Proc., *5*: 585–587, 1973.

14. Smith, R. T. Potentials for immunologic intervention in cancer. *In;* B. Amos (ed.), Progress in Immunology, pp. 1115–1129, Academic Press, New York and London, 1971.

15. Alexander, P. Foetal antigens in cancer. Nature, *235*: 137–140, 1972.

16. Coggin, J. H., Jr., Ambrose, K. R., and Anderson, N. G. Fetal antigen capable of inducing transplantation immunity against SV40 hamster tumor cells. J. Immunol., *105*: 524–526, 1970.

17. Coggin, J. H., Jr., Ambrose, K. R., and Anderson, N. G. Immunisation against tumors with fetal antigens. *In;* Proceedings of the First Conference and Workshop on Embryonic and Fetal Antigens in Cancer, Oak Ridge National Laboratory, Oak Ridge, Tennessee, May 24–26, 1971, USAEC Report CONF-710527, United States Department of Commerce, pp. 185–202, Springfield, Va., 1971.

18. Ghose, T. and Nigam, S. P. Antibody as a carrier of Chlorambucil. Cancer, *29*: 1398–1400, 1972.

19. Perlmann, P., O'toole, C., and Unsgaard, B. Cell mediated immune mechanism of tumour destruction. Fed. Proc., *32*: 153–155, 1973.

20. Currie, G. A. and Basham, C. Serum mediated inhibition of the immunological reactions of the patient to his own tumour: A possible role for circulating antigen. Brit. J. Cancer, *26*: 427–437, 1972.

21. Baldwin, R. W. and Embleton, M. J. Demonstration by colony inhibition methods of cellular and humoral immune reaction to tumour specific antigens associated with aminoazo-dye induced rat hepatomas. Int. J. Cancer, *7*: 17, 1971.

22. Turk, J. L. and Poulter, L. W. Selective depletion of lymphoid tissue by cyclophosphamide. Clin. Exp. Immunol., *10*: 285–296, 1972.

23. Raff, M. C., Nase, S., and Mitchison, N. A. Mouse specific bone marrow derived lymphocyte antigens as a marker for thymus independent lymphocytes. Nature, *230*: 50–51, 1971.

24. Baum, M. and Fisher, B. Macrophage production by the bone marrow of tumour bearing mice. Cancer Res., *32*: 2813, 1972.

25. Old, L. J., Benacerraf, B., Clarke, D. A., Carswell, E. A., and Stockert, E. The role of the reticuloendothelial system in host reaction to neoplasia. Cancer Res., *21*: 1281–1300, 1961.

26. Klamschmidt, R. F. and Pulliam, L. A. Changes in the opsonin and cellular influences on phagocytosis during the growth of transplantable tumours. J. Reticuloendothel. Soc., *11*: 1, 1972.

27. Old, L. J., Benacerraf, B., Clarke, D. A., Carswell, E. A., and Stockert, E. The role of the reticuloendothelial system in host reaction to neoplasia. Cancer Res., *21*: 1281–1300, 1961.

28. Salvin, S. B., Sell, S., and Nishio, J. Activity *in vitro* of lymphocytes and macrophages in delayed hypersensitivity. J. Immunol., *107*: 655–662, 1971.

29. Askonas, B. A. and Rhodes, J. M. Immunogenicity of antigen containing ribonucleic acid preparations from macrophages. Nature, *205*: 470–474, 1965.

30. Evans, R. and Alexander, P. Mechanisms of immunologically specific killing of tumour cells by macrophages. Nature, *236*: 168, 1972.

31. Levis, W. R. and Robbins, J. H. Effect of glass adherent cells on the blastogenic response of ' purified ' lymphocytes to phytohaemagglutinin. Exp. Cell Res., *61*: 153–158, 1970.

32. Unanue, E. R. and Cerottini, J. C. The immunogenicity of antigen bound to the plasma membrane of macrophages. J. Exp. Med., *131*: 711–725, 1970.

33. Halpern, B. N., Prevot, A. R., Blozzi, G., Stiffel, C., Mouton, D., Morard, J. C., Bouthillier, Y., and Decreuseford, C. Stimulation de l'activite phagocytaire du systeme reticuloendothelial provaquee par *Corynebacterium parvum*. J. Reticuloendothel. Soc., *1*: 77, 1964.

34. Castro, J. E. The effect of *Corynebacterium parvum* on the structure and function of the lymphoid system in mice. Eur. J. Cancer, *10*: 115–120, 1974.

35. Smith, L. H. and Woodruff, M. F. A. Comparative effects of two strains of *Corynebacterium parvum* on phagocytic activity and tumour growth. Nature, *219*: 345, 1968.

36. Smith, S. E. and Scott, M. J. Biological effects of *Corynebacterium parvum*: III. Amplification of resistance and impairment of active immunity to murine tumours. Brit. J. Cancer, *26*: 361–367, 1972.

37. Woodruff, M. F. A. and Boak, J. L. Inhibitory effect of injection of *Corynebacterium parvum* on the growth of tumour transplants in isogenic hosts. Brit. J. Cancer, *20*: 345–355, 1966.

38. Castro, J. E. Antitumour effects of *Corynebacterium parvum*. Eur. J. Cancer, *10*: 121–126, 1974.

39. Sadler, T. E. and Castro, J. E. Treatment of a metastasising murine tumour with *Corynebacterium parvum*. Brit. J. Surg., in press.

40. Woodruff, M. F. A., Dunbar, N., and Ghaffar, D. The growth of tumours in T cell deprived mice and their response to treatment with *Corynebacterium parvum*. Proc. Roy. Soc., Ser. B, *184*: 97–102, 1973.

41. Howard, J. G., Scott, M. T., and Christie, G. H. Cellular mechanisms underlying the adjuvant activity of *Corynebacterium parvum*: Interaction of activated microphages

with T and B lymphocytes. *In;* G. E. W. Wolstenholme and J. Knight (eds.), Immunopotentiation (Ciba Foundation Symposium), vol. 18, pp. 101–116, Elsevier / Excerpta Medica / North Holland, Amsterdam / London / New York, 1973.

42. Sadler, T. E. and Castro, J. E. The immunological and antitumour effects of orally administered *Corynebacterium parvum* in mice. Brit. J. Cancer, *31*: 359–363.

43. Wexler, H. Accurate identification of experimental pulmonary metastases. J. Natl. Cancer Inst., *36*: 641–643, 1966.

44. Castro, J. E. Orchidectomy and the immune response. I. The effect of orchidectomy on lymphoid tissues of mice. Proc. Roy. Soc., Ser. B, *185*: 425–436, 1974.

45. Castro, J. E. Orchidectomy and the immune response. II. Response of orchidectomised mice to antigens. Proc. Roy. Soc., Ser. B, *185*: 437–451, 1974.

46. Graff, R. J., Lappe, M., and Snell, G. D. The influence of gonads and adrenal glands on the immune response to skin grafts. Transplantation, *7*: 105–111, 1969.

47. Kaplan, H. A. and Rosston, B. H. Amelioration by adrenalectomy of the homologous "wasting disease" induced in irradiated hybrid mice by injections of parental lymphoid cells. Transplant. Bull., *6*: 107, 1959.

48. Campbell, P. A. T cells; the limiting cells in the initiation of immune responses in normal mouse spleen. Cell. Immunol., *5*: 338–340, 1972.

49. Davies, A. J. S., Carter, R. L., Leuchars, E., and Wallis, V. The morphology of immune reaction in normal, thymectomised and reconstituted mice. II. The response to oxazolone. Immunology, *17*: 111–126, 1969.

50. Hopewell, J. W. The effects of castration in the induction of experimental gliomas in male rats. Brit. J. Cancer, *24*: 187–190, 1970.

51. Bertram, J. S. and Craig, A. W. Specific induction of bladder cancer in mice by butyl-nitrosamine and effects of hormonal modifications on the sex difference in response. Eur. J. Cancer, *8*: 587–593, 1972.

52. Old, L. J., Boyse, E. A., Clarke, D. A., and Carswell, E. A. Antigenic properties of chemically induced tumours. Ann. N.Y. Acad. Sci., *101*: 80–106, 1962.

53. Washburn, T. C., Medearis, D. N., and Childs, B. Sex differences in susceptibility to infections. Paediatrics, *35*: 57–64, 1965.

54. Galton, M. Factors involved in the rejection of skin transplanted across a weak histo-incompatibility barrier: Gene dosage, sex of recipient and nature of expression of histo-incompatibility genes. Transplantation, *5*: 154–168, 1967.

55. Castro, J. E. Orchidectomy and the immune response. III. The effect of orchidectomy on tumour induction and transplantation in mice. Proc. Roy. Soc., Ser. B, *186*: 387–397, 1974.

56. Murphy, J. B. Effect of adrenal cortical and pituitary adrenocorticotrophic hormones on transplanted leukaemia of rats. Science, *99*: 303–307, 1944.

57. Murphy, J. B. and Sturm, E. Adrenals and susceptibility to transplanted leukaemia of rats. Science, *98*: 568–570, 1943.

58. McEndy, D. P., Boon, M. C., and Furth, J. On the role of the thymus, spleen and gonads in the development of leukaemia in high leukaemia stock mice. Cancer Res., *4*: 377–383, 1944.

59. Blamey, R. W. Experiments in tumour immunology. Brit. J. Surg., *55*: 769–771, 1968.

60. Curtis, J. E. Adoptive immunotherapy in the treatment of advanced malignant melanoma. Proc. Am. Assoc. Cancer Res., *12*: 52, 1971.

61. Buckley, R. and Rowlands, D. T. Proceedings of Symposium on Tissue Typing and Organ Transplantion, Minneapolis, Minn., May, 1970.

62. Lawrence, H. S. Immunotherapy with transfer factor. New Engl. J. Med., *287*: 1092–1095, 1972.

63. Brandes, L. J., Galton, D. A. G., and Wiltshaw, E. New approach to immunotherapy of melanoma. Lancet, *II*: 293–295, 1971.

64. Chihara, G. The nature of immunopotentiation by the antitumour polysaccharide lentinan and significance of serotonin, histamine and catecholamines in its action. *In;* G. E. W. Wolstenholme and J. Knight (eds.), Immunopotentiation (Ciba Foundation Symposium), vol. 18, pp. 259–282, Elsevier / Excerpta Medica / North Holland, Amsterdam / London / New York, 1973.

65. Prager, M. D., Derr, I., Swann, A., and Cotropia, J. Immunisation with chemically modified cancer cells. Proc. Am. Assoc. Cancer Res., *12*: 2, 1971.

66. Bekesi, G., Arneault, G. St., and Holland, J. F. Increased immunogenicity of leukaemic L. 1210 cells after vibrio cholerae neuraminidase. Proc. Am. Assoc. Cancer Res., *12*: 47, 1971.

67. Sanderson, C. J. and Frost, P. The induction of tumour immunity in mice using glutaraldehyde-treated tumour cells. Nature, *248*: 690–691, 1974.

68. Lindenmann, J. and Klein, P. A. *In;* Immunological Aspects of Viral Oncogenesis. Springer, New York, 1967.

69. Lindenmann, J. The use of viruses as immunological potentiators. *In;* G. E. W. Wolstenholme and J. Knight (eds.), Immunopotentiation (Ciba Foundation Symposium), vol. 18, pp. 197–210, Elsevier / Excerpta Medica / North Holland, Amsterdam / London / New York, 1973.

70. Lindenmann, J. Viral oncolysis with host survival. Proc. Soc. Exp. Biol. Med., *113*: 85–91, 1963.

71. Sanford, B. H. An alteration in tumour histocompatibility induced by Neuraminidase. Transplantation, *5*: 1273–1279, 1967.

72. Loor, F. Comparative immunogenicities of Tobacco Mosaic virus, protein subunits and re-aggregated protein subunits. Virology, *33*: 215–219, 1967.

73. Prehn, R. T. and Lappe, M. A. An immunostimulation theory of tumour development. Transplant. Rev., *7*: 26–49, 1971.

74. Sheagren, J. N. and Monaco, A. P. Protective effect of antilymphocyte serum on mice infected with *Plasmodium berghei*. Science, *164*: 1423–1425, 1969.

75. Attia, M. A. M. and Weiss, D. W. Immunology of spontaneous mammary carcinomas in mice. V. Acquired tumor resistance and enhancement in strain A mice infected with mammary tumor virus. Cancer Res., *26*: 1787–1800, 1966.

76. Prehn, R. T. The immune reaction as a stimulator of tumour growth. Science, *176*: 170–171, 1972.

77. Jeejeebhoy, H. F. Stimulation of tumour growth by the immune response. Int. J. Cancer, *13*: 665–678, 1974.

78. Stonehill, E. H. and Benditch, A. Retrogenetic expression: The reappearance of embryonal antigens in cancer cells. Nature, *228*: 370–372, 1970.

79. Gold, P. and Freedman, S. O. Demonstration of tumour specific antigens in human colonic carcinomata by immunological tolerance and absorption techniques. J. Exp. Med., *121*: 439–459, 1964.

80. Baldwin, R. W., Glaves, D., and Pimm, M. V. Tumor-associated antigens as expressions of chemically induced neoplasia and their involvement in tumor-host interactions. *In;* B. Amos (ed.), Progress in Immunology, vol. 1, pp. 907–920, Academic Press, New York, 1971.

81. Castro, J. E., Lance, E. M., Medawar, P. B., Zanelli, J., and Hunt, R. Foetal antigens and cancer. Nature, *243*: 225–226, 1973.

82. Oettgen, H. F., Old, L. J., McLean, E. P., and Carswell, E. A. Delayed hypersensitivity and transplantation immunity elicited by soluble antigens of chemically induced tumours in inbred guinea pigs. Nature, *220*: 295–297, 1968.

83. Old, L. J. and Boyse, E. A. Antigens of tumors and leukaemias induced by viruses. Fed. Proc., *24*: 1009, 1965.

84. Castro, J. E., Hunt, R., Lance, E. M., and Medawar, P. B. Implications of the fetal antigen theory for fetal transplantation. Cancer Res., *34*: 2055–2060, 1974.

85. Coggin, J. H., Jr., Ambrose, K. R., Bellomy, B. B., and Anderson, N. Tumor immunity in hamsters immunized with fetal tissues. J. Immunol., *107*: 526–533, 1971.

86. Coggin, J. H. and Anderson, N. R. Cancer, differentiation and embryonic antigens: Some central problems. Cancer Res., *19*: 105, 1974.

87. Burnet, F. M. *In;* Cellular Immunology, Cambridge Univ. Press, London, 1969.

Discussion of Paper of Dr. Castro

Dr. Dresser: You noted that some of your cytotoxic antibodies might be active against foetal antigens. I wonder if those are appropriate targets for such a model. D. B. Thomas (Eur. J. Immunol., 4: 820, 1974) has proposed that foetal antigens are manifested in the adult during certain stages of the cell cycle and that the difference between normal adult and foetal or tumour-bearing individuals is that the latter are subject to much greater periods of cell cycling. The presence of such foetal antigens in tumour-bearing animals would not therefore be a consequence of a tumour-induced dedifferentiation or foetalization.

Dr. Castro: We have completed various experiments, published between 1971 and 1973, suggesting that an adult animal is capable of mounting a cell-mediated immune response against its own foetal tissues. We injected first trimester syngeneic tissues under the kidney capsules of normal mice as well as thymectomized and bone marrow-reconstituted mice. Growth of these tissues was superior in the immunologically deprived animals. It has been shown by Coggin that the age of foetal tissues which can be rejected by normal adults is critical. In mice this is between 10 1/2 and 11 days of gestation but the exact period varies between species.

Dr. S. Hayashi (National Cancer Center Research Institute, Tokyo):   Have you investigated the immunologic capacity of orchidectomized mice following androgen replacement, or the effects of anti-androgens on normal animals?

   Secondly, how do you rationalize the discrepancy between your first series of experiments, in which *Corynebacterium parvum* appears to suppress thymic activity accompanied by decreased tumourigenesis, with the latter series of results in which decreased activity of the thymus appeared in the face of increased tumour incidence.

Dr. Castro: All the tumours we examined were ostensibly non-endocrine dependent. In skin graft studies, androgen therapy abrogated the effect of orchidectomy, while in large doses androgen appears to be immunosuppressive to normal mice, producing thymic atrophy. We were unable to detect any effect of Cyproterone acetate, an anti-androgen, on skin graft survival. However, we did not employ a wide dosage range and have not looked at possible disturbances of other parameters of immunologic function.

Dr. S. Hayashi: Do you believe that the effects you observed following orchidectomy are based solely on androgen depletion?

DR. CASTRO: Yes. With regard to your second point, in our first model using *C. parvum* we produced thymic atrophy and protection against neoplasia, while in the second situation involving orchidectomy there was thymus enlargement and an increase in the total number of θ-positive cells. This also was accompanied by a decrease of tumourigenesis. This paradox was a basic part of our paper and suggests several antitumour mechanisms may be effective. It is possible that orchidectomy has a greater effect on solid tumours, while *C. parvum* acts mainly on dissociated tumour cells.

DR. H. MITSUI (National Cancer Center Research Institute, Tokyo):   In a system employing the Donryu rat and Sato lung carcinoma, we recorded results similar to yours based on the combined therapy of killed *Corynebacterium* and surgical excision. We achieved both a significant reduction in metastases and prolongation of survival. Were survival rates affected in your experiments?

DR. CASTRO: Our experiments are still in progress but to date about one-third of our tumour-bearing animals have survived for 100 days completely tumour-free following *C. parvum* therapy plus surgery.

DR. H. OKADA: There are at least two possible explanations for the suppression of lung metastases which you secured upon *Corynebacterium* administration. One involves a decrease in the incidence of metastasis from the original tumour mass, and the other offers an effect of *C. parvum* on already disseminated tumour cells, perhaps related to some alteration in the host's immunologic capacity produced by a sudden decrease in the level of antigenic stimulation upon resection of the primary tumour. If this second possibility is operative, the interval between tumour resection and the administration of *C. parvum* might be critical. What do you think is the mechanism of action of *C. parvum* in your system?

DR. CASTRO: *C. parvum* does not have the capacity to prevent liberation of cells from a primary subcutaneous tumour, as circulating tumour cells are always detectable in treated or non-treated animals. It apparently is able to stimulate mechanisms that "mop up" circulating cells, as well as effect non-vascularized metastatic deposits. I do not think it produces much effect on an established tumour. It may delay the rate of growth of metastases but does not affect established metastases. In combination with surgery, the fact that protection is observed with *C. parvum* administered 6, 7, or 8 days following surgery but less so on days 9 or 10 is probably because *C. parvum* requires a certain period to stimulate the mechanisms that exert an effect against tumour. There is an apparent correlation between the anti-tumour capacity of *C. parvum* and an increase in spleen size which take 5 or 6 days to reach a maximum.

DR. HOBBS: You've demonstrated an immunologic effect of orchidectomy, but I don't believe you've satisfactorily excluded a concomitant hormone-dependent effect. A group in Australia has shown that both dimethylbenzanthracene and methylcholanthrene (MCA) act as carcinogens by replacing steroid receptors in their interaction with DNA, thereby frequently giving rise to hormone-dependent tumours.

DR. CASTRO: Our MCA-induced tumour is a sarcoma, such tumours not usually being considered hormone-dependent, and can be propagated in tissue culture without the addition of hormones. It does grow slightly better in male than female mice, but this may be a reflection of the fact that females are more immunologically competent than males. In our tumour transplantation system, anti-lymphocyte serum and thymectomy abrogate, the anti-tumour effect of orchidectomy, again suggesting that it has primarily an immunologic effect on tumour growth.

DR. HOBBS: Have you combined *C. parvum* administration with orchidectomy?

DR. CASTRO: Not as yet. We would also like to test the effects of lentinan together with *C. parvum* in our systems.

DR. FACHET: You noted a significant decrease in thymus weight following *C. parvum* injection. Do you believe this was a direct effect of *Corynebacterium* on the thymus, or was it perhaps mediated through activation of the adrenocortical system. We have demonstrated that zymosan and various types of endotoxin can activate this system and thereby suppress the thymus.

DR. CASTRO: We have administered *C. parvum* to adrenalectomized mice but unfortunately the animals were exquisitely susceptible to the *C. parvum* and died.

HOST DEFENSE AGAINST CANCER AND ITS POTENTIATION, D. MIZUNO ET AL. (EDS.),
UNIV. OF TOKYO PRESS, TOKYO / UNIV. PARK PRESS, BALTIMORE, PP. 181–197, 1975

Antitumour Polysaccharides and Host Defence against Cancer

Yukiko Y. Maeda, Kazuko Ishimura, Nobuo Takasuka,
Takuma Sasaki, and Goro Chihara

National Cancer Center Research Institute, Tokyo, Japan

Abstract: Antitumour effect of numerous basidiomycetes belonging to Polyporaceae family and Tricholomataceae family was examined and a polysaccharide,
lentinan, was isolated from one of the edible mushrooms, *Lentinus edodes*. Lentinan
was found to almost completely regress solid-type tumour of sarcoma-180 in mice.
Higher structure or the micelle structure of the polysaccharide seemed important
for the correlation between the polysaccharide structure and its antitumour activity.

The action of lentinan and other antitumour polysaccharides is not a direct
cytotoxicity against tumour cells and there exists a characteristic optimal dose in
their antitumour effect, and there is a marked difference in their antitumour effect
according to mouse strains. Antitumour activity of polysaccharides is highly inhibited by thyroxine or hydrocortisone.

Lentinan and other polysaccharides do not show any antitumour activity in
neonatally thymectomized mice, and the thymus or thymus-derived lymphocytes
(T-cells) are taking part in this activity. These polysaccharides do not stimulate
the conventional immune responses, including the reticuloendothelial system. Lentinan may therefore be termed as a T-cell adjuvant with characteristics markedly
different from the action of BCG, *Corynebacterium parvum*, endotoxin, and many
other immunopotentiators.

In an early period after the administration of antitumour polysaccharides,
there is a marked increase in three kinds of serum proteins, and such a phenomenon
cannot be observed in polysaccharides not possessing an antitumour activity and in
the strains of mice which do not react to the antitumour activity of polysaccharides.
These proteins may be a new factor in the action mechanism of lentinan as a T-
helper cell stimulant or restorer. The fact that antitumour polysaccharides show
other interesting characteristics, such as the increase in histamine or serotonin sensitivity of mice and anticomplimentary activity, and these points should be noted in
considering the host's defence against cancer and its potentiation.

Action mechanism of numerous immunopotentiators is extremely varied, and
the most effective application range of lentinan and the possibility of their co-opera-

tion with other kinds of immunopotentiators or immunopotentiating methods will be discussed from this point.

There are some evidences that suggest that the host is resistant to cancer. There is also an experimental evidence that indicates that the host excites a cell-mediated immune reaction even against an autochthonous tumour (1, 2). It seems that elucidation of such intrinsic defence mechanism of an animal body against cancer and to find a biologically active substance that promotes this mechanism would be one of important means for breaking the difficulty now confronting cancer chemotherapy and for opening a new way for cancerostasis.

In the present paper, some new observations gained in our laboratory in recent years, and our studies on the antitumour polysaccharides and host defence against cancer will be reviewed.

Antitumour Activity of Basidiomycetes Polysaccharides

1. Basidiomycetes extracts

There is a strong tradition in Japan from olden times that basidiomycetes belonging to the Polyporaceae family is effective against cancer. We have re-examined a large number of these folk remedies and found that the hot water extracts of *Ganoderma applanatum* (PERS.) PAT., *Coriolus versicolor* (FR.) QUÉL., and numerous

TABLE 1. Antitumour Activity of the Extract from Various Basidiomycetes against Sarcoma-180

Basidiomycetes	Dose (mg/kg × days)	Average tumour weight (g)	Tumour inhibition ratio (%)	Complete regression
Polyporaceae				
Coriolus versicolor (FR.) QUÉL.	200×10	1.5	77.5	4/8
Control		6.4		0/7
Coriolus hirsutus (FR.) QUÉL.	200×10	4.0	65.0	2/10
Control		11.5		0/9
Lenzites betulina FR.	200×10	10.6	23.9	0/8
Control		13.9		0/8
Ganoderma applanatum (PERS.) PAT.	200×10	2.4	64.9	5/10
Control		6.9		0/10
Phellinus linteus (BERK. et CURT)	200×10	0.2	96.7	7/7
Control		6.8		0/8
Tricholomataceae: edible mushroom				
Lentinus edodes (BERK.) SING.	200×10	2.2	80.7	6/10
Flammulina velutipes (CURT ex FR.)	200×10	2.1	81.1	3/10
Control		11.4		0/10
Agaricaceae: edible mushroom				
Agaricus bisporus (LANGE) SING.	200×10	9.3	12.7	0/10
Control		10.6		0/10

Sarcoma-180 (8×10^6 cells) were inoculated subcutaneously in Swiss albino mice. Hot water extract of the basidiomycetes was injected intraperitoneally daily from one day after the inoculation. Tumour inhibition ratios were determined at 5 weeks after tumour transplantation.

other basidiomycetes, and the edible mushroom, *Lentinus edodes* (BERK.) SING., strongly suppressed the growth of sarcoma-180 solid tumour transplanted subcutaneously in Swiss albino mice *(3–5)* (Table 1). These extracts were entirely ineffective against the ascites form of sarcoma-180.

2. *Lentinan*

Six kinds of polysaccharide were isolated from *L. edodes*, the most popular edible mushroom grown in Japan, by the scheme shown in Fig. 1, and the effective principle that had the strongest antitumour activity was named lentinan *(6, 7)*. This substance was able to almost completely regress sarcoma-180 transplanted subcutaneously in Swiss or ICR mice, in a minute quantity.

Chemical structure of lentinan has not been completely elucidated yet but it is a β-1,3-glucan having several β-1,6-glucopyranoside branching, with a molec-

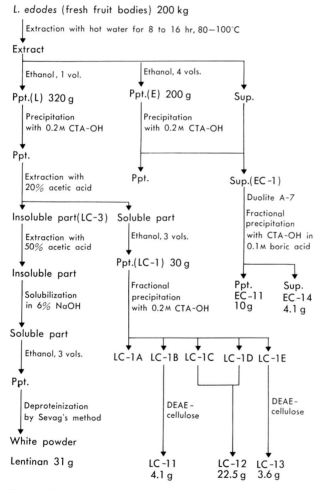

FIG. 1.   Extraction of polysaccharides from *L. edodes* and fractionation of water-soluble extract into 6 polysaccharide preparations, lentinan, LC-11, LC-12, LC-13, EC-11, and EC-14. CTA-OH: cetyltrimethylammonium hydroxide.

ular weight of about one million. It does not contain nitrogen, phosphorus, and sulphur.

3.   Other antitumour polysaccharides and structure activity relationship

We have also found many polysaccharides with antitumour activity besides lentinan, including carboxymethylpachymaran, chemically derived from pachyman, a polysaccharide of the Chinese crude drug, Hoelen (*Poria cocos* (SCHW. ex FR.) WOLF) (*8–10*). Table 2 lists the relationship between primary structure and antitumour activity of some polysaccharides, including the effect of lichen polysaccharide found by Shibata and others (*11*).

It will be seen from this table that even in polysaccharides with the main chain of β-1,3-glucopyranoside linkage, there are some that have antitumour activity like lentinan and those without an antitumour activity, like pachyman, while in the polysaccharides with β-1,6-glucan, pusturan (GE-3) (*11*) has an antitumour activity. These facts suggest that a higher structure or micelle formation of the polysaccharide is an important factor in the correlation between the structure and activity in the antitumour polysaccharides. This is strongly suggested by the fact that pachyman, the polysaccharide without antitumour activity, can be derived to U-pachyman with a strong antitumour activity simply by treatment with urea, without any conversion in its primary structure (*7*). It may be possible to surmise that there is some substance, either humoral or cellular, in the living organism that interacts directly with the antitumour polysaccharide, besides the fact that antitumour polysaccharides produce changes in the α-helix content of the proteins (*10*).

TABLE 2.   The Primary Structure and Antitumour Activity of the Polysaccharides

Polysaccharides	Primary structure	Antitumour activity against S-180			
		Dose (mg/kg × days)	Inhibition ratio (%)	Complete regression	Reference
Lentinan	β-(1, 6)(1, 3)-glucan[a]	1×10	100	10/10	*6*
Pachyman	β-(1, 6)(1, 3)-glucan	5×10	0	0/8	*8*
U-pachyman	β-(1, 6)(1, 3)-glucan	5×10	91.4	5/10	*7*
Hydroxyethylpachyman	β-(1, 6)(1, 3)-glucan	5×10	100	9/10	*10*
Screloglucan	β-(1, 6)(1, 3)-glucan	3×10	89.3	6/10	*42*
Debranched lentinan	β-(1, 3)-glucan	2×5	90.0	3/5	—[b]
Laminaran	β-(1, 3)-glucan	25×10	1.5	0/10	—[b]
Pachymaran	β-(1, 3)-glucan	5×10	88.0	2/6	*8*
Pusturan (GE-3)[c]	β-(1, 6)-glucan	200×10	99.1	8/10	*11*
LC-12[d]	α-(1, 6)-glucan	5×10	-17.6	0/10	*6*
Dextran	α-(1, 6)-glucan	10×10	-21.2	0/10	*38*
CM-cellulose[e]	β-(1, 4)-glucan	10×10	4.5	0/10	*38*
AR[f]	β-(1, 2)-glucan	5×10	0	0/7	—[b]
EC-11[d]	Mannofucogalactan	50×10	-1.6	0/10	*6*

[a] Main structure is underlined.   [b] Our unpublished data.   [c] Lichen polysaccharide.   [d] A polysaccharide from *L. edodes*.   [e] CM-cellulose : carboxymethylcellulose.   [f] A polysaccharide from *Agronobacterium radiogenesis*.

Characteristics of the Antitumour Activity of Lentinan and Other Polysaccharides

1. No direct cytotoxicity against tumour cells

The characteristic of the antitumour activity of lentinan and many other polysaccharides is that they do not show any direct cytotoxicity against tumour cells. The viability of sarcoma-180 ascites cells cultured for 24 hr in the medium containing a high concentration of lentinan or carboxymethylpachymaran is no different from that of the same cells cultured in a medium not containing the polysaccharide (*12*) (Table 3). This is a direct evidence that the antitumour action of polysaccharides is host-mediated.

TABLE 3. The Viability of Sarcoma-180 Cells in a Culture Medium Containing Lentinan, Carboxymethylpachymaran, or Mitomycin C

Samples	Dose (mg/5 ml medium)	Number of Petri dishes	Average viability of tumour cells (%)
Lentinan	0.1	3	96.0
Lentinan	0.5	3	97.5
Control		3	98.0
Lentinan	1	3	94.5
Lentinan	5	3	95.3
Control		3	96.4
Carboxymethylpachymaran	5	3	92.0
Carboxymethylpachymaran	25	3	91.7
Control		3	96.4
Mitomycin C	0.15	3	0.9
Control		3	98.0

TABLE 4. The Antitumour Activity and Optimal Dose of Lentinan against Sarcoma-180 in ICR or SWM/Ms Mice

Mice	Dose (mg/kg × days)	Body weight change (g)	Average tumour weight (g)	Tumour inhibition ratio (%)	Complete regression
ICR-JCL	1 × 10	+4.5	0	100	10/10
	2 × 10	+4.3	0.0	100	9/10
	Control	+7.7	11.6		0/10
ICR-JCL	25 × 10	+3.0	3.0	66.2	0/8
	Control	+3.0	8.8		0/8
ICR-JCL	80 × 5	+1.1	6.6	−8.5	0/7
	Control	+4.1	6.1		0/7
SWM/Ms	1 × 10	+4.8	0	100	7/7
	Control	+1.7	9.5		0/10
SWM/Ms	0.1 × 10	+4.6	8.9	19.1	0/9
	0.5 × 10	+1.9	0.6	94.7	8/10
	5 × 10	+5.0	6.2	44.0	0/9
	Control	+4.5	11.0		0/10

2. Presence of optimal dose in antitumour action

In the antitumour action of polysaccharides, there is an interesting phenomenon of an optimal dose, differing from the action of cytotoxic agents in general. As shown in Table 4, lentinan can completely regress sarcoma-180 transplanted in ICR mice in a dose of 1–2 mg/kg for 10 days but in a larger dose of 80 mg/kg for 5 days, lentinan no longer shows any antitumour activity and the tumour grows as in control mice.

3. Difference in antitumour activity according to mouse strains

Lentinan shows a strong antitumour activity against sarcoma-180 transplanted in Swiss or ICR mice but is entirely ineffective against the same tumour transplanted in C3H/f mice, as shown in Table 5. Further, lentinan is effective in BALB/c (13) and A mice but ineffective in CBA (13) mice.

It has been reported that the reason for this strain difference may be the genotype of the host animal, and the polysaccharides are effective in mice lacking the histocompatibility antigen, H-2^d (14). However, our experimental result seems to indicate that the absence of H-2^d has no relation to it. For example, BALB/c mice have H-2^d locus but lentinan is effective in them while C3H/f mice have H-2^k but lentinan is ineffective. Therefore, it seems necessary to examine the reason for the difference in antitumour activity of lentinan according to mouse strains from a wider point of view.

TABLE 5.   Lacking of the Antitumour Effect of Lentinan against Sarcoma-180 in C3H/f (H-2^k) Mice

Dose of lentinan (mg/kg × days)	Average tumour weight (g)	Tumour inhibition ratio (%)	Complete regression
4×5	7.16	−16.4	0/7
20×5	7.02	−14.1	0/8
80×5	6.75	−9.7	0/6
Control	6.15		0/6

Lentinan also fails to the effect in CBA (H-2^k) mice, but not in BALB/c (H-2^d), SWM/Ms, or ICR mice.

4. Inhibition of antitumour activity of lentinan by thyroxine or hydrocortisone

As by zymosan (15), antitumour activity of lentinan is slightly inhibited by hydrocortisone acetate (16). Action of cortisol is synergetic with the action of anti-lymphocyte serum, and the hormone is known to specifically attach the thymus-derived lymphocytes (T cells) (17, 18). Therefore, it is natural that the antitumour action of lentinan is inhibited by hydrocortisone acetate.

What is most interesting is that the antitumour activity of lentinan is strongly inhibited by thyroxine (Table 6), the activity lowering from 96 to 22% by the administration of thyroxine. Since thyroxine tends to enhance the growth of a tumour, there remains a possibility that this inhibition may be the result of antagonism between the actions of lentinan and thyroxine. In any case, it is interesting that thyroid gland takes part in tumour growth. There is a report that cancer incidence is high in myxoedema patients and low in hyperthyroidemia (19), so that the role

TABLE 6. The Effect of L-Thyroxine or Hydrocortisone on the Antitumour Activity of Lentinan

Samples	Dose	Tumour inhibition ratio (%)	Complete regression
Lentinan	1 mg/kg × 10	96.6	8/9
Lentinan Thyroxine	1 mg/kg × 10 10 µg/kg × 25	53.0	0/6
Lentinan Thyroxine	1 mg/kg × 10 100 µg/kg × 25	22.4	0/6
Thyroxine Thyroxine	10 µg/kg × 25 100 µg/kg × 25	2.5 −77.9	0/6 0/6
Lentinan Hydrocortisone acetate	1 mg/kg × 10 50 mg/kg × 10	73.0	1/10
Hydrocortisone acetate	50 mg/kg × 10	42.2	0/10

of the thyroid gland in tumour invasion is an important problem to be considered in future studies on the host's defence against cancer and its potentiation.

Immunological and Biological Properties of Lentinan and Other Antitumour Polysaccharides

Lentinan and other antitumour polysaccharides have interesting characteristics differing from those of known immunopotentiators, such as BCG (*20, 21*), *Corynebacterium parvum* (*22*), endotoxin (*23*), and dextran sulphate (*24*).

1. Lentinan and other antitumour polysaccharides as T-cell adjuvant

The antitumour action of lentinan, carboxymethylpachymaran, or zymosan does not appear in neonatally thymectomized mice (*12, 25*), and is markedly decreased by the administration of anti-lymphocyte serum (*26*) (Table 7).

TABLE 7. Antitumour Activity of Lentinan, Carboxymethylpachymaran and Zymosan on Sarcoma-180 in Normal and Neonatally Thymectomized Mice

Mice	Samples	Dose (mg/kg × days)	Average weight of tumour (g)	Tumour inhibition ratio (%)	Complete regression
Normal mice	Lentinan	1 × 10	0.1	99.2	9/10
Normal mice	Control		10.3		0/10
TX mice[a]	Lentinan	1 × 10	7.3	6.6	0/5
TX mice	Control		7.8		0/5
Normal mice	CM-pachymaran[b]	25 × 10	0.1	99.0	9/10
Normal mice	Control		9.1		0/7
TX mice	CM-pachymaran	25 × 10	8.7	6.6	0/5
TX mice	Control		9.3		0/6
Normal mice	Zymosan	5 × 10	1.8	83.9	5/10
Normal mice	Control		10.9		0/10
TX mice	Zymosan	5 × 10	10.7	−4.0	0/4
TX mice	Control		10.2		0/5

[a] TX mice: neonatally thymectomized SWM/Ms mice.　[b] CM-pachymaran: carboxymethylpachymaran.

This fact indicates that the thymus or T cells are taking an important part in the mechanism of tumour regression by lentinan or zymosan, and that this action mechanism differs markedly from that of *C. parvum* or BCG whose antitumour activity does not change in athymic mice (*27,28*).

In recent years, many researchers have examined the nature of lentinan as an immunopotentiator, such as Dresser and Phillips (*29, 30*), Kitagawa and others (*31*), and Dennert and Tucker (*32*), and it has been revealed that the characteristic of lentinan as an immunopotentiator is that it is a T-oriented adjuvant or a T-helper cell restorer or stimulant. In other words, lentinan may be termed a best immuno-potentiator in humoral immune responses against T-dependent antigen. Such a characteristic of lentinan should be taken into consideration in the future development of studies on preclinical trial, combined use with other immunopotentiators, and combination with radiotherapy.

2.   *No stimulation of reticuloendothelial system and conventional immune responses by antitumour polysaccharides*

Lentinan and other antitumour polysaccharides do not stimulate conventional immune responses such as the increase in peripheral lymphocytes and phagocytic activity. Table 8 indicates that lentinan and carboxymethylpachymaran do not increase the phagocytic index at all when examined by the carbon clearance test (*33*). These polysaccharides also do not stimulate the reticuloendothelial system, differing from BCG (*34*), *C. parvum* (*35*), or zymosan (*36*).

Lentinan and carboxymethylpachymaran have no action of increasing the number of circulating leucocytes (Table 9), so that their biological activity is different from those of dextran sulphate or heparin (*24*).

TABLE 8.   No Effect of Lentinan or Carboxymethylpachymaran on the Carbon Clearance Activity and Spleen Weight

Samples	Dose (mg/kg × days)	Average spleen weight (% body weight)	Average phagocytic index (K)
Lentinan	1 × 10	0.53%	0.0243±0.0019
Lentinan	10 × 1	0.78	0.0289±0.0065
CM-pachymaran	25 × 10	0.56	0.0258±0.0052
Control		0.55	0.0213±0.0019

TABLE 9.   The Effect of Lentinan or Carboxymethylpachymaran on the Numbers of Circulating Leukocyte in Mice

Samples	Dose (mg/kg × days)	Average numbers of total leukocytes (cells/mm³)			
		Day[a] 1	2	3	4
Lentinan	10 × 1	7,000	6,600	7,700	7,700
Lentinan	1 × 10	7,100	9,100	8,700	7,800
CM-pachymaran	25 × 10	7,200	9,300	7,100	8,900
Control		7,200	9,700	8,800	7,600

[a] Days after the last injection of polysaccharides.   Twelve mice are divided into 4 groups of 3 mice each.

3. Antitumour polysaccharides and unique increase of serum protein components

It has been shown in the foregoing that lentinan is an interesting immuno-potentiator with a unique characteristic, but it is still entirely obscure with what kind of a substance (molecule) or cell the antitumour polysaccharides affect *in vivo* in the initial step before any immunological or biological reaction is produced. However, there are still some suggestive evidences that there is a substance in the animal body that interacts directly with the polysaccharide immediately at the early period after its administration (*37*), such as the presence of an optimal dose in the antitumour activity of polysaccharides and importance of higher or micelle structure of polysaccharides in the structure-activity relationship.

In connection with this problem, we have found that there is a marked increase in three kinds of serum protein components by the administration of anti-tumour polysaccharides, with a peak 4 to 7 days later (*38*). Figure 2 shows the pattern of serum protein components separated by gradient acrylamide gel PAA 4/30 (Pharmacia Fine Chemicals, Uppsala) from the serum of ICR mice 4 days after the administration of 4 mg/kg of lentinan for 5 days. Compared to the pattern of serum obtained from control mice, dramatic increase in three kinds of protein components, LA, LB, and LC, are observed. The use of this method allows separation of serum protein components into more than 21 and their assignment has not been established to date. With reference to the results of polyacrylamide gel electrophoresis of other serum proteins reported to date (*39*), LA is considered to be β-globulin, and LB and LC must be one of α-globulins. Pillemer and others (*40, 41*) reported that pro-

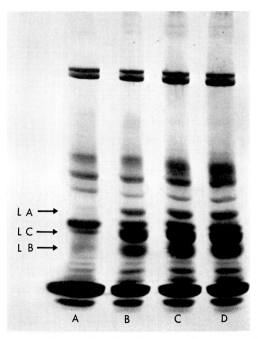

Fig. 2.   The acrylamide gel pattern of serum samples from lentinan-treated ICR mice. A, contol (4th day after saline injection); B, 4th day after the last injection of lentinan, C, serum B after the adsorption by lentinan; D, serum B after the adsorption by zymosan.

TABLE 10. The Correlation between the Serum Protein Components, LA, LB, and LC, and the Antitumour Activity of Polysaccharides

Polysaccharides	Dose (mg/kg × 5 days)	Increase of serum proteins						Tumour inhibition ratio (%)
		LA	Date[a] of peak	LB	Date of peak	LC	Date of peak	
Lentinan	4	₩	4	₩	4	₩	4	98.0
Pachymaran	10	₩	7	₩	7	₩	7	95.3
CM-pachymaran	75	₩	7	₩	7	₩	10	98.4
Zymosan	20	₩	7	₩	7	₩	7	91.5
Control (saline)	0.1 (ml)	—	—	—	—	—	—	—
Pachyman	10	+	1	₩	1	₩	1	−7.0
Laminarin	10	—	—	—	—	—	—	−7.0
Starch	10	—	—	—	—	—	—	NE[b]
Dextran	10	—	—	—	—	—	—	−21.2
Cellulose	10	—	—	—	—	—	—	10.1

The mice were ICR female mice.   [a] Date of peak was counted after the last injection of polysaccharides.   [b] NE: not effective.

perdin, one of β-globulins, in the serum increases after the injection of zymosan, and that this protein is adsorbed by zymosan. The serum proteins isolated as above are not adsorbed on incubation with lentinan or zymosan by Pillemer's method, as shown in Fig. 2, and appear in far larger amounts than properdin, indicating that these protein components are not properdin.

There is a clear parallelism between the antitumour activity of polysaccharides and the unique increase in these serum protein components (Table 10). Although there is a marked increase in serum proteins LA, LB, and LC after the administration of antitumour polysaccharides like lentinan, such a phenomenon is entirely absent by the administration of polysaccharides lacking in antitumour activity. Lentinan has an optimal dose for its antitumour activity to appear and the activity does not appear at all when a large dose of 80 mg/kg is used. In the later case, there is no increase in the serum protein components.

As was stated earlier, antitumour activity of polysaccharides differs markedly according to mouse strains and, when lentinan is administered to C3H/f mice, in which lentinan is completely ineffective, there is slight increase in serum protein components compared with Swiss or ICR mice (Fig. 3).

It is clear from above facts that there is a very close relation shipbetween the unique increase of these three kinds of serum protein components in the early period after the administration of the polysaccharide and the antitumour activity of these polysaccharides. The function and role of these serum proteins are obscure at present but they may be one of new factor that take some part in a series of mode of action of lentinan which potentiates humoral immune responses as a T-cell adjuvant. On the other hand, antitumour polysaccharides have various interesting biological activities such as the anticomplementary activity (42), generation of anaphylatoxin (42), and increased sensitivity of mice to histamine or serotonin (7, 43) which is also observed in C. parvum (44). In the mode of these actions, participation of various biogeneic amines such as epinephrine, histamine, and 5-hydroxytryptamine, and the

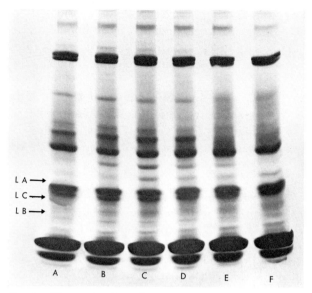

LA →
LC →
LB →

A   B   C   D   E   F

FIG. 3.   The acrylamide gel pattern of serum samples from lentinan-treated C3H/f mice. A, contol (4th day after saline injection); B, 1st day; C, 4th day; D, 7th day; E, 10th day; F, 14th day after the last injection of lentinan.

participation of the functions of the adrenal gland and hypothalamus may also be considered in the mechanism of host's defence against cancer. The increase of serum proteins by the polysaccharide may also be considered as one of the phenomena that appears in connection with the above facts.

CONCLUSION

As has been iterated above, many researchers have confirmed that lentinan and other polysaccharides have many interesting and varied immunological and biological properties, including the fact that the application of their antitumour activity is relatively narrow but that they are a powerful T-oriented adjuvant. These facts will prove them to be a powerful and useful tool in the immunological studies of cancer.

On the other hand, we must always consider the potentiation of host's defence against human autologous cancer. It has been revealed recently that a cytotoxic antibody plays an important role in the host-tumour relationship in some tumours such as melanoma (45, 46). It may, therefore, be of value to consider the characteristic of antitumour polysaccharides as a restorer or a stimulant of humoral immune response against T-dependent antigen. It seems possible that such properties of polysaccharide, PS-K are taking part in the increased reaction of the host to tumours when the antigen has been modified by X-irradiation (47). Lentinan is known to have the ability to restore the host's immune response which had been suppressed by cyclophosphamide (48).

It is now known that the nature of immunopotentiators and immunopotentiating methods are extremely numerous and varied, such as T-oriented or B-oriented immunopotentiation (*29, 31*), macrophage-mediated immunopotentiation (*49, 50*), hormone-mediated immunopotentiation (*51*), *etc.* It seems possible that their action mechanisms are interwoven in a complex manner or cooperate closely to display the appropriate mechanism in correspondence to the varied mode of the host-tumour relationship, thereby potentiating the activity of host's resistant against cancer (*16*). Possibility of the co-operative action of these various immunopotentiators and immunopotentiation methods from such an angle, and development of a new anticancer substances along such a line seem to be required in future.

REFERENCES

1. Foley, E. J. Antigenic properties of methylcholanthrene induced tumors in mice of the strain of origin. Cancer Res., *13*: 835–873, 1953.
2. Klein, G., Sjögren, H. O., Klein, E., and Hellström, K. E. Demonstration of resistance against methylcholanthrene-induced sarcomas in the primary autochthonous host. Cancer Res., *20*: 1561–1572, 1960.
3. Ikekawa, T., Nakanishi, M., Uehara, N., Chihara, G., and Fukuoka, F. Antitumor action of some basidiomycetes, especially *Phellinus linteus*. Gann, *59*: 155–157, 1968.
4. Chihara, G., Maeda, Y. Y., Hamuro, J., Sasaki, T., and Fukuoka, F. Inhibition of mouse sarcoma-180 by polysaccharides from *Lentinus edodes* (BERK.) SING. Nature, *222*: 687–688, 1969.
5. Ikekawa, T., Uehara, N., Maeda, Y. Y., Nakanishi, M., and Fukuoka, F. Antitumor activity of aqueous extracts of edible mushrooms. Cancer Res., *29*: 734–735, 1969.
6. Chihara, G., Hamuro, J., Maeda, Y. Y., Arai, Y., and Fukuoka, F. Fractionation and purification of the polysaccharides with marked antitumor activity, especially lentinan, from *Lentinus edodes* (BERK.) SING. (an edible mushroom). Cancer Res., *30*: 2776–2781, 1970.
7. Maeda, Y. Y., Hamuro, J., Yamada, Y. O., Ishimura, K., and Chihara, G. The nature of immunopotentiation by the anti-tumour polysaccharide lentinan and the significance of biogeneic amines in its action. *In;* G. E. W. Wolstenholme and J. Knight (eds.), Immunopotentiation (Ciba Foundation Symposium), vol. 18, pp. 259–286, Elsevier / Excerpta Medica / North Holland, Amsterdam / London / New York, 1973.
8. Chihara, G., Hamuro, J., Maeda, Y. Y., Arai, Y., and Fukuoka, F. Antitumour polysaccharide derived chemically from natural glucan (pachyman). Nature, *225*: 943–944, 1970.
9. Hamuro, J., Yamashita, Y., Ohsaka, Y., Maeda, Y. Y., and Chihara, G. Carboxymethylpachymaran, a new water soluble polysaccharide with marked antitumour activity. Nature, *233*: 486–487, 1971.
10. Hamuro, J. and Chihara, G. Effect of antitumour polysaccharides on the higher structure of serum protein. Nature, *245*: 40–41, 1973.
11. Fukuoka, F., Nakanishi, M., Shibata, S., Nishikawa, Y., Takeda, T., and Tanaka, M. Antitumor activities on sarcoma-180 of the polysaccharide preparations from *Gyrophora esculenta* Miyoshi, *Cetraria islandica* (L.) Ach. *var. orientalis* Asahina, and some other lichens. Gann, *59*: 421–432, 1968.
12. Maeda, Y. Y. and Chihara, G. The effects of neonatal thymectomy on the antitumour

activity of lentinan, carboxymethylpachymaran and zymosan, and their effects on various immune responses. Int. J. Cancer, *11*: 153–161, 1973.

13. Davies, A. J. S. Discussion on site of action of adjuvants. *In;* G. E. W. Wolstenholme and J. Knight (eds.), Immunopotentiation (Ciba Foundation Symposium), vol. 18, pp. 335, Elsevier/Excerpta Medica/North Holland, Amsterdam/London/New York, 1973.

14. Tarnowski, G. S., Mountain, I. M., and Stock, C. C. Influence of genotype of host on regression of solid and ascitic forms of sarcoma 180 and effect of chemotherapy on the solid form. Cancer Res., *33*: 1885–1888, 1973.

15. Bradner, W. T. and Clarke, D. A. Stimulation of host defense against experimental cancer. II. Temporal and reversal studies of the zymosan effect. Cancer Res., *19*: 673–678, 1959.

16. Ishimura, K., Maeda, Y. Y., and Chihara, G. A possibility of synergism between *Corynebacterium parvum*, lentinan, and serotonin or thyroid hormones in potentiation of host resistance against cancer. *In;* B. Halpern (ed.), *Corynebacterium parvum* in Experimental and Clinical Oncology, pp. 300–315, Plenum Publishing, New York, 1975.

17. Gunn, A., Lance, E. M., Medawar, P. B., and Nehlsen, S. L. Synergism between cortisol and antilymphocyte serum. Part I. Observation in murine allograft systems. *In;* G. E. W. Wolstenholme and J. Knight (eds.), Hormones and the Immune Response (Ciba Foundation Study Group, No. 36), pp. 66–72, Churchill, London, 1970.

18. Lance, E. M. and Cooper, S. Synergism between cortisol and antilymphocyte serum. Part II. Effect of cortisol and antilymphocyte serum on lymphoid populations. *In;* G. E. W. Wolstenholme and J. Knight (eds.), Hormones and the Immune Response (Ciba Foundation Study Group, No. 36), pp. 73–99, Churchill, London, 1970.

19. Spencer, J. G. C. The influence of the thyroid in malignant disease. Brit. J. Cancer, *8*: 393–411, 1954.

20. Biozzi, G., Stiffel, C., Halpern, B. N., and Mouton, D. Effet de l'inoculation du *Bacille de Calmette-Guérin* sur le devéloppement de la tumeur ascitique d'Ehrlich chez la souris. C. R. Séances Soc. Biol., *153*: 987–989, 1959.

21. Old, L. J., Clarke, D. A., and Benacerraf, B. Effect of Bacillus Calmette-Guérin infection on transplanted tumours. Nature, *184*: 291–292, 1959.

22. Halpern, B. N., Biozzi, G., Stiffel, C., and Mouton, D. Inhibition of tumour growth by administration of killed *Corynebacterium parvum*. Nature, *212*: 853–854, 1966.

23. Benacerraf, B. and Sebestyen, M. M. Effect of bacterial endotoxins on the reticuloendothelial system. Fed. Proc., *16*: 860–867, 1957.

24. Sasaki, S. and Suchi, T. Mobilization of lymphocytes from lymph nodes and spleen by polysaccharide polysulphates. Nature, *216*: 1013–1014, 1967.

25. Maeda, Y. Y. and Chihara, G. Lentinan, a new immunoaccelerator of cell-mediated responses. Nature, *229*: 634, 1971.

26. Maeda, Y. Y., Hamuro, J., and Chihara, G. The mechanisms of action of antitumour polysaccharides. I. The effect of antilymphocyte serum on the antitumour activity of lentinan. Int. J. Cancer, *8*: 41–46, 1971.

27. Castro, J. E. Antitumour effects of *Corynebacterium parvum* in mice. Eur. J. Cancer, *10*: 121–127, 1974.

28. Pimm, M. V. and Baldwin, R. W. BCG immunotherapy of rat tumours in athymic nude mice. Nature, *254*: 77–78, 1975.

29. Dresser, D. W. and Phillips, J. M. The cellular targets for the action of adjuvants: T-adjuvants and B-adjuvants. *In;* G. E. W. Wolstenholme and J. Knight (eds.), Immunopotentiation (Ciba Foundation Symposium), vol. 18, pp. 3–28, Elsevier/ Excerpta Medica/North Holland, Amsterdam/London/New York, 1973.

30. Dresser, D. W. and Phillips, J. M. The orientation of the adjuvant activities of *Salmonella typhosa* lipopolysaccharide and lentinan. Immunology, *27*: 895–902, 1974.

31. Haba, S., Takatsu, K., Masaki, H., and Kitagawa, M. Immunosuppression by cancerous ascites and the restoration with antitumor agent. Proc. Japan. Cancer Assoc., *32*: 249, 1973.

32. Dennert, G. and Tucker, D. Antitumor polysaccharide lentinan—a T-cell adjuvant. J. Natl. Cancer Inst., *51*: 1727–1729, 1973.

33. Biozzi, G., Benacerraf, B., and Halpern, B. N. Quantitative study of the granulopectic activity of the reticuloendothelial system. II. A study of the kinetics of the granulopectic activity of the R. E. S. in relation to the dose of carbon injected. Relationship between the weight of the organs and their activity. Brit. J. Exp. Pathol., *34*: 441–457, 1953.

34. Halpern, B. N., Biozzi, G., Stiffel, C., and Mouton, D. Effet de la stimulation du systéme réticulo-endothélial par l'inoculation du bacille de Calmette-Guérin sur le développement de l'épithelioma atybique T-8 de Guérin chez le rat. C. R. Séances Soc. Biol., *153*: 919, 1959.

35. Halpern, B. N., Prévot, A. R., Biozzi, G., Stiffel, C., Mouton, D., Morard, J. C., Bouthiller, Y., and Decreusefond, C. Stimulation de l'activité phagocytaire du systéme réticuloendothélial provoquée par *Corynebacterium parvum*. J. Reticuloendothel. Soc., *1*: 77–96, 1964.

36. Riggi, S. J. and DiLuzio, N. R. Identification of a reticuloendothelial stimulating agent in zymosan. Am. J. Physiol., *200*: 297–300, 1961.

37. Maeda, Y. Y. and Chihara, G. Periodical consideration on the establishment of antitumor action in host and activation of peritoneal exudate cells by lentinan. Gann, *64*: 351–357, 1973.

38. Maeda, Y. Y., Chihara, G., and Ishimura, K. Unique increase of serum proteins and action of antitumour polysaccharides. Nature, *252*: 250–252, 1974.

39. Maurer, H. R. and Allen, R. C. Polyacrylamide gel electrophoresis in clinical chemistry: Problems of standardization and performance. Clin. Chim. Acta, *40*: 359–370, 1972.

40. Pillemer, L. and Ross, O. A. Alterations in serum properdin levels following injection of zymosan. Science, *121*: 732–733, 1955.

41. Todd, E. W., Pillemer, L., and Lepow, I. H. The properdin system and immunity. IX. Studies on the purification of human properdin. J. Immunol., *83*: 418–427, 1959.

42. Okuda, T., Yoshioka, Y., Ikekawa, T., Chihara, G., and Nishioka, K. Anticomplementary activity of antitumour polysaccharides. Nature New Biol., *238*: 59–60, 1972.

43. Homma, R. and Kuratsuka, K. The histamine-sensitizing activity of lentinan, an antitumour polysaccharide. Experientia, *29*: 290–293, 1973.

44. Adlam, C., Broughton, E. S., and Scott, M. T. Enhanced resistance of mice to infection with bacteria following pretreatment with *Corynebacterium parvum*. Nature New Biol., *235*: 219–220, 1972.

45. Lewis, M. G. Possible immunological factors in human malignant melanoma in Uganda, Lancet, *II*: 921–922, 1967.

46. Lewis, M. G., Ikonopisov, R. L., Nairn, R. C., Phillips, T. M., Fairley, G. H., Boden-ham, D. C., and Alexander, P. Tumour specific antibodies in human malignant melanoma and their relationship to the extent of the disease. Brit. Med. J., *3*: 547–551, 1969.

47. Ohmi, K., Kasamatsu, T., Nakanishi, T., and Seto, T. Relationship of radiosensi-tivity to histological type of uterine carcinoma, with a special reference to PS-K combination therapy. Proc. Japan. Cancer Assoc., *33*: 641, 1974.

48. Shiio, T. and Yugari, Y. Studies of antitumour polysaccharide lentinan. Proc. Japan. Cancer Assoc., *33*: 390, 1974.

49. Howard, J. G., Scott, M. T., and Christie, G. H. Cellular mechanisms underlying the adjuvant activity of *Corynebacterium parvum*: Interactions of activated macrophages with T and B lymphocyte. *In;* G. E. W. Wolstenholme and J. Knight (eds.), Immuno-potentiation (Ciba Foundation Symposium), vol. 18, pp. 101–120, Elsevier/Excerpta Medica/North Holland, Amsterdam/London/New York, 1973.

50. Alexander, P. The role of macrophage in the host defence against cancer. *In;* D. Mizuno *et al.* (eds.), Host Defense against Cancer and Its Potentiation, pp. 113–130, Univ. of Tokyo Press, Tokyo, 1975.

51. Castro, J. E., Medawar, P. B., and Hamilton, D. N. H. Orchidectomy as a method of immunopotentiation in mice. *In;* G. E. W. Wolstenholme and J. Knight (eds.), Immunopotentiation (Ciba Foundation Symposium), vol. 18, pp. 237–258, Elsevier/Excerpta Medica/North Holland, Amsterdam/London/New York, 1973.

Discussion of Paper of Drs. Chihara et al.

DR. DRESSER: You offered a long list of hot water polysaccharide extracts of fungi which have antitumour effects on sarcoma-180 in susceptible ICR mice. Are there any polysaccharide isolates of any fungus which does not have an effect against sarcoma-180 in these mice?

DR. CHIHARA: We have several extracts from the fungus such as *A. bisporus* (Champinion), or *P. cocos*, which do not have any antitumour effect. Pachyman, a polysaccharide isolated from *P. cocos*, is a β-1,3-glucan with some β-1,6-branching, which lacks an antitumour activity. After stirring in 8 M urea solution at 70°C for 4 hr and removing the urea through a Millipore filter, pachyman (U-pachyman) responds in a manner similar to lentinan. Apparently the higher or micelle structure of the polysaccharide is here critical.

DR. STOCK: I was very interested in the three serum proteins which appear in those mice susceptible to the antitumour effect of lentinan, as they may be similar to a factor which was isolated by Dr. Green, one of my colleagues, in the serum of mice sensitized with BCG and then given endotoxin. Did you directly examine possible antitumour activities of three elevated serum fractions?

DR. CHIHARA: I have not directly examined the antitumour activity of the three elevated serum proteins. I feel it will be very interested if the serum factors obtained by Dr. Green *et al.* would be identified to ours, as I considered that the mode of action of lentinan differs from that of BCG or endotoxin. However, at present, I think that it is necessary to examine whether these serum proteins are identified or not.

DR. CASTRO: We have used the lentinan you have kindly supplied and discovered that it is without effect on thymus size, skin graft survival or growth of methylcholanthrene-induced tumors in BALB/c mice. Can you suggest why lentinan is effective only in particular strains of mice and with certain tumours? Also, did you look at the vascular pattern of the various tumours to determine whether lentinan has a similar mode of action to a substance described by Hellman which alters tumour vascularization?

DR. CHIHARA: We have also observed that lentinan does not have any effect on thymus weight in normal mice, and on skin graft survival in the combination of donor and recipient mouse strains such as $AKR \rightarrow C3H/f$, or $(C3H/f \times DDD)$ $F_1 \rightarrow C3H/f$. However, we found a complete restoration and considerable increase of thymus weight decreased in tumour-bearing hosts, by lentinan. I cannot well explain at present why lentinan is effective in the particular situation only. However, I believe that the differential effect of lentinan is not based on the presence or absence of a certain histocompatibility locus, but rather possibly on the various manner in a multiplicity of immunologic responses of the host-including hormonal and other physiological characters. The three serum proteins which increase in susceptible mice might play some role in this regard. We have not noted a change in vascular pattern of tumours after administration of lentinan comparing immediately with 1, 2-bis (3, 5-dioxopiperazin-1-yl) propane (ICRF) which was described by Hellmann and his colleagues. But, I think that the mode of action of lentinan perhaps differs from that of ICRF, as lentinan does not cause any haemorrhages reaction at all, though lentinan increase a histamine or serotonin sensitivity in mice which may be concerned with vascular permeability.

DR. DUKOR: Is lentinan active after oral administration? Also, does the mushroom from which you isolated these various polysaccharides have any use in Japanese folk medicine?

DR. CHIHARA: Lentinan has no antitumour activity after oral administration in mice differed from PS-K, which will be offered by Dr. Tsukagoshi in this Symposium, although the mode of action of PS-K seems similar to that of lentinan. The use of the Polyporaceae, especially *G. applanatum* or *C. versicolor*, in Japanese folk remedies is oral administration of hot water extract of the dried fungus.

DR. H. HIRAI (Hokkaido University School of Medicine, Sapporo):   After the immunization of rats with allogeneic tumour cells we noted the elevation of an α-globulin in the serum, which was also observed during an inflammatory process in otherwise normal rats of the same strain. Some of the elevated protein fractions you recorded may therefore be related to a non-specific host response to inflammation.

HOST DEFENSE AGAINST CANCER AND ITS POTENTIATION, D. MIZUNO ET AL. (EDS.),
UNIV. OF TOKYO PRESS, TOKYO / UNIV. PARK PRESS, BALTIMORE, PP. 199–211, 1975

Xenogenized Cell and Allogeneic Cell: Possible Relation to Immunotherapy for Cancer*

Hiroshi Kobayashi, Takao Kodama, Masuo Hosokawa, Fujiro Sendo,
Noritoshi Takeichi, Noboru Kuzumaki, Eiko Gotohda, Tsuneyuki Oi-
kawa, Masayuki Nakayama, and Masahiro Imamura

Laboratory of Pathology, Cancer Institute, Hokkaido University School of Medicine, Sapporo, Japan

Abstract: There may be many ways to stimulate the immune responses of the host
against cancer by specific and nonspecific means. A strong immunizing effect may
be brought by the immunization with viable cells. The authors established the ways
by viable cell-immunization with xenogenized rat tumor cells artificially infected
with murine leukemia virus and by allogeneic normal and malignant cells both
in inhibiting the growth of rat tumor cells immunologically. The xenogenized cell-
immunity relates to specific immunity to tumor-specific transplantation antigen and
the allogeneic cell-immunity relates to nonspecific immunity of the host. Viable
cells may be useful in part for the new approach to immunotherapy for cancer
without biohazard.

Both xenogenized tumor cells infected with murine leukemia virus and allogeneic normal and malignant cells in rat are viable cells to be used as a strong live-
vaccine which may result in producing specific immunity in xenogenized cells and
nonspecific immunity in allogeneic cells both for inhibiting the growth of tumor
cells. The authors will describe the experiments on the xenogenized cell and of allogeneic cell in relation to immunotherapy for cancer.

Xenogenized Cell

"Xenogenization" is immunological regression of rat tumor cells after infection
with murine leukemia virus (*1–14*).

Friend virus is infectious to mice but not to rats. However, newborn rats were
susceptible to Friend virus infection and produced leukemia in approximately 6
months.

---

* This work was supported in part by a research grant for cancer research from the Princess Takamatsu
Cancer Research Fund and the Ministry of Education of Japan.

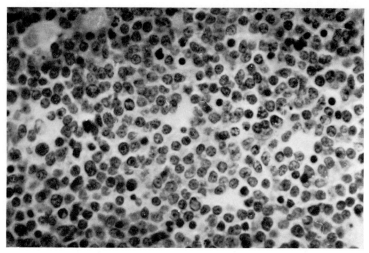

FIG. 1. Histopathology of Friend virus-induced lymphoma in spleen of rat.

Figure 1 shows the histological pattern of Friend virus-induced leukemia developed from spleen revealing typical lymphosarcoma or reticulum cell sarcoma. However, these tumors are very difficult to maintain in normal adult rats.

The transplantation of tumors developed from spleens of rats suffering from Friend leukemia produced the following results. In our laboratory we now have 13 lines which can be transplanted in 2- to 3-month-old Friend-tolerant Wistar King Aptekman (WKA) rats injected with Friend virus at birth (Table 1). In normal rats, however, there is no successful growth of tumors. This is very strange and different from the usual results in our transplantation experiments. The question then arose as to why such histologically typical malignant tumors were not

TABLE 1. Growth of Friend Virus-induced Tumors (Inoculated i.p.)

Tumor	Lethal growth in	
	Friend tolerant rat	Normal rat
WFT-1	128/129	3/38
WFT-2	113/113	0/53
WFT-3	84/84	0/26
WFT-4	25/25	0/9
WFT-5	9/12	—
WFT-6	9/9	0/4
WFT-7	7/13	0/3
WFT-8	11/11	0/5
WFT-9	13/13	0/4
WFT-10	2/2	—
WFT-11	2/2	—
WFT-12	2/2	—
WFT-13	50/50	0/26
Total	455/465 (97.8%)	3/168 (1.8%)

TABLE 2. Lethal Growth of Various Rat Tumors Artificially Infected with Murine Leukemia Viruses in the Syngeneic or Autochthonous Rat[a]

| Tumors infected with virus | | Lethal growth in | |
Tumor	Virus	Normal rats (%)	Tolerant or immunosuppressed rats (%)
Spont.-sarcoma-(WST-5)	Friend	0/26 (0)	7/8 (88)
„ -(Takeda)	„	6/23 (23)	— —
MCA-sarcoma-(primary)	„	0/4 (0)	4/4 (100)
„ -(KMT-17)	„	0/43 (0)	30/30 (100)
„ -(KMT-17)	Gross	0/9 (0)	12/12 (100)
„ -(KMT-68)	Friend	0/24 (0)	28/28 (100)
NBU-breast-(KBT-1)	„	0/12 (0)	9/9 (100)
„ -(KBT-2)	„	0/8 (0)	10/10 (100)
4NQO-lung-(Sato-LT)	„	0/28 (0)	11/12 (92)
DAB-hepatoma-(AH109)	„	2/8 (25)	— —
Total		8/185 (4)	125/127 (98)

[a] Gross-tolerant rats were used.

capable of growing and killing the normal adult host but only the Friend-tolerant host or immunologically suppressed host (3, 8).

In the second step in our experiments, the authors attempted to convert commonly transplanted rat tumors induced by causes other than viruses from lethal to non-lethal tumors after an artificial infection with Friend virus (Table 2). We used more than 10 different transplantable lines of tumors which we divided into 5 groups according to the cause of the tumor. The groups were spontaneously developed sarcomas, methylcholanthrene (MCA)-induced sarcomas, N-nitrosobutylurea (NBU)-induced breast cancers, 4-nitroquinoline N-oxide (4NQO)-induced lung cancer, and dimethylaminoazobenzene (DAB)-induced liver cancers.

They were incapable of growing and killing the normal rats after infection with Friend virus. Even if the tumors grew initially, most of them regressed by themselves later. That the tumors are actually neoplasms even after the virus infection is evidenced by the fact that the virus-infected tumors were capable of growing and killing rats tolerant to Friend virus and rats immunologically suppressed by chemicals or X irradiation. We tentatively referred to this phenomenon as "xenogenization." We also succeeded in producing xenogenization of autologously transplanted primary tumors as well as that of transplanted syngeneic tumors after infecting them with Friend virus. Rauscher virus and Gross virus were also used for the xenogenization experiment. These were all successful in producing the xenogenization of rat tumors.

Figure 2 is one of the methods of infection of tumors with Friend virus. There are several ways to infect the tumors with the virus, but this one is commonly used because of its simplicity and effectiveness. When the tumor was transplanted into the rats injected with Friend virus at birth for one or two generations, the tumor cells were infected with Friend virus while the tumor was growing in the host suf-

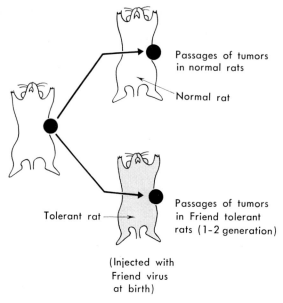

FIG. 2.   One of the methods of artificial infection of rat tumors with virus for xenogenization.

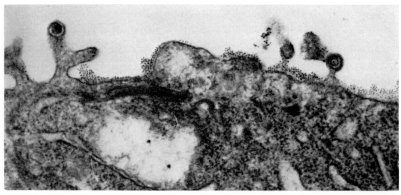

FIG. 3.   Budding of C-type virus particles from the surface of tumor cell and ferritin granules indicating virus-specific membrane antigens.

fering from Friend virus leukemia. Cultured tumor cells were also easily infected with Friend virus.

Figure 3 proves that the tumor cell was actually infected with Friend virus. The electron micrograph indicates the budding of the Friend virus from the surface of the cell and also fine ferritin granules on the surface of the cell indicating the virus-specific membrane antigen newly formed by the virus infection after xenogenization. In the normal host there were no hazardous effects of virus released from the virus-infected xenogenized tumor cell. Even in the Friend virus-tolerant rat neonatally infected with the virus no particular symptoms appeared when the virus was a high dose, and the rat grew as well as the normal rat.

Now, we will explain the mechanism of xenogenization. We think that the

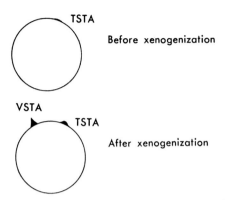

FIG. 4. Increase of antigenicity of tumor cell after xenogenization.

major reason why the tumor cells infected with Friend virus were not capable of growing even in the normal syngeneic rat is because the virus-specific transplantation antigen (VSTA) which appeared on the cell surface after xenogenization may be highly antigenic and easily recognized as foreign and thus be rejected by the rat (Fig. 4). Please note that the tumor cells in mice even after infection with Friend virus were not highly antigenic to the mouse. Thus the Friend virus-infected mouse tumors did not regress by themselves and were only slightly inhibited by the previous immunization with Friend virus.

Another possible reason is that the tumor-specific transplantation antigen (TSTA) existing on the cell surface which is weakly antigenic before xenogenization becomes moderately antigenic after xenogenization. This was proved both by *in vivo* and *in vitro* experiments. In the experiment involving active immunization with dead virus-infected or noninfected tumor cells the growth of identical types of tumors was more evidently inhibited in the rats immunized with virus-infected cells. In cytotoxicity tests using antitumor antiserum virus-infected cells were highly sensitive. These results suggest that both immunogenicity and immunosensitivity of tumor-specific antigen increased after xenogenization.

Next we tried to treat transplanted tumor and its metastasis first by only active immunization with virus-infected xenogenized tumor cells, then by surgical removal of the tumor alone, and finally by a combination of surgical operation and active immunization (Table 3). The survival rate was shown in the rats transplanted in the footpad with KMT-17 tumor which grew rapidly and developed metastasis only 3 to 4 days after transplantation. In the first experiment of single treatment with

TABLE 3. Active Immunization against Metastasis after Surgical Operation

Treatment	Survivors (%)
Active immunization	0/25 (0)
Surgical operation	18/56 (32.0)
Surgical operation Active immunization	37/65 (57.0)
None	0/30 (0)

TABLE 4.   Effect of Single or Combination Treatment on KMT-17

Treatment	Survivors (%)
Active immunization	4/21 (19.0)
Passive immunization	4/22 (18.2)
Chemotherapy	4/23 (17.4)
Active immunization } Chemotherapy }	14/25 (56.0)
Active immunization } Passive immunization }	14/23 (60.9)
Active immunization } Passive immunization } Chemotherapy }	28/33 (84.8)
None	0/33 (0)

active immunization performed 3 days after transplantation of the tumor, there were no survivors. This suggests that immunotherapy alone, even when xenogenized tumor cells are used, is not effective in treating tumors already growing visibly. Second, surgical removal of the tumor also performed 3 days after transplantation of the tumor resulted in a degree of inhibition of metastasis. However, the survival rate of 32% was still not statisfactory. Then we combined surgical removal of the tumor with active immunization of xenogenized tumor cells resulting in a definitely higher rate of survivors, 37 out of 65 rats which is 57% (15).

Table 4 summarizes the results of experiments for immunotherapy under conditions different from those in experiments described previously. Single treatments, namely, by active immunization with xenogenized tumor cells, passive immunization with anti-tumor syngeneic immune lymphocytes and chemotherapy represented by Mitomycin C were not satisfactory. However, when we combined active immunization with chemotherapy, or active immunization with passive immunization, a higher rate of survival was observed.

When we combined active immunization with both passive immunization and chemotherapy, much higher rate of survival was attained, 28 out of the 33 rats or 85% survived (16, 17).

In all of our experiments we used transplanted tumors, so we have to admit the possibility of different results in experiments using primary or human tumors. However, I would like to say that if it were permitted to transplant xenogenized cells into human patients it might be possible to expect a certain degree of inhibition to the growth of tumor, because viable cells with increased antigenicity of TSTA may produce a strong immunity in inhibiting the growth of the original tumor. Of course, this should be used together with other treatments.

Allogeneic Cell

In the course of the previous xenogenization experiments we used AH-66 hepatoma cells from allogeneic Donryu strain rats as a control for the xenogenized cell-immunity. This is because both xenogenized tumor cells and allogeneic tumor cells are viable cells and regress by themselves in the WKA rat. However, we were surprised when we looked at the unexpected results summarized in Table 5. A strong

TABLE 5. Reduced Transplantability of Tumors in WKA Rat Immunized with Allogeneic Tumors of Donryu Rat

Immunized with allogeneic Donryu tumor	Challenging WKA tumors (10^6–10^8)	Lethal growth of tumors	
		In immune rat	In nonimmune rat
AH-66	KMT-17	1/106 (6/106)[a]	20/20
AH-272	,,	0/4 (1/4)	,,
Sato-LT	,,	0/4 (1/4)	,,
AS-D653	,,	0/7 (0/7)	,,
AH-66	KST-1	0/4 (0/4)	4/4
,,	NRT	0/7 (0/7)	5/5
,,	KBT-10	0/4 (0/4)	8/8
,,	KMT-50	0/4 (0/4)	8/8

[a] Number in parentheses indicates temporary growth of tumor more than 10×10 mm in size.

inhibition to the growth of transplanted syngeneic KMT-17 tumor was observed 2–3 weeks after the previous immunization with viable AH-66 hepatoma cells. Even when we observed a temporary growth of KMT-17, no rats were killed by the tumor. All nonimmune rats died of the tumor. Even when the WKA rats were immunized with various types of Donryu tumor other than AH-66 hepatoma such as AH-272, Sato-LT and AS-D653, the host resisted the growth of KMT-17 tumor. The AH-66 immune rats also resisted the growth of other transplanted tumors such as KST-1, NRT, KBT-10, and KMT-50. There are a number of experiments supporting the same result, but we will skip the details at this time (*18*). The only exceptions were lymphomas and leukemias, which were less capable of producing inhibition to the growth of syngeneic tumors and also less responsive to immunization with allogeneic tumors. The reason for this has not been clarified yet.

The inhibition to the growth of transplanted syngeneic tumors was not only observed in the rats immunized with allogeneic tumors but also observed in the rats immunized with normal tissues from Donryu strain (Table 6). In the WKA rats immunized with more than one hundred million Donryu normal cells, growth of KMT-17 tumor was strongly inhibited and only half of the rats immunized with liver cells were killed. The same was true in those immunized with spleen, kidney

TABLE 6. Reduced Transplantability of KMT-17 Tumor in WKA Rat Immunized with Allogeneic Normal Tissues of Different Organs

Immunized with allogeneic Donryu normal tissues	Lethal growth of KMT-17
Liver	2/4 (4/4)[a]
Spleen	1/7 (4/7)
Kidney	1/4 (2/4)
Embryo	1/5 (2/5)
Skin graft	0/31 (2/31)
Whole blood	2/9 (3/9)
White blood cell	12/28 (16/28)
None	12/12

[a] Number in parentheses indicates temporary growth of tumor more than 10×10 mm in size.

TABLE 7. Allogeneic Cell-immune Effect (Why Is This Not a Syngeneic or Xenogeneic Cell-immune Effect?)

Immunized with	Lethal growth of KMT-17
Syngeneic tumor[a]	2/20
„ skin	10/10
(WKA)	
Allogeneic tumor	0/20
„ skin	0/18
(Donryu)	
Xenogeneic tumor	3/6
„ skin	5/5
(ddy)	

[a] Immunized with identical tumor after xenogenization.

and embryonic cells: for only one out of seven in the spleen, one out of four in the kidney, and one out of five in the embryonic cell were killed. The most striking inhibition to the growth of KMT-17 tumor was observed in the WKA rats immunized with skin grafts from Donryu rats. None of the 31 rats were killed and only two of them tolerated temporary growth of the tumor to more than 10×10 mm in size. Even in the rat immunized with whole blood or white blood cells from Donryu rats, a moderate inhibition to the KMT-17 tumor was observed.

Table 7 explains why we referred to the above-mentioned phenomenon as allogeneic cell immunity or allogeneic cell-immune effect. The most striking inhibitions to the transplanted syngeneic tumors were observed only in the rats immunized with either tumors or normal cells both from allogeneic Donryu rats. This was weakly observed in syngeneic rats and xenogeneic animals. Although a comparatively strong inhibition to the KMT-17 tumor was observed in the rat immunized with xenogenized syngeneic KMT-17 tumors, this may be due to specific immunity of TSTA which was common to the immunizing cell and challenging cell, a fact which must be taken into account when comparing the result with others.

Table 8 is a comparison between xenogenized cell-immunity and allogeneic cell-immunity. Xenogenized cell-immunity was specific to the TSTA, while allogeneic cell-immunity did not seem to be specific to the TSTA. The inhibition to the syngeneic tumors was observed more widely in allogeneic cell-immunity. Allogeneic cell-immunity seemed to be much stronger and more quickly developed than xenogenized cell-immunity. However, the immunizing effect in allogeneic cells seemed to be more unstable than in xenogenized cells in the treatment by X irradia-

TABLE 8. Comparison between Xenogenized Cell and Allogeneic Cell as an Immunizing Material

	Xenogenized cell-immunity	Allogeneic cell-immunity
Specificity of immunity	Yes	No
Range for target tumor		Wider
Immunizing effect		Stronger, quicker, but unstable
Durability of immunity	5–6 months	2–3 months

tion. For example, allogeneic cell-immunity was destroyed by a low dose of X irradiation of 250 rads, but xenogenized cell-immunity was not destroyed by the 250 rads and only destroyed by a sublethal dose of X irradiation of 600 rads. The duration of the immune effect was much longer in xenogenized cell-immunity than in allogeneic cell-immunity. We were careful to take note of the differences between the two types of immunity.

Concerning the mechanism of allogeneic cell-immunity, there is no decisive explanation available at this moment. One possible explanation seems to be that common antigens exist between immunizing cells and challenging tumor cells. In fact, there are many types of common antigens which possibly play a part in inhibition of syngeneic tumor. Although it is very difficult to exclude any possibility, a more plausible explanation is that allogeneic cell-immunity might be related to nonspecific immunity such as that to BCG and *Corynebacterium*.

One of the reasons is that there was no sign at all of common antigens detected by cytotoxicity in either direct or absorption tests. For example, serum from the WKA rat immunized with AH-66 hepatoma cells was not cytotoxic to KMT-17 tumor cells and was also not absorbed by the KMT-17 cells. The immune serum of anti-KMT-17 tumor cells prepared by immunization with xenogenized Friend virus-infected KMT-17 tumor cells in the WKA rat was also not absorbed by AH-66 hepatoma cells.

Other reason for this is the radiosensitivity of the immunity. It has been said that nonspecific immunity can be easily destroyed by a low dose of X irradiation such as in Dr. Klein's bolstering effect. In fact, our allogeneic cell-immunity was also sensitive to the low dose of X irradiation of 250 rads.

Transfer of immunity by lymphocytes has been successful in the specific immunity of xenogenized tumor cells, but it has not been successful in the allogeneic cell-immunity under ordinary conditions. In spite of the fact that we observed a fairly strong inhibition in *in vivo* experiments, we failed to achieve satisfactory results in the transfer experiment. This is very peculiar.

These results suggest that allogeneic cell-immunity may be due not to common antigen, but rather to nonspecific immunity or immunopotentiation of the host. However, much remains to be studied about the mechanism.

Concerning the possible application of allogeneic cells to immunotherapy of cancer, we do not have data that we can share with you at the present time. However, one of the merits of allogeneic cell-immunity as compared with xenogenized cell-immunity is that it may be possible to use normal tissues such as skin graft in human beings. As it is described above an allogeneic skin graft of 1.5 cm in diameter is capable of producing a strong resistance to the transplantation of syngeneic tumors. We were also surprised to note that a blood transfusion from allogeneic origin was capable of moderately inhibiting the growth of syngeneic tumors.

The inhibition effect of allogeneic skin graft against syngeneic tumor growth is not always strongly observed in skin graft obtained from all allogeneic strains of rats (Table 9). The most striking inhibition to KMT-17 tumor was observed in the rats immunized with skin grafts from Donryu or Kyoto. None of the rats were killed. In the rats immunized with skin grafts from either Sprague Dawley or

TABLE 9.   Reduced Transplantability of KMT-17 Tumor in WKA Rat Immunized with Allogeneic Skin Graft of Different Strains

Immunized with skin graft from	Lethal growth of KMT-17	
Donryu strain	0/31	(2/31)[a]
Kyoto strain	0/10	(0/10)
Long Evans strain	1/7	(4/7)
Buffalo strain	2/5	(4/5)
ACI strain	10/24	(21/24)
Fischer strain	6/14	(14/14)
Sprague Dawley strain	3/6	(6/6)
Tokyo strain	7/10	(9/10)
None	29/29	(29/29)

[a] Numbers in parentheses indicate temporary growth of tumor.

Tokyo strain, the inhibition to syngeneic tumors was not so definite. This indicated that the inhibition effect of allogeneic skin graft varies with the strain used as donor skin graft. Experiments using rats of strains other than WKA as recipients were not conducted, so at this point we can not prove that allogeneic skin graft immunity is a universal phenomenon in all experimental animals.

REFERENCES*

1. Kobayashi, H., Sendo, F., Shirai, T., Kaji, H., Kodama, T., and Saito, H. Modification in growth of transplantable rat tumors exposed to Friend virus. J. Natl. Cancer Inst., 42: 413–419, 1969.
2. Kobayashi, H. Growth of rat tumor cells infected with Friend virus: An approach to the immunological treatment of cancer. Immunity and Tolerance in Oncogenesis (IV Perugia Quadrennial International Conference on Cancer 1969), 637–659, 1969.
3. Kobayashi, H., Hosokawa, M., Takeichi, N., Sendo, F., and Kodama, T. Transplantable Friend virus-induced tumors in rats.   Cancer Res., 29: 1385–1392, 1969.
4. Sendo, F., Kaji, H., Saito, H., and Kobayashi, H. Antigenic modification of rat tumor cells artificially infected with Friend virus in the primary autochthonous host. Gann, 61: 223–226, 1970.
5. Kobayashi, H., Sendo, F., Kaji, H., Shirai, T., Saito, H., Takeichi, N., Hosokawa, M., and Kodama, T. Inhibition of transplanted rat tumors by immunization with identical tumor cells infected with Friend virus. J. Natl. Cancer Inst., 44: 11–19, 1970.
6. Takeichi, N., Kuzumaki, N., Kodama, T., Sendo, F., Hosokawa, M., and Kobayashi, H. Runting syndrome in rats inoculated with Friend virus. Cancer Res., 32: 445–449, 1972.
7. Kodama, T., Kuzumaki, N., and Takeichi, N. Immuno-electron microscopic studies on cell surface antigens of Friend virus-induced tumor in the rat. Gann, 64: 273–276, 1973.
8. Kobayashi, H., Kuzumaki, N., Gotohda, E., Takeichi, N., Sendo, F., Hosokawa,

* Restricted to references available in the Laboratory of Pathology, Cancer Institute, Hokkaido University School of Medicine, Sapporo.

M., and Kodama, T. Specific antigenicity of tumors and immunological tolerance in the rat induced by Friend, Gross and Rauscher viruses. Cancer Res., *33*: 1598–1603, 1973.

9. Kobayashi, H. Relationship between carcinogenesis and immunity. *In*; W. Nakahara, T. Hirayama, K. Nishioka, and H. Sugano (eds.), Analytic and Experimental Epidemiology of Cancer, pp. 381–388, Univ. of Tokyo Press, Tokyo, 1973.

10. Kuzumaki, N., Takeichi, N., Sendo, F., Kodama, T., and Kobayashi, H. Correlation between various cell-surface antigens induced by murine leukemia virus in the rat: Serological analysis. Int. J. Cancer, *11*: 575–585, 1973.

11. Kodama, T., Gotohda, E., and Kobayashi, H. Morphological aspects of xenogenization of tumors by artificial infection with virus. GANN Monograph on Cancer Research, *16*: 167–181, 1974.

12. Takeichi, N., Kuzumaki, N., and Kobayashi, H. Suppression of specific and nonspecific immune responses in rats infected with Friend or Gross virus. GANN Monograph on Cancer Research, *16*: 27–35, 1974.

13. Takeichi, N., Kaji, H., Kodama, T., and Kobayashi, H. Breakdown of Friend virus-induced tolerance and development of runting syndrome in rats. Cancer Res., *34*: 543–550, 1974.

14. Kobayashi, H. Lymphomas and immunological tolerance in the rat induced by murine leukemia viruses. *In;* Y. Ito and R.M. Dutcher (eds.), Comparative Leukemia Research 1973, pp. 291–300, Univ. of Tokyo Press, Tokyo, 1975.

15. Kobayashi, H., Gotohda, E., Hosokawa, M., and Kodama, T. Inhibition of metastasis in rats immunized with xenogenized autologous tumor cells after excision of the primary tumor. J. Natl. Cancer Inst., 1975, in press.

16. Hosokawa, M., Sendo, F., Gotohda, E., and Kobayashi, H. Combination of immunotherapy and chemotherapy to experimental tumors in rats. Gann, *62*: 57–60, 1970.

17. Gotohda, E., Sendo, F., Hosokawa, M., Kodama, T., and Kobayashi, H. Combination of active and passive immunization and chemotherapy to transplantation of methylcholanthrene-induced tumor in WKA rats. Cancer Res., *34*: 1947–1951, 1974.

18. Kobayashi, H., Gotohda, E., Kuzumaki, N., Takeichi, N., Hosokawa, M., and Kodama, T. Reduced transplantability of syngeneic tumors in rats immunized with allogeneic tumors. Int. J. Cancer, *13*: 522–529, 1974.

Discussion of Paper of Drs. Kobayashi et al.

DR. AMOS: Have you investigated the capacity of other viruses besides Friend virus, especially non-oncogenic types, to modify the antigenicity of tumor cells for use in your system?

DR. KOBAYASHI: We have also observed tumor regression following xenogenization using Rauscher and Gross leukemia viruses. We have as yet employed only oncogenic viruses, but the effect appears to be a general principle applicable to those viruses which bud from cell surfaces to become membrane coated.

DR. KENNEDY: In susceptible hosts Friend virus is very immunosuppressive. Were such effects noted in your system? Secondly, do the infected tumor cells produce Friend virus?

DR. KOBAYASHI: Xenogenization following virus exposure here seems to be the dominant effect, overshadowing any immunodepressive effect such treatment may evoke. This virus produces a persistent infection, and viral progeny can be observed both microscopically and biologically for long periods subsequent to tumor cell infection.

DR. KENNEDY: Are your studies compatible with similar experiments performed using influenza viruses as a carrier-hapten system?

DR. KOBAYASHI: Influenza virus causes a productive infection with lysis of tumor cells. In our scheme, viable antigenically modified tumor cells remain as immunogens.

DR. FROST: Is your "allogeneic immune effect" similar to the one defined by D. H. Katz? What is your proposed mechanism for the inhibition of the growth of a syngeneic tumor following allogeneic cell-immunization?

DR. KOBAYASHI: Although the terms are similar, our phenomenon is totally different from Dr. Katz's allogeneic effect. Ours may be the result of a non-specific immunostimulation of the host upon allogeneic tumor cell transplantation.

DR. AMOS: Often a tumor may fail to implant when inoculated intradermally and still provoke good systemic immunity, while the same dose administered by another route may kill the host. Have you any data offering why your immunization procedure was greatest following grafting of normal skin?

DR. KOBAYASHI: No.

DR. T. TANAKA (National Cancer Center Research Institute, Tokyo):   Have you rechallenged with tumor those rats whose neoplasms were suppressed by your allogeneic immune effect?

DR. KOBAYASHI: We have not as yet performed that experiment.

DR. NAKAHARA: Did you examine histologically the areas about the xenogenized tumors? The cellular reactions surrounding allogeneic tumors and foreign bodies may be quite different. For example, a host may simply disregard xenogeneic implants by the lack of vascular proliferation.

DR. KOBAYASHI: The xenogeneic neoplasms are surrounded by a tremendous number of cells. We have never histologically compared allogeneic tissue *vs.* xenogenized tissue graft rejection processes.

HOST DEFENSE AGAINST CANCER AND ITS POTENTIATION, D. MIZUNO ET AL. (EDS.), UNIV. OF TOKYO PRESS, TOKYO / UNIV. PARK PRESS, BALTIMORE, PP. 213-226, 1975

Suppression of Autochthonous Tumor Grafts by Mixed Implantation with Allogeneic Tissues

Reiko Tokuzen and Waro Nakahara

National Cancer Center, Tokyo, Japan

Abstract: That a characteristic local cellular reaction is associated with the destruction of transplanted allogeneic tumors is well known; also well known is that grafts always take and grow in autochthonous tumor-host system. These facts led us to wonder what would happen to autografts if they were implanted in the location where the mechanism of destruction of transplanted tumors may be actively at work.

Autografts used were those of spontaneous mammary adenocarcinoma and of methylcholanthrene-induced primary sarcoma in mice. These were implanted back to their original hosts mixed with allogeneic tissues, including leukemia L1210 and C1498, which are histoincompatible to Swiss albino strain, sarcoma 180, which can be suppressed with the aid of an immunopotentiator (lentinan), and normal spleens from two strains of mice. AH130 hepatoma of the rat was also used.

Suppression of autochthonous tumor grafts occurred in association with reaction to tumor-specific transplantation antigen, and to far less extent to xenogeneic tumor antigen, but not to normal alloantigen. However, the destruction of an autochthonous tumor grafts *in loco* did not induce systemic immunity, as evidenced by the occurrence of local recurrence at the site of operation and also, in the case of the spontaneous mammary tumor, by the development of new tumors in the mammary gland away from the site of operation. It was concluded that in the strictly autochthonous tumor-host system the tumor has at best only a feeble antigenicity.

Much has been done and written concerning the so-called tumor immunity, but the bulk of our knowledge on the subject is derived from immunological studies using transplanted tumors, be they syngeneic or allogeneic. There has always been a doubt as to how far can the reaction mechanism to tumor-specific transplantation antigen be extrapolated to the resistance mechanism in the autochthonous tumor-host system. We are reasonably confident that the host does put up some sort of resistance against tumor cells of its own (*i.e.*, autochthonous tumor cells), and more recent studies utilizing finer immunologic *in vitro* techniques, with the aid of syngeneic transplantation methods, yielded indications of the existence of antigenicity in autochthonous tumor cells. The presence of blocking antibody and possibility of unblocking its action have been suggested. The state of immunodepression on the part of tumor-bearing host must also be considered. The fact remains, however, that it has not been possible to bring about the destruction of an autochthonous tumor within the body of the host by the mobilization or potentiation of immune mechanisms.

The experiments to be reported here represent attempts to construct a bridge between our knowledge of allogeneic tumor transplantation and that of autochthonous tumor grafting by utilizing local reaction to allogeneic tumor grafts.

Local Cellular Reaction Accompanying Allogeneic Tumor Graft Rejection

Since the early days of Da Fano (*1*) it has been known that lymphoid cell infiltration forms the main feature of the local histological reaction in the rejection mechanism of allogeneic tumor grafts. We re-confirmed this fact with our own eyes, in our attempt to elucidate the so-called antitumor effect of some non-cytotoxic plant polysaccharides. In these experiments we used three kinds of polysaccharides, namely, wheat straw hemicellulose B (*2*), lichen polysaccharide termed GE-3 (partially acetylated β-1,6-glucan) isolated from *Gyrophora esculenta* (*3*), and lentinan,

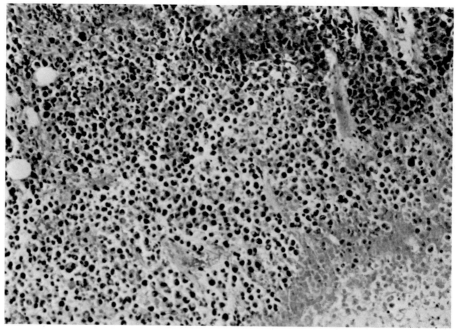

FIG. 1. Outpouring of lymphoid cells around an island of sarcoma 180 cells, one week after implantation in a mouse treated with wheat straw hemicellulose B.

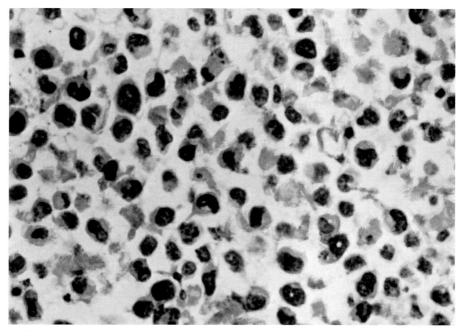

FIG 2. A high-power view of the above, showing the character of cell types participating in the reaction.

β-1$\rightarrow$3-glucan, isolated from edible mushroom, *Lentinus edodes* (*4*). It is well documented that intraperitoneal injections of these polysaccharides bring about very high percent of complete regression of sarcoma 180, implanted subcutaneously in mice 24 hr before starting the injections. Sarcoma 180 is a well-known long-term transplanted allogeneic tumor, but its grafts take and progressively grow in 100% in the mice of our Swiss albino strain.

We found that one week after implantation the bulk of sarcoma 180 graft was in the state of necrosis, with many islands of intact tumor cells in the peripheral part (*5*). In the polysaccharide-treated mice, there was at this period an extensive outpouring of lymphoid cells in the immediate vicinity of the tumor cell masses (Fig. 1 and Fig. 2). The lymphoid cells were mostly of macrophage or histiocyte type; small lymphocytes were not prominent. This characteristic local cell reaction was no longer present in later periods, when only a few isolated tumor cells may be seen encircled by connective tissue cells, as the last remains of failing tumor graft. The entire granulation tissue was eventually completely absorbed and left no scar.

In untreated mice as well as in mice treated with antitumor-inactive polysaccharides (wheat straw hemicellulose A, sunflower stalk hemicellulose B, for example), the histologic reaction to sarcoma 180 grafts conformed to the well-known picture of successful allogeneic tumor grafts in general. Tumor cells were at first loosely spread out or infiltrating into surrounding tissue but they soon became established as solid tumors, with supporting stromal tissue and adequate

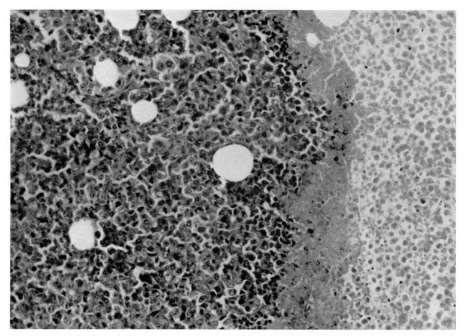

FIG. 3. A sarcoma 180 graft in untreated mouse, showing the absence of cellular reaction between the border of growing tumor mass and the necrotic area. One week after implantation.

vascular supply. The lymphoid cell reaction around the tumor cell masses was entirely absent throughout the whole process (Fig. 3).

From these findings we are strongly inclined to believe that the characteristic local lymphoid cell reaction may be a morphological expression of resistance to allogeneic tumor grafting, and that the polysaccharides concerned may be considered as immunopotentiators.

The Case of Autochthonous Tumor Grafts

In strong contrast to allogeneic tumor grafts (sarcoma 180), autochthonous tumor grafts were not at all influenced by injections of any of the polysaccharides (6). Using autografts of spontaneous mammary adenocarcinoma of mice, which grew in 100% of cases, we found that these autografts did not call forth any lymphoid cell reaction, such as observed constantly in the inhibition and regression of allogeneic tumor grafts under the influence of immunopotentiators. The autografts of spontaneous mammary adenocarcinoma always grew in the usual acinous form, with supporting stromal tissue and abundant vascularization (Fig. 4).

At this point we posed to ourselves a question: what happen to autografts if they were placed in the field of local lymphoid cell reaction such as is induced around sarcoma 180 grafts under the influence of an immunopotentiator? This question we attempted to answer in the first place by implanting autografts mixed with sarcoma 180, followed by the treatment of the mice with one of the immuno-

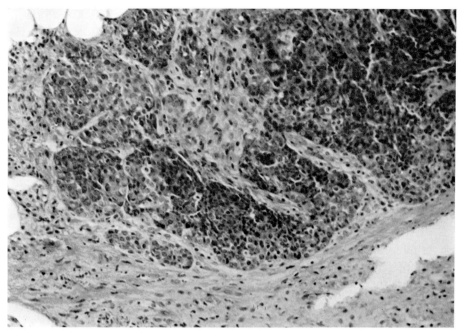

FIG. 4. Growing edge of an autograft of spontaneous mammary tumor in a mouse treated with wheat straw hemicellulose B, showing the acinus-type structure of the graft with stromal and vascular reaction but without lymphoid infiltration.

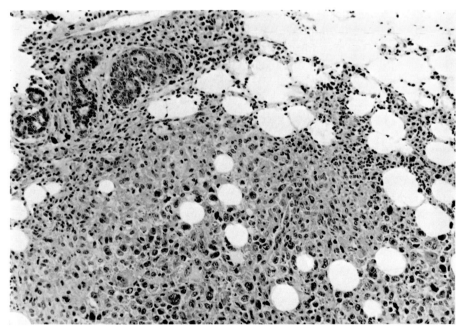

FIG. 5. Granulation tissue containing remains of autograft of spontaneous mammary tumor, 3 weeks after mixed implantation with sarcoma 180 in a mouse under treatment with lentinan.

potentiators (lentinan). The object of the proposed experiment, restated in another way, was to determine whether or not the induced allogeneic graft rejection mechanism discriminated the autochthonous cells from allogeneic cells. Somewhat to our surprise it was found that when autochthonous tumor grafts were implanted mixed with sarcoma 180 the autografts were suppressed and many underwent complete regression (7). This showed that within the area of the granulomatous reaction to allogeneic tumor grafts (Fig. 5), the host failed to recognize the autografts as "self" and to tolerate them; instead the host acted toward the autograft as though they were "not self," same as allogeneic tumor grafts. It was this finding that served as the immediate starting point of the experiments to be reported next.

Method of Mixed Implantation of Tumor Autografts with Other Tissues

Using spontaneous mammary adenocarcinoma of Swiss albino mice, kindly supplied by Dr. H. Nagasawa of our Institute, we first removed the tumor surgically as completely as possible. A mouse sometimes bore more than one tumor, and these were removed at the same time. The size of the tumor at the time of operation varied from that of small fingertip to thumtip. These tumors have never shown any spontaneous regression in our experience, and autografts always showed 100% takes.

The mixed implantation was accomplished by aspirating 0.05 ml of the material to be tested into a small syringe fitted with an injection needle of caliber large enough to accommodate a small solid autochthonous tumor graft, about 1 mm in diameter, which was inserted at the end of the needle. The whole material was then delivered under the skin of the mouse by simply pushing the plunger.

Materials used for mixed implantation with tumor autografts were as follows: (1) allogeneic normal spleens from ddY and BDF_1 mice; (2) allogeneic normal embryos of ddY mice, at about second week of gestation.

Sarcoma 180, leukemia L1210, and leukemia C1498 were used as allogeneic tumors, all in ascites form but implanted subcutaneously. Sarcoma 180 is readily accepted by Swiss albino mice, producing lethal tumors, but is rejected in the majority of the mice if mice were given intraperitoneal injections of immunopotentiator. Leukemia L1210 is highly strain specific to BDF_1 mice, and is consistently rejected when implanted subcutaneously into Swiss albino mice. C1498 produced very large tumors during the first week but the tumors gradually disappeared in the course of 3–4 weeks.

Xenogeneic tumor was also tested, using rat ascites hepatoma AH130.

As immunopotentiator we used lentinan (β-1→3-glucan) isolated from an edible mushroom, *L. edodes*. The sample of it was kindly donated by Dr. G. Chihara.

Autografts of Spontaneous Mammary Tumors Implanted Mixed with Allogeneic Tissues

Experiments were carried out according to the methods described above, and the results, partly already published (8), are summarized in Table 1. The main point considered is naturally the fate of autografts.

TABLE 1. Fate of Autografts of Spontaneous Mammary Tumors Implanted Mixed with Various Allogeneic Tissues, with or without Lentinan Treatment of the Host

Experimental groups	Mice with tumor[a]/ total No. of mice	%
1. Autograft mixed with ddY spleen Host untreated	19/20	95
2. Autograft mixed with BDF$_1$ spleen Host untreated	7/7	100
3. Autograft mixed with ddY spleen Host sensitized with ddY spleen	8/9	88
4. Autograft mixed with ddY spleen Host treated with lentinan	8/8	100
5. Autograft mixed with embryo cells Host untreated	15/15	100
6. Autograft alone Host treated with lentinan	15/15	100
7. Autograft mixed with sarcoma 180 Host treated with lentinan	14/37	38
8. Autograft mixed with sarcoma 180 Host untreated	6/6	100
9. Autograft mixed with L1210 Host untreated	6/21	29
10. Autograft mixed with L1210 Host treated with lentinan	4/9	44
11. L1210 alone Host untreated	0/5	0
12. Autograft mixed C1498 Host untreated	8/16	50
13. C1498 alone Host untreated	0/5	0
14. Autograft mixed with AH130 Host untreated	10/14	71
15. Autograft alone Host untreated	26/26	100

[a] Tumors resulting from the growth of the autografts, except in groups 7 and 8 where tumors were sarcoma 180.

The time between the implantation of autograft and the first day when it became palpable showed considerable individual variation. However, no difference was apparent on this point among different experimental groups, and hence was not cited in the table. It may also be mentioned in passing that the number of mice with lung metastasis was not given, nor data on the postoperative longevity. In the present experiments recurrent or new tumors grew to such large sizes that the mice were killed when the fate of autografts was definitely established. This rendered the postoperative survival and metastasis incidence in different groups not rationally comparable.

The following annotations may be appropriate to the data presented in Table 1.

First, tumor autografts were not suppressed when implanted mixed with normal allogeneic spleen. In one of the groups the mice were previously sensitized by implantation of normal spleen, with an interval of 10 days between the sensitizing (first) implantation on the back and the second implantation mixed with tumor autograft in the inguinal region. Normal allogeneic spleen transplants were rapidly destroyed and only traces of them were palpable, if at all, at the time of the second mixed implantation with autograft. Attempted immunopotentiation with the aid of lentinan injection did not change the matter. The evidence seems complete that the local immunological reaction to normal alloantigen does not participate in the destruction of autochthonous tumor graft.

Mixed implantation with allogeneic normal embryonic tissue did not suppress the tumor autografts. This may rule out the active role of carcinoembryonic antigen in the destruction of tumor autograft.

The case of sarcoma 180 is somewhat complicated. This tumor grows actively and constantly in all normal mice, but is rejected if the mice were given lentinan injections; that is, susceptible to immunopotentiation. The tumor autografts were destroyed if implanted mixed with sarcoma 180 under the lentinan treatment. Without the lentinan injections the autografts become overwhelmed by the rapid growth of sarcoma 180; it is then impossible to trace the fate of the autografts.

In contrast to sarcoma 180, leukemia L1210, and C1498 are histoincompatible to Swiss albino mice. It was remarkable that autografts, when implanted simply mixed with L1210 or C1498 cells showed a very high rate of complete regression without the aid of immunopotentiator. We interpret this fact to mean that L1210 and C1498 cells have very efficient tumor-specific transplantation antigen, far more so than sarcoma 180. Transplantation antigen of sarcome 180 requires the aid of immunopotentiator in order to act in Swiss mice.

Somewhat to our surprise reaction to xenogeneic tumor antigen apparently took part in the process of autograft destruction, though far less effectively than allogeneic tumor antigen.

Autografts of Methylcholanthrene (MCA)-induced Sarcoma

In addition to spontaneous mammary tumors, we carried out similar experiments using autografts of MCA-induced primary sarcoma for comparison. A single subcutaneous injection of 0.5 mg of this carcinogen in olive oil was sufficient to

TABLE 2. Fate of Autografts of MCA-induced Sarcoma Implanted Mixed with Allogeneic Tumors, with or without Lentinan Treatment of the Host

Experimental groups	Mice with tumor/ total No. of mice	%
1. Autograft alone Host untreated	38/40	95
2. Autograft alone Host treated with lentinan	16/19	84.2
3. Autograft mixed with sarcoma 180 Host treated with lentinan	4/16	25
4. Autograft mixed with L1210 Host untreated	0/5[a]	0

[a] Nine other mice died with hepatomegaly and splenomegaly during from 7 to 10 days after implantation mixed with L1210, too early to determine the fate of the autograft. Those livers and spleens were invaded with L1210 and the cause of death was L1210.

yield sarcoma of adequate sizes for our purpose in the course of 100–180 days in the majority of the mice.

Autografts of these sarcomas took almost always but not exactly in 100% of the cases. However, they behaved essentially in the same way as the mammary tumor autografts when implanted mixed with allogeneic tissues. Experimental results are shown in Table 2.

Failure to Induce Systemic Immunity

One thing stood out very clearly in the experimental results, and that was that the destruction of autochthonous tumor grafts *in vivo* failed to induce any recognizable systemic immunity to the same respective tumor. This was evidenced by the occurrence of local recurrence at the site of operation and also, in the case of spontaneous mammary tumors, by the development of new tumors in the mammary gland away from the site of operation. These recurrent or new tumors served the role of challenge test in the entirely natural manner, without resorting to the artificial system of transplanting the original tumor to a syngeneic mouse and challenging the mouse, which rejected autografts, by retransplanting to it the syngeneically transplanted tumor. We presented the pertinent data in Table 3 in order specifically to compare the rate of systemic immunity between the mice which accepted autografts and those which rejected them.

The result that the suppression of autografts under our experimental conditions was apparently a local affair and there was no induction of systemic tumor immunity is contradictory to the reports of previous workers who showed the induction of systemic immunity after the suppression of the first grafts. There is no doubt in our minds that the discrepancy here is due to the difference between the strictly autochthonous tumors in our experiments and allogeneic (or syngeneic) transplanted tumors used by other workers. Syngeneic tumor-host system is not the same as the autochthonous system.

It must be pointed out also that mice bearing large autochthonous tumors are in the state of immunodepression, which may have something to do with the failure of systemic immunity induction. This state of immunodepression in mice with autochthonous tumors cannot be remedied by an immunopotentiator (lentinan), which can greatly increase the resistance of normal mice to allogeneic tumor transplants (sarcoma 180) but not of spontaneous tumor mice to autochthonous grafts. Here a search for a new immunopotentiator capable of restoring to normal the decreased immune responsiveness of tumor-bearing animals is strongly indicated.

If we are to consider immunotherapy in cancer it would be necessary to discover new immunotherapeutic agents which can induce systemic immunity in autochthonous tumor-host system.

Mechanism of Autograft Destruction

How does it happen that autochthonous tumor grafts are not recognized as

TABLE 3. Incidence of Local Recurrences and New Tumors in Mice in Which Autografts Grew or Suppressed

Experimental groups	Total No. of mice in which	
	Autograft grew	Autograft suppressed
Mammary tumors: local recurrences		
1. Autograft mixed with ddY spleen Host untreated	13/19	0/1
2. Autograft mixed with BDF$_1$ spleen Host untreated	5/7	—
3. Autograft mixed with ddY spleen Host sensitized with ddY spleen	3/8	0/1
4. Autograft mixed with ddY spleen Host treated with lentinan	6/8	—
5. Autograft mixed with embryo cells Host untreated	12/15	—
6. Autograft alone Host treated with lentinan	5/15	—
7. Autograft mixed with sarcoma 180 Host treated with lentinan	10/14	17/23
8. Autograft mixed with L1210 Host untreated	4/6	11/15
9. Autograft mixed with L1210 Host treated with lentinan	3/4	2/5
10. Autograft mixed with C1498 Host untreated	4/8	5/8
11. Autograft mixed with AH130 Host untreated	8/10	3/4
12. Autograft alone Host untreated	15/26	—
Total	88/140 (62.9%)	38/57 (66.7%)
Mammary tumor: new tumors		
1. Autograft mixed with ddY spleen Host untreated	9/19	1/1
2. Autograft mixed with BDF$_1$ spleen Host untreated	3/7	—
3. Autograft mixed with ddY spleen Host sensitized with ddY spleen	3/8	1/1
4. Autograft mixed with ddY spleen Host treated with lentinan	3/8	—
5. Autograft mixed with embryo cells Host untreated	9/15	—
6. Autograft alone Host treated with lentinan	4/15	—
7. Autograft mixed with sarcoma 180 Host treated with lentinan	5/14	14/23
8. Autograft mixed with L1210 Host untreated	6/6	9/15
9. Autograft mixed with L1210 Host treated with lentinan	3/4	3/5
10. Autograft mixed with C1498 Host untreated	5/8	6/8
11. Autograft mixed with AH130 Host untreated	8/10	3/4
12. Autograft alone Host untreated	12/26	—
Total	70/140 (50%)	37/57 (64.9%)

TABLE 3.   (Continued)

Experimental groups	Total No. of mice in which	
	Autograft grew	Autograft suppressed
MC-sarcoma : local recurrences		
1. Autograft alone Host treated with lentinan	15/16	2/3
2. Autograft mixed with sarcoma 180 Host treated with lentinan	3/4	9/12
3. Autograft mixed with L1210 Host untreated	—	2/5
4. Autograft alone Host untreated	32/38	2/2
Total	50/58 (86.2%)	13/22 (59.1%)

"self" and are destroyed when implanted mixed with allogeneic tumors? No ready explanation is forthcoming.

It is easy to say that activated macrophages destroyed tumor cells, but to define the exact roles of cellular and humoral factors involved may be a difficult task. It may be that the specific lymphoid cells entering the allogeneic tumor grafts react with the target antigens and the toxic substance(s) produced may incidentally injure the autochthonous tumor cells, which are not directly involved in the process. If so, one may reasonably attempt to isolate and identify the hypothetical cytotoxic factor.

In the present study we have been able to show that the host reaction to tumor-specific transplantation antigen, but not to normal alloantigen is in some way implicated in the mechanism of autograft destruction. In this connection it was of considerable interest that xenogeneic tumor antigen (rat ascites hepatoma AH130) participated in the destruction of autografts, though far less effectively than allogeneic tumor antigens. This means that there may exist tumor antigen which is non-species specific. We believe that the elucidation of this relative specificity may lead to better understanding of the mechanism.

REFERENCES

1. Da Fano, C. Zellulare Analyse der Geschwulstimmunitatsreaktionen. Z. Immunitaetsforsch., *5*: 1–75, 1910.
2. Nakahara, W., Tokuzen, R., Fukuoka, F., and Whistler, R. L. Inhibition of mouse sarcoma 180 by a wheat hemicellulose B preparation. Nature, *216*: 374–375, 1967.
3. Shibata, S., Nishikawa, Y., Tanaka, M., Fukuoka, F., and Nakanishi, M. Antitumor activities of lichen polysaccharides. Z. Krebsforsch., *71*: 102–104, 1968.
4. Chihara, G., Maeda, Y., Hamuro, J., Sasaki, T., and Fukuoka, F. Inhibition of mouse sarcoma 180 by polysaccharides from *Lentinus edodes* (BERK.) SING. Nature, *222*: 687–688, 1969.
5. Tokuzen, R. Comparison of local cellular reaction to tumor grafts in mice treated with some plant polysaccharides. Cancer Res., *31*: 1590–1593, 1971.

6. Tokuzen, R. and Nakahara, W. Die Wirkung einiger pflanzliches Polysaccharide auf das spontane Mamma-Adenocarcinom der Maus. Arzneimittel-Forschung, *21*: 269–271, 1971.

7. Tokuzen, R. and Nakahara, W. Suppression of autochthonous grafts of spontaneous mammary tumor by induced allogeneic grafts rejection mechanism. Cancer Res., *33*: 645–647, 1973.

8. Tokuzen, R. and Nakahara, W. Autochthonous grafts of spontaneous mammary tumors implanted together with allogeneic tissues. Z. Krebsforsch., *81*: 239–242, 1974.

Discussion of Paper of Drs. Tokuzen and Nakahara

DR. AMOS: It is gratifying to see that your system encompasses the problem of local tumor immunity, which is often overlooked. Similar studies by Kayliss, in which tumor growth was enhanced on one side of an animal in the presence of local immunity on the contralateral side, have never been completely resolved. I believe that it is unlikely that you will find a toxic factor responsible for the suppression of autochthonous tumor grafts.

DR. TOKUZEN: As yet we have been unable to demonstrate such a substance.

DR. KENNEDY: Dr. T. Jones and I found that semi-allogeneic one-way mixed spleen cell cultures in which the only immunologically specific reaction should have been that of parent against hybrid in actual fact generated cells capable of inhibiting colony formation by fibrosarcoma cells of parental origin. Up to 70% colony inhibition was produced by semi-allogeneic mixtures cultured for 3 days. The effector cells belong to an adherent cell population.

DR. AMOS: Have you checked for specificity in this system? Dr. Thistlethwaite in my laboratory has noted that rat lymphoid cells cultured alone *in vitro* for several days often develop a non-specific reactivity.

DR. KENNEDY: After 3 days of culture, both parental and F_1 hybrid spleen cells produced approximately 20% inhibition of colony formation by malignant cells of parental origin. The 70% colony inhibition by cells from semi-allogeneic mixed spleen cell cultures is an additional 70%, calculated on the basis that the inhibition caused by cells from pure cultures of parental or F_1 hybrid spleen cells is taken as zero.

DR. NAKAHARA: I think it is often difficult if not misleading to attempt to correlate findings in tissue culture with apparently similar *in vivo* systems, for in the former case one is working with very simplified conditions. Our scheme is, of course, much more complex than the *in vitro* system you've outlined.

DR. HOBBS: Fakhri and I demonstrated in a xenogeneic adoptive immunity experiment that specific rat antibody could assist mouse macrophage and lymphocytes in tumor killing. By such passively transferred antibody one could cure a C3H mouse of its autologous neoplasm but after one month it is again susceptible to this tumor, showing that acquired immunity was not produced.

DR. SIMMONS: The fact that you did not observe a decrease in the incidence of second primary tumors, for example additional mammary adenocarcinomas, may be because the animals were non-responsive to the mammary tumor virus antigen common to both tumors. However, you also observed local recurrences, indicating that immunity to the private or very weak specific tumor antigens was also not evoked.

HOST DEFENSE AGAINST CANCER AND ITS POTENTIATION, D. MIZUNO ET AL. (EDS.),
UNIV. OF TOKYO PRESS, TOKYO / UNIV. PARK PRESS, BALTIMORE, PP. 227–244, 1975

Active Specific Immunotherapy of Cancer in Experimental Animals*

Richard L. Simmons and Angelyn Rios

Department of Surgery, University of Minnesota, Minneapolis, Minnesota, U.S.A.

Abstract: Firmly established transplantable C3H/HeJ mammary carcinomas can
be inhibited by host challenge with *Vibrio cholerae* neuraminidase (VCN)-treated
tumor cells. The effect is totally immunospecific; even VCN-treated tumors bearing
shared mammary tumor virus (MTV) antigen cannot induce the regression. Thus,
VCN is capable of increasing the immunogenicity of the private, unique-unshared
tumor antigens on mammary carcinomas; VCN is incapable of increasing the
immunogenicity of the shared MTV-associated tumor antigen even in syngeneic
C3HeB/FeJ MTV-free mice. The immunoregressive effect of VCN-treated tumor
cells can be augmented by subtotal or total surgical excision of large transplantable
tumors.

Spontaneous mammary tumors in retired breeder C3H/HeJ female mice can
be made to regress by two immunological maneuvers: (1) repeated intratumor
injections of VCN and/or BCG, (2) total excision and immunotherapy with VCN-
treated autochthonous mammary tumor cells. The use of VCN-treated transplantable mammary tumor cells sharing the MTV-associated antigen was not better
than excision alone. The evidence supports the idea that active specific immunotherapy of spontaneous tumors with VCN-altered tumor cells may require the use
of autochthonous cells.

We previously demonstrated that methylcholanthrene (MCA)-induced fibrosarcomas transplanted into syngeneic C3H/HeJ female recipients could be made
to regress if the mice are challenged with tumor cells treated *in vitro* with *Vibrio
cholerae* neuraminidase (VCN) (*1*). The regression is immunospecific (*1*). The
immunoregressive effect could be augmented by simultaneous inoculations of non-
specific immunostimulants, *e.g.*, *Mycobacterium bovis* (strain BCG) (*2, 3*) and the
effect was not abrogated by pretreatment of the challenging tumor cells with

---

* Supported by USPHS Grant No. CA 11605 and Grant IM-20A from American Cancer Society.

mitomycin C to prevent the growth of the challenging inoculum. The present studies were designed to determine whether the immunoregression of transplantable and spontaneous mammary tumors could be induced by challenge with VCN-treated tumor cells.

Mice: C3H/HeJ and C3HeB/FeJ female mice were obtained from Jackson Laboratory, Bar Harbor, Maine. The animals were housed separately in covered plastic cages, 10 or less per cage and provided with tap water and a standard laboratory diet (Purina chow checkers) *ad libitum.* C3H/HeJ mice are infested with a mammary tumor virus (MTV) and will develop a high incidence of spontaneous mammary tumors in the second year of life. C3HeB/FeJ is a strain of mice derived from C3H/HeJ ova-transferred to C57 BL/6 mice by Fekete in 1949. C3HeB/FeJ mice are believed not to contain the same MTV virus which infests the C3H/HeJ strain since they have a low incidence of mammary tumors (*4*). Heppner has recently noted a higher incidence of mammary tumors in this strain, but she also has evidence that the mammary tumor viral associated antigen of C3H/HeJ mice and that C3HeB/FeJ mice do not cross-react with each other (*5*).

Tumors: Several spontaneous mammary adenocarcinomas (M-1, M-2) appearing in aged C3H/HeJ mice were maintained by serial transplantation in syngeneic C3H/HeJ female mice. Sterile tumor cells for inoculation were prepared from tumors (1.0–1.4 cm diameter) growing in C3H/HeJ female mice 3–4 weeks following inoculation. Cells were pressed through #45 mesh stainless steel screens in Medium 199 (M199) (Grand Island, New York) without addition of trypsin. Cell clumps were then allowed to settle and the supernatant single cell suspensions were washed three times in M199 and counted in hemocytometers. Viability was determined by trypan blue exclusion (*6*).

In transplanted tumor experiments, the living tumor cells were injected into the subcutaneous (s.c.) tissue of the lateral posterior flank of recipient C3H/HeJ or C3HeB/FeJ mice. The largest diameter of the growing tumor was measured by calipers three times weekly and the day of death was also recorded.

Neuraminidase: VCN obtained from Behring Diagnostics (Somerville, New Jersey), is stated to contain 500U enzyme/ml. (One unit of activity is equivalent to the release of 1 μg of N-acetylneuraminic acid from a glycoprotein substrate at 37°C in 15 min at pH 5.5.) VCN is inactivated by heating to 65°C for 30 min or 100°C for 10 min. Sialic acid is released from cell surfaces of normal and malignant cells by VCN at neutral pH without affecting cell viability (*7–13*). Tumor cells in M199 (pH 7.2) were incubated for one hour at 37°C with 25U VCN/ml/10^6 cells, with heat-inactivated VCN, or with M199. The cells were washed three times prior to injection as a challenging inoculum into tumor-bearing hosts.

Mitomycin C: Mitomycin C was obtained from Sigma Chemical Co. (St. Louis, Missouri) and incubated with tumor cells in a concentration of 25 μg/ml/10^6 cells in the same incubation mixture with VCN or heat-inactivated VCN. We have previously demonstrated that mitomycin C has no adverse effect on the efficacy of VCN-treated cells to induce immunospecific regression of firmly established MCA fibrosarcomas in C3H/HeJ mice. Mitomycin C treatment of tumor cells does not increase the uptake of trypan blue by such tumor cell suspensions, but effectively prevents the growth of palpable tumors from the treated cells.

Transplantable tumor experimental protocol: The basic experimental design in transplantable tumor experiments was to inoculate adult female C3H/HeJ mice or C3HeB/FeJ mice with viable tumor cells s.c. into the left lateral posterior flanks. The tumors usually reached palpable size by day 6 and measured 0.3–0.9 cm by day 15. The tumors were then either left untreated or excised, and the host was challenged with VCN-treated cells into the s.c. tissues of the right flank. The challenging inoculum was then repeated on alternate days to a total of 6 inoculations. The effect of VCN-treated tumor cells on the growth of the firmly established mammary tumors was then determined.

Spontaneous tumor experimental protocol: Our experiments utilizing spontaneous tumors were somewhat different. Adult female C3H/HeJ mice naturally infected with the MTV were utilized. Mice were purchased when they were 9–15 months old and after having delivered multiple litters at the Jackson Laboratories. The mice were examined twice weekly for the appearance of spontaneous mammary adenocarcinomas. When the tumors were found (0.7–0.9 cm in diameter) the mice were individually placed in precoded cages. A second investigator then utilized the code to determine the tumor treatment to be administered.

Two experiments were designed. In the first, the tumor treatment consisted of intratumor injections every fourth day with 0.1 ml sterile solution containing M199, 50 U of VCN, heat-inactivated VCN, 1 mg *M. bovis* (strain BCG), or a combination of VCN, heat-inactivated VCN, and/or BCG. Tumor diameter was measured every 4 days just prior to next treatment, and the date of death recorded.

In the second set of experiments designed to treat spontaneous mammary tumors in retired breeding C3H/HeJ female mice, surgical excision was combined with VCN or inactivated VCN-treated autochthonous or M-1 cells. When the spontaneous tumors were found the mice were individually placed in pre-coded cages. Fourteen days later, when progressive tumor growth was assured, tumor excision and immunotherapy was carried out according to the cage code. The immunotherapeutic code was not revealed until after excision was performed in order to eliminate bias in the performance of the surgery.

Effect of VCN-treated Mammary Carcinoma Cells on Growth of Established Transplantable Mammary Adenocarcinomas in Syngeneic C3H/HeJ Hosts

In the left flank of recipient syngeneic C3H/HeJ mice, 40,000 M-1 transplantable mammary adenocarcinoma cells were injected s.c. Fifteen days thereafter, when the tumor nodules measured 0.3–0.8 cm in diameter, recipient mice were inoculated with 10^6 M-1 tumor cells that had been incubated either with VCN (plus mitomycin) or heat-inactivated VCN (plus mitomycin). Results are summarized in Table 1. The injection of 10^6 M-1 tumor cells exposed to heat-inactivated VCN did not affect the progressive fatal growth of the tumors. In contrast, injection of 10^6 VCN-treated M-1 cells markedly slowed tumor growth and produced total regression of 4/40 firmly established M-1 mammary adenocarcinomas. Animals whose tumors totally disappeared survived indefinitely, and life was significantly

TABLE 1. Effect of VCN-treated M-1 Mammary Adenocarcinoma Cells on Regression of M-1 Tumors in C3H/HeJ Mice

Group	Treatment of cellular challenge[a]	Fraction 1° tumor undergoing total regression	Mean tumor diameter day 30 (cm±SE)	Mean day of death (±SE)[b]
1	—	0/30	1.89±0.09	49.4±2.2
2	VCN	4/40	1.06±0.10[c]	60.4±3.3[c]
3	Inactive VCN	0/40	1.79±0.07	49.3±2.1

[a] Challenging inocula consisted of 6 injections of 10^6 M-1 cells incubated with VCN (25 U/ml/10^6 cells) or heat-inactivated VCN (plus mitomycin C). First challenge was given 15 days after tumor inoculation and subsequent challenges at 2-day intervals. [b] Does not include mice whose tumors totally regressed. [c] $P \leq 0.05$ when compared to groups 1 and 3 by Student's t test.

TABLE 2. Effect of VCN-treated M-2 Mammary Adenocarcinoma Cells on Regression of M-2 Tumors in C3H/HeJ Mice

Group	Treatment of cellular challenge[a]	Fraction 1° tumors undergoing total regression	Mean tumor diameter day 30 (cm±SE)	Mean day of death (±SE)[b]
1	—	0/10	1.24±0.04	78.0±2.3
2	VCN	1/10	0.51±0.08[c]	94.3±3.7[c]
3	Inactive VCN	0/10	1.07±0.04	72.4±2.2

[a] Challenging inocula consisted of 6 injections of 10^6 M-2 cells incubated with VCN (25 U/ml/10^6 cells) or heat-inactivated VCN (plus mitomycin C). First challenge was given 15 days after tumor inoculation and subsequent challenges at 2-day intervals. [b] Does not include mice whose tumors totally regressed. [c] $P \leq 0.05$ when compared to groups 1 and 3 by Student's t test.

TABLE 3. Effect of VCN-treated M-1 or M-2 Cells on Regression of M-1 Tumors in C3H/HeJ Mice

Group	Challenging tumor	Treatment of cellular challenge[a]	Fraction 1° tumors undergoing total regression	Mean tumor diameter day 30 (cm±SE)	Mean day of death (±SE)[b]
1	—	—	0/20	1.73±0.10	51.0±3.8
2	M-1	VCN	1/20	1.03±0.12[c]	66.8±4.8[c]
3	M-1	Inactive VCN	0/20	1.79±0.10	52.7±3.3
4	M-2	VCN	0/20	1.81±0.08	53.5±3.2
5	M-2	Inactive VCN	0/20	1.82±0.09	51.4±3.2

[a] Challenging inocula consisted of 6 injections of M-1 or M-2 cells incubated with VCN (25 U/ml/10^6 cells) or heat-inactivated VCN (plus mitomycin C). First challenge was given 15 days after tumor inoculation and subsequent challenges at 2-day intervals. [b] Does not include animals whose tumors totally regressed. [c] $P \leq 0.05$ when compared to groups 1, 3, 4 and 5 by Student's t test.

prolonged even in those animals whose tumors did not totally disappear. A similar experiment was carried out with a second mammary adenocarcinoma (M-2) (Table 2).

Two experiments were then done to determine the immunospecificity of the regression induced by VCN-treated mammary adenocarcinoma cells. The first such experiment is summarized in Table 3. Into the left flank of syngeneic C3H/HeJ mice, 40,000 M-1 mammary adenocarcinoma cells were injected s.c. Fifteen days later, tumor-bearing mice were challenged with 10^6 M-1 or 10^6 M-2 mammary adenocarcinoma cells that had been exposed to VCN (plus mitomycin) or heat-inactivated VCN (plus mitomycin). Slowing of tumor growth and prolongation of life in mice with M-1 tumors were seen only when injections of M-1 tumor exposed to VCN were given. Total regression in this series occurred in 1 of 20 animals. Tumor growth was not inhibited in recipients challenged with M-2 tumors or recipients challenged with M-1 tumors treated with inactivated VCN (Table 3).

Cross-immunization of M-1 Tumors with M-2 Tumors in C3HeB/FeJ Mice

These results suggested that M-1 and M-2 did not share the same tumor-specific transplantation antigens. We needed to confirm this fact before proceeding further. 10^6 M-1 or M-2 viable tumor cells from C3H/HeJ mice were injected s.c. in the left

TABLE 4.   Growth of M-1 or M-2 Mammary Carcinomas in C3HeB/FeJ Mice Pre-exposed to M-1 or M-2 Tumors

Primary inoculum	Challenging tumor	No. of cells	Fraction of mice supporting secondary tumor
None	M-1	5×10^3	3/20
		5×10^4	14/20
		5×10^5	20/20
	M-2	5×10^3	3/20
		5×10^4	15/20
		5×10^5	20/20
C3H/HeJ spleen cells	M-1	5×10^3	1/10
		5×10^4	6/10
		5×10^5	10/10
	M-2	5×10^3	1/10
		5×10^4	7/10
		5×10^5	10/10
C3HeB/FeJ spleen cells	M-1	5×10^3	1/10
		5×10^4	7/10
		5×10^5	10/10
	M-2	5×10^3	1/10
		5×10^4	8/10
		5×10^5	10/10
M-1	M-1	5×10^3	2/10
		5×10^4	1/10
		5×10^5	4/10
	M-2	5×10^3	2/10
		5×10^4	3/10
		5×10^5	4/10
M-2	M-1	5×10^3	0/20
		5×10^4	1/20
		5×10^5	1/20
	M-2	5×10^3	0/20
		5×10^4	0/20
		5×10^5	1/20

posterior flank of adult female C3HeB/FeJ mice. All injected mice developed tumors. Control mice received 10^6 C3H/HeJ or C3HeB/FeJ spleen cells or an equal volume (0.1 ml) of M199. Two weeks following the injection, when the tumors ranged in size from 0.8 to 1.6 cm diameter the tumor masses were totally excised, and excision of normal tissues were performed in mice not bearing tumors. Two weeks after tumor excision (1 month after tumor inoculation), all mice were challenged in the s.c. tissues of the right posterior flank with 5×10^3, 5×10^4, or 5×10^5 M-1 or M-2 viable tumor cells. The results are recorded in Table 4. C3HeB/FeJ mice who had not received previous injections of M-1 or M-2 tumor cells developed tumors from the challenging inocula which progressed to death (Table 4). C3HeB/FeJ mice pre-exposed to nonmalignant C3H/HeJ or C3HeB/FeJ spleen cells supported a similar proportion of either M-1 or M-2 tumors. C3HeB/FeJ mice immunized with either M-1 or M-2 tumors failed to support both M-1 or M-2 tumors ($P \leq 0.05$) although it seemed that mice pre-exposed to M-2 tumors supported a significantly smaller proportion of either M-1 or M-2 tumors, than did mice pre-exposed to M-1 tumors ($P \leq 0.05$). These results strongly suggest that M-1 and M-2 tumors share the same MTV antigen, and that C3HeB/FeJ mice can be immunized by the MTV antigen from the C3H/HeJ mammary tumors (Table 4).

Effect of VCN-treated Mammary Carcinoma Cells on the Growth of Simultaneous Established M-1 and M-2 Tumors in Syngeneic C3H/HeJ or C3HeB/FeJ Mice

Forty thousand viable M-1 tumor cells were injected s.c. in the left flank of

TABLE 5. Immunospecificity of Mammary Tumor Regression in Viral-infested (C3H/HeJ) or Viral-free (C3HeB/FeJ) Mice Bearing Both M-1 and M-2 Tumors

Tumor bearing host	Group	Treatment of challenging inoculum[a]		Fraction tumors regressing		Mean tumor diameter day 30 (cm $\pm$ SE)	
				M-1[b]	M-2[b]	M-1	M-2
C3H/HeJ	1	None	M199	0/14	0/14	0.90±0.07	1.20±0.06
	2	M-1	VCN	3/20	0/20	0.40±0.05[c]	1.32±0.06
	3	M-1	Inactive VCN	0/17	0/17	0.86±0.04	1.19±0.06
	4	M-2	VCN	0/19	1/19	1.07±0.06	0.52±0.08[d]
	5	M-2	Inactive VCN	0/15	0/15	1.11±0.05	1.46±0.07
C3HeB/FeJ	6	None	M199	0/10	0/19	1.09±0.05	1.06±0.03
	7	M-1	VCN	6/19	0/19	0.37±0.06[e]	1.11±0.04
	8	M-1	Inactive VCN	0/18	0/18	0.87±0.03	1.03±0.04
	9	M-2	VCN	0/20	4/20	0.96±0.04	0.42±0.07[f]
	10	M-2	Inactive VCN	0/19	0/19	0.94±0.04	1.22±0.04

[a] Challenging inocula consisted of 6 injections of M-1 or M-2 cells which had been incubated with 25 U/ml/10^6 cells of VCN or heat-inactivated VCN (plus mitomycin C). The first challenge was given 12 days after tumor inoculation and subsequent challenges at 2-day intervals. [b] Does not include animals whose tumors blended so that each could not be separately distinguished. [c] $P \leq 0.05$ when compared to groups 1, 3, 4, 5, and contralateral tumor. [d] $P \leq 0.05$ when compared to groups 1, 2, 3, 5, and contralateral tumor. [e] $P \leq 0.05$ when compared to groups 6, 8, 9, 10, and contralateral tumor. [f] $P \leq 0.05$ when compared to groups 6, 7, 8, 10, and contralateral tumor.

C3H/HeJ or C3HeB/FeJ mice. Simultaneously 40,000 M-2 tumors were injected in the right flank of the same mice. Thus, separate M-1 and M-2 tumors were established in both the MTV-infested C3H/HeJ mice and in the MTV-free C3HeB/FeJ mice. Twelve days thereafter, after separate tumors were palpable, the mice were challenged at a third site with either 10^6 M-1 or M-2 tumor cells which had been exposed to VCN (plus mitomycin) or inactivated VCN (plus mitomycin). The regression of the pre-existing tumors was then determined. The results are shown in Table 5. Inhibition of growth and regression of firmly established M-1 tumors took place only in animals challenged with VCN-treated M-1 tumors. M-1 tumors did not regress when mice were challenged with M-1 tumors exposed to inactivated VCN, nor did the M-1 tumor regress when treated with M-2 cells exposed to VCN or inactivated VCN. Conversely, M-2 tumors did not regress if mice were challenged with M-2 tumors exposed to inactivated VCN, or to M-1 cells in any form. The strain of the host mouse had no effect on this response. Even the C3HeB/FeJ mice free of the MTV virus failed to reject M-1 tumors when challenged with VCN-treated M-2 cells, and *vice versa.*

Effect of Neuraminidase-treated Mammary Adenocarcinoma Cells on the Regression of Partially and Totally Excised Adenocarcinomas in C3H/HeJ Mice

Eighty thousand M-2 mammary adenocarcinoma cells were injected s.c. into the left flank of recipient C3H/HeJ mice. Fifteen or 25 days thereafter, wedge excision, enucleation or total tumor excision was carried out and the mice challenged with 10^6 living M-2 tumor cells which had been incubated either with VCN or heat-inactivated VCN (plus mitomycin). The results are tabulated in Table 6. Mice challenged on either day 15 or day 25 with VCN-treated tumor cells demonstrated significant slowing of tumor growth. Wedge excision of the tumor on day 15 added nothing to the immunoregressive effect of VCN-treated tumor cells. One of 10 tumors disappeared even without tumor excision.

When treatment was delayed until day 25, tumor regrowth was significantly inhibited by a combination of partial, subtotal, or attempted total excision plus challenge with VCN-treated tumor cells. Seven of 10 animals were cured by attempted total tumor excision plus VCN-treated tumor cells. Partial tumor excision plus challenge with heat-inactivated VCN-treated tumor cells did not significantly inhibit tumor regrowth, and total excision plus inactivated VCN-treated tumor cells cured only three of 10 animals.

Effect of Direct Intratumor Injections of Neuraminidase and/or BCG into Spontaneous Mammary Adenocarcinomas in C3H/HeJ Mice

It is possible that transplantable mammary tumors do not resemble spontaneous mammary tumors in their responses to immunotherapy with neuraminidase-treated cells. Since we had shown that the repeated intralesional injection of VCN into transplantable fibrosarcomas led to the immunospecific rejection of these

TABLE 6. Effect of Tumor Excision and Immunotherapy on the Growth of M-2 Tumors in C3H/

Group No.	Interval between 1° and excision (days)	Excision	Treatment of cellular challenge[a]	Fraction 1° tumors totally regressing
1[c]	—	None	—	0/10
2	15	None	VCN	1/10
3	15	None	Inactive VCN	0/10
4	15	Wedge	VCN	0/10
5	15	Wedge	Inactive VCN	0/10
6[c]	—	None	—	0/10
7	25	None	VCN	0/10
8	25	None	Inactive VCN	0/10
9	25	Enucleation	VCN	1/10
10	25	Enucleation	Inactive VCN	0/10
11	25	Total	VCN	7/10
12	25	Total	Inactive VCN	3/10

[a] Challenging inocula consisted of 6 injections of 10^6 M-2 cells; the first challenge was given 15 or 25 whose tumors totally regressed.   [c] Groups 1 and 6 refer to the same animals, tumors being measured test).   [e] $P \leq 0.05$ when compared to groups 6, 8, and 10 (Student's t test).   [f] $P \leq 0.05$ when compared

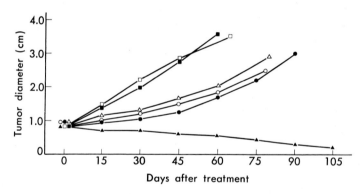

Fig. 1. Response of spontaneous mammary adenocarcinomas to repeated intratumor injections of VCN and/or BCG. Half the animals in each group were dead at the termination of the growth lines. ○ BCG; ● VCN; △ inactivated VCN+BCG; ▲ VCN+BCG; □ inactivated VCN; ■ M-199.

tumors (14), we attempted to determine if such treatment would have a similar effect on spontaneous mammary tumors.

Figure 1 illustrates the mean tumor diameter of tumors treated by intralesional injections of VCN and/or BCG. Neither M-199 nor heat-inactivated VCN injected directly into the spontaneous mammary adenocarcinoma had any effect on the progressive growth and early death of the mice. Metastases were found in the livers and the lungs of such mice by 60 days after treatment. The intratumor injection of 1 mg of viable BCG, however, led to tumor regression. Four of 13 tumors disappeared in recipients of intratumor injections of 50 U of VCN plus 1 mg of

HeJ Mice

Mean tumor diameter (cm±SE)			Mean day of death[b] (±SE)
24 hr prior to excision	24 hr post excision	2 weeks post excision	
0.27±0.03	0.29±0.03	1.47±0.09	60.9± 4.9
0.26±0.03	0.30±0.03	0.56±0.10[d]	65.9± 5.9
0.28±0.03	0.31±0.03	1.44±0.08	64.0± 4.2
0.25±0.02	0.27±0.02	0.86±0.15[d]	61.0± 5.7
0.28±0.03	0.30±0.02	1.03±0.21	59.7± 5.1
0.96±0.05	1.19±0.06	2.61±0.19	60.9± 4.9
0.95±0.04	1.08±0.06	1.85±0.17[e,f]	74.7± 3.1[e,f]
0.91±0.04	1.11±0.04	2.78±0.09	59.8± 3.0
0.95±0.05	0.61±0.05	0.98±0.13[e,f]	87.0± 4.4[e,f]
0.90±0.03	0.63±0.06	2.22±0.18	65.0± 3.5
0.91±0.03	0.00±0.00	0.14±0.07[e]	103.7±13.0[e,f]
0.92±0.03	0.00±0.00	0.33±0.16[e]	77.6±13.5[e]

days after tumor inoculation with subsequent challenges at 2-day intervals.   [b] Does not include mice at differing intervals after implantation.   [d] $P \leq 0.05$ when compared to groups 1, 3, and 5 (Student's t with mice challenged with inactive VCN-treated cells (Student's t test).

BCG every 4 days. The life in these animals was significantly prolonged when compared with those that received the intratumor injections of VCN or BCG alone.

Table 7 demonstrates that second mammary adenocarcinomas frequently developed in mice treated with VCN and/or BCG. These tumors developed only in animals that demonstrated some slowing of the growth of the first tumor. The more effective the treatment, the more often did secondary tumors arise. Three animals even developed a third tumor, and one of these animals developed a fourth. Regression could be induced by the same treatment used for treatment of the primary tumor in 2 of 9 tumors and the growth of most was inhibited by the local injection of the substance which had induced regression of the primary tumor.

TABLE 7.   Development of Second Spontaneous Mammary Adenocarcinomas in C3H/HeJ Mice Bearing Primary Tumors Treated by Intralesional Injections of Neuraminidase (VCN) and/or BCG

Intratumor Rx	Mean day of death	Second tumor	Day of second tumor
M199	66.5	0/11	—
Inactive VCN	50.8	0/11	—
VCN	88.4	4/10	28, 35, 47, 51
BCG	79.5	1/10[a]	32
Inactive VCN+BCG	83.1	2/10[a]	24, 118
VCN+BCG	107.0	9/13[a]	27, 28, 50, 52, 54, 57, 62, 83

[a] One developed 3rd or 4th tumors.

Effect of Neuraminidase-treated Tumor Cells on the Regression of Totally Excised Spontaneous Mammary Carcinomas

C3H/HeJ retired breeding female mice were randomly assigned to treatment categories after development of spontaneous tumors. Fourteen days after tumor appearance, total excision of the tumors with narrow margins was carried out and the mice re-randomized to treatment cages. Immunotherapy in these mice was then carried out utilizing VCN-treated autochthonous or M-1 mammary adeno-carcinoma cells or inactivated VCN-treated autochthonous tumor cells. Untreated mice died from progressively growing tumor in all cases (Fig. 2). Total excision without immunotherapy cured the local tumor in 7 of the 15 mice and significantly prolonged life. Total excision, plus VCN-treated, M-1 cells locally cured 7 of the 15 mice. Life was significantly prolonged in this group when compared with the untreated mice but the survival was not significantly different when compared with excision alone. Mice treated with total excision plus inactivated VCN-treated autochthonous tumor cells survived significantly longer than did untreated mice but not longer than did mice treated with total excision without immunotherapy. Only one of these mice was cured of the local tumor. The longest survival was seen in mice treated by total excision and VCN-treated autochthonous tumor cells. Here, 8 of the 15 mice were totally cured of the primary tumor. The survival of this group as a whole was significantly better than mice treated by total excision plus VCN-treated M-1 tumor cells or mice treated with total excision plus in-activated VCN-treated autochthonous cells.

A number of observations have suggested that VCN increases the immuno-genicity of cells exposed to it *in vitro*. (a) Fetal tissue incubated in VCN and injected into allogeneic recipients results in a greater degree of sensitization of those recipients than animals injected with fetal tissue exposed to heat-inactivated VCN (*15*). (b) When small nonimmunogenic doses of lymphoid cells were injected into allogeneic

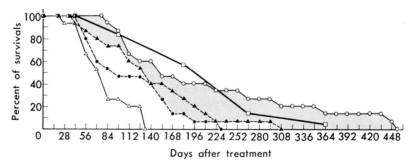

FIG. 2. Effect of treatment on the cumulative survival of C3H/HeJ female mice bearing spontaneous mammary tumors. The tumors were treated by total excision and VCN-treated tumor cells. Excision plus VCN-treated transplantable mammary tumor cells (M-1) prolong-ed life no longer than excision alone. Excision plus VCN-treated autochthonous cells led to prolongation of survival equal to that enjoyed by cohort mice of the same age who did not develop tumors at all. 15 mice per group. ○ excision+VCN-treated autoch-thonous cells; ● excision+VCN-treated M-1 cells; △ no excision; ▲ excision; □ no tumor.

recipients, donor skin grafts were rejected significantly more rapidly (*16*). (c) Cyclophosphamide-prepared mice do not become tolerant of VCN-treated bone marrow cells (*17*). (d) Human lymphocytes treated with VCN and mitomycin are severalfold more stimulating to allogeneic lymphocytes in one-way mixed lymphocyte culture than are lymphocytes treated with mitomycin alone (*18, 19*). (e) TA-3 tumor (*20*), Landschutz ascites tumor (*8*), L1210 leukemia (*7*), MCA-induced fibrosarcoma (*1, 21, 22*), and Ehrlich ascites tumors (*23*) grow less well in normally susceptible recipients if the tumor cells have been incubated in VCN. Recipients that survive the primary tumor inoculum are rendered immune to subsequent inocula of untreated cells (*21–23*). We have shown that total immunospecific regression of firmly established MCA fibrosarcomas can be induced by challenging the tumor-bearing animals with syngeneic tumor cells treated *in vitro* with VCN. The effect was shown to be due to the enzymatic action of VCN on the sialic acid residues of the tumor cell surfaces since heat-inactivation of the VCN or incubation of VCN and tumor cells with an excess of sialic acid or neuraminilactose (*24*) destroyed the ability of such cells to induce tumor regression (*1*). Similar results in murine leukemia systems have been obtained by Bekesi *et al.* (*12*), and by Kollmorgen (*25*).

Subsequent experiments demonstrated that immunospecific regression of tumors can be induced by injecting VCN directly into the tumor mass even after it has become firmly established and is growing actively (*14*). With injections of VCN beginning on day 15 when the tumors were small (0.6–0.9 cm), complete disappearance of the tumor could be achieved in a number of treated animals. The treatment was totally immunospecific and regression of untreated tumor nodules could be induced by injecting VCN into immunologically identical tumors on the opposite side. Tumors which were not identical to the treated tumor, however, continued to grow and kill the animal. Indeed, it was possible to induce tumor regression by immunologic means in animals that were simultaneously dying of an immunologically distinct tumor (*14*). Intralesional BCG will induce the regression of syngenic hepatomas in guinea pigs (*26*), a few melanomas in man (*27*) and, if used repeatedly, will induce the regression of a few MCA-induced fibrosarcomas in mice (*28*). By itself, however, BCG is not very effective in mice.

The present results demonstrate that the immunospecific regression of firmly established solid syngeneic transplantable tumors by VCN-treated cells is not restricted to MCA-induced fibrosarcomas. The growth of transplantable mammary tumors in C3H/HeJ mice is also inhibited if their hosts are challenged with VCN-treated tumor cells of the same tumor line. The curative effect can be augmented by total or near-total excision of advanced transplantable mammary tumors.

The immunospecificity of this effect appears to be remarkable. Both M-1 and M-2 tumors appear to share tumor antigens—presumably the MTV antigen shared by all known (C3H/HeJ) mammary tumors (*27, 29*). The C3HeB/FeJ mouse is capable of being immunized to this shared antigen. However, once established, M-1 tumor cannot be inhibited by VCN-treated M-2 tumor, or *vice versa*. This inability of the neonatally MTV-infested C3H/HeJ host to respond might be expected since tolerance to the MTV antigen has been postulated in this strain

(*27*). However, even the C3HeB/FeJ host appears to be unresponsive to immuno-therapy with a VCN-treated MTV cell. The deficit in response does not appear to rest with the tumor host or the tumor itself, since immunoregression of both tumors in either host can be induced with VCN-treated cells of the specific tumor type. Thus, VCN appears capable of increasing the immunogenicity of specific private tumor antigens without increasing the immunogenicity of the shared MTV antigen on mammary carcinomas. Such "private" tumor antigens have been detected in some murine mammary carcinomas but they are very weak (*27, 29*). These results may help to explain the results of subsequent experiments utilizing spontaneous tumors in C3H/HeJ mice. The growth of such spontaneous tumors can be inhibited by intratumor injections of VCN or BCG. New mammary adeno-carcinomas histologically identical with the regressing tumor appear in untreated mammary glands. These tumors were similar to those appearing in C3H/HeJ mice if the primary tumors were excised (*28*). Therefore, the induction of im-munity to the primary tumor is unaccompanied by immunity to the MTV-asso-ciated antigen present on mammary tumors arising in this strain. If immunity had been induced to the MTV-associated antigen, new tumors would not have arisen. The best hypothesis to explain the appearance of new MTV tumors in mice cured of the primary MTV tumor by immunotherapy is that the immunotherapeutic response is a result of immunization to "private" tumor-specific antigens coexisting on the surface of MTV tumors. Why VCN is incapable of increasing the im-munogenicity of the relatively strong MTV antigen in C3H/HeJ mice is not sur-prising since these mice are infected with the virus since birth. Although true tolerance may not be present, effective immunity might be difficult to establish. Why VCN is incapable of increasing the immunogenicity of the MTV-associated antigen in the viral-free C3HeB/FeJ mouse is less clear. It is possible that VCN actually damages the MTV antigen as it does the M and N antigens on human red blood cells (*30*).

Whatever the mechanism, these findings stimulated us to perform the last experiment involving the treatment of spontaneous mammary tumors with surgical excision plus immunotherapy with autochthonous or syngeneic M-1 tumor cells. Here again more prolonged survival was obtained after total tumor excision and immunotherapy with VCN-treated autochthonous cells than with M-1 cells which share the MTV-associated antigen.

These findings may be of particular importance in the experimental practice of immunotherapy. Many human tumors are thought to share antigens (*31*) perhaps because of their common viral etiology. If it were possible to use vaccines of homol-ogous tumors bearing cross-reacting antigens, clinical immunotherapy would be simplified. The present study suggests that autochthonous tumor cells might have unsuspected advantages in some cases.

How VCN increases the immunogenicity of cellular antigens is unknown but several correlates exist.

VCN acts on both synthetic substrates (*33, 34*) and cell surfaces to release sialic acid residues (*7–12, 31, 32*). Removing these sialic acid residues from the cell surface reduces the negative charge of the cell (*35*), increases cell deformability

(*36*), and increases the susceptibility of the cell to phagocytosis (*37, 38*). All these factors might increase the availability of tumor-specific antigenic sites on the cell surface to immunoreactive cells in the host. Some investigators (*30, 39–41*) have even demonstrated the unmasking of various antigens on cells treated with VCN, though this may not be true for all antigens (*9*). That such a variety of normal and malignant cells can be made more immunogenic by treatment with VCN suggests that VCN acts nonspecifically to render cells more susceptible to immunologic processing by the recipient. Such a process is analogous to changing the immunogenicity of a haptene by changing the characteristics of the carrier molecule.

Most interesting in this regard is the suggestion by Rosenberg and Schwarz (*42*) that mice may have a natural antibody to cellular antigens (distinct from tumor antigens) unmasked by VCN. Rosenberg and Rogentine (*43*), Rogentine and Plocinik (*44*), and Reisner (*40*) have independently demonstrated similar natural antibodies in man. It is possible that the binding of the natural antibody to VCN-treated tumor cells in some way renders tumor antigens on the cells more immunogenic.

REFERENCES

1. Simmons, R. L., Rios, A., and Lundgren, G. Immunospecific regression of methylcholanthrene fibrosarcoma using neuraminidase. Surgery, *70*: 38–46, 1971.
2. Simmons, R. L. and Rios, A. Immunotherapy of cancer: Immunospecific rejection of tumors in recipients of neuraminidase-treated tumor cells plus BCG. Science, *174*: 591–593, 1971.
3. Simmons, R. L. and Rios, A. Immunospecific regression of methylcholanthrene fibrosarcoma using neuraminidase. III. Synergistic effect of BCG and neuraminidase treated tumor cells. Ann. Surg., *176*: 188–194, 1972.
4. Jax Notes (Jackson Laboratory, Bar Harbor, Maine), No. 410, February, 1972.
5. Heppner, G. H. Personal communication.
6. Boyse, E. A., Old, L. J., and Chouroulinkov, I. Cytotoxic test for demonstration of mouse antibody. *In;* H. N. Eisen (ed.), Methods in Medical Research, vol. 10, pp. 39–47, Year Book Medical Publishers Inc., Chicago, 1964.
7. Bagshawe, K. D. and Currie, G. A. Immunogenicity of L1210 murine leukemia cells after treatment with neuraminidase. Nature, *218*: 1254–1255, 1968.
8. Currie, G. A. and Bagshawe, K. D. The role of sialic acid in antigenic expression: Further studies of the Landschutz ascites tumour. Brit. J. Cancer, *22*: 843–853, 1968.
9. Ray, P. K. and Simmons, R. L. Failure of neuraminidase to unmask allogeneic antigens on cell surfaces. Proc. Soc. Exp. Biol. Med., *138*: 600–604, 1971.
10. Sanford, B. H. and Codington, J. F. Further studies on the effect of neuraminidase on tumor cell transplantability. Tissue Antigens, *1*: 153–161, 1971.
11. Woodruff, J. J. and Gesner, B. M. The effect of neuraminidase on the fate of transfused lymphocytes. J. Exp. Med., *129*: 551–567, 1969.
12. Bekesi, J. G. St., Arneault, G., and Walter, L. Immunogenicity of leukemia L1210 cells after neuraminidase treatment. J. Natl. Cancer Inst., *49*: 107–118, 1972.
13. Rosenberg, S. A. and Einstein, A. B. Sialic acids on the plasma membrane of cul-

tured human lymphoid cells: Chemical aspects and biosynthesis. J. Cell Biol., *53*: 466–473, 1972.

14. Simmons, R. L. and Rios, A. Immunospecific regression of methylcholanthrene fibrosarcoma using neuraminidase. II. Intratumor injections of neuraminidase. Surgery, *71*: 556–564, 1972.

15. Simmons, R. L., Lipschultz, M. L., and Rios, A. Failure of neuraminidase to unmask histocompatibility antigens on trophoblast. Nature New Biol., *231*: 111–112, 1971.

16. Simmons, R. L., Rios, A., and Ray, P. K. Immunogenicity and antigenicity of lymphoid cells treated with neuraminidase. Nature New Biol., *231*: 179–181, 1971.

17. Im, H. M. and Simmons, R. L. Modification of graft-*versus*-host disease by neuraminidase treatment of donor cells. Decreased tolerogenicity of neuraminidase treated cells. Transplantation, *12*: 472–478, 1971.

18. Lundgren, G., Jeitz, L., and Lundin, L. Increased stimulation by neuraminidase treated cells in mixed lymphocyte cultures. Fed. Proc., *30*: 395, 1971.

19. Lundgren, G. and Simmons, R. L. Effect of neuraminidase on the stimulatory capacity of cells in human mixed lymphocyte cultures. Clin. Exp. Immunol., *9*: 915–926, 1971.

20. Sanford, B. H. An alteration in tumor histocompatibility induced by neuraminidase. Transplantation, *4*: 1273–1279, 1967.

21. Currie, G. A. and Bagshawe, K. D. Tumour specific immunogenicity of methylcholanthrene-induced sarcoma cells after incubation in neuraminidase. Brit. J. Cancer, *23*: 141–149, 1969.

22. Simmons, R. L., Rios, A., and Ray, P. K. Effect of neuraminidase on the growth of a 3-methylcholanthrene induced fibrosarcoma in normal and immunosuppressed syngeneic mice. J. Natl. Cancer Inst., *47*: 1087–1094, 1971.

23. Lindemann, J. and Klein, P. A. Immunological aspects of viral oncolysis. Recent Results Cancer Res., *9*: 66, 1967.

24. Simmons, R. L. and Rios, A. Immunospecific regression of methylcholanthrene fibrosarcoma with the use of neuraminidase. V. Quantitative aspects of the experimental immunotherapeutic model. Israel J. Med. Sci., *10*: 925–938, 1974.

25. Kollmorgen, G. M., Erwin, D. N., and Killion, J. J. Combination chemotherapy and immunotherapy of transplantable murine leukemia. Proc. Am. Assoc. Cancer Res., *14*: 69, 1973.

26. Zbar, B. and Tanaka, T. Immunotherapy of cancer: Regression of tumors after intralesional injection of living *Mycobacterium bovis*. Science, *172*: 271–273, 1971.

27. Morton, D. L., Goldman, L., and Wood, D. A. Acquired immunological tolerance and carcinogenesis by the mammary tumor virus. II. Immune responses influencing growth of spontaneous mammary adenocarcinomas. J. Natl. Cancer Inst., *42*: 321–329, 1969.

28. Rios, A. and Simmons, R. L. Comparative effect of *Mycobacterium bovis*- and neuraminidase-treated tumor cells on the growth of established methylcholanthrene fibrosarcomas in syngeneic mice. Cancer Res., *32*: 16–22, 1972.

29. Heppner, G. H. Studies on serum-mediated inhibition of cellular immunity to spontaneous mouse mammary tumors. Int. J. Cancer, *4*: 608–615, 1969.

30. Kassulke, J. T., Stutman, C., and Yunis, E. J. Blood group isoantigens in leukemic cells: Reversibility of isoantigenic changes by neuraminidase. J. Natl. Cancer Inst., *46*: 1201–1208, 1971.

31. Morton, D. L. and Malmgren, R. A. Human osteosarcomas: Immunological evidence suggesting an associated infectious agent. Science, *162*:1279–1281, 1968.

32. Morton, D. L., Goldman, L., and Wood, D. A. Acquired immunological tolerance and carcinogenesis by the mammary tumor virus. II. Immune responses influencing growth of spontaneous mammary adenocarcinomas. J. Natl. Cancer Inst., *42*: 321–329, 1969.

33. Drzeniek, R. Differences in splitting capacity of virus and *Vibrio cholerae* neuraminidases on sialic acid type substrates. Biochem. Biophys. Res. Commun., *26*: 631–638, 1967.

34. Drzeniek, R. and Gaube, A. Differences in substrate specificity of myxovirus neuraminidases. Biochem. Biophys. Res. Commun., *38*: 651–654, 1970.

35. Simon-Reuss, I., Cook, C. M., and Seaman, C.V.F. Electrophoretic studies on some types of mammalian tissue cells. Cancer Res., *24*: 2038–2043, 1964.

36. Weiss, L. Studies on cell deformability. I. Effect of surface charge. J. Cell Biol., *26*: 735–744, 1965.

37. Weiss, L., Mayhew, E., and Ulrich, K. The effect of neuraminidase on the phagocytic process in human monocytes. Lab. Invest., *15*: 1304–1309, 1966.

38. Lee, A. Effect of neuraminidase on the phagocytosis of heterologous red cells by mouse peripheral macrophages. Proc. Soc. Exp. Biol. Med., *128*: 891–894, 1968.

39. Ray, P. K. and Simmons, R. L. Unmasking of xenogeneic neoantigens on mouse lymphoid cell surfaces by *Vibrio cholerae* neuraminidase. Proc. Soc. Exp. Biol. Med., *142*: 217–222, 1973.

40. Reisner, E. G. and Amos, D. B. The complement-binding and absorptive capacity of human white blood cells treated with neuraminidase. Transplantation, *14*: 455–451, 1972.

41. Rosenberg, S. A., Plocinik, B. A., and Rogentine, G. N., Jr. "Unmasking" of human lymphoid cell heteroantigens by neuraminidase treatment. J. Natl. Cancer Inst., *48*: 1271–1276, 1972.

42. Rosenberg, S. A. and Schwarz, S. Murine antibodies to a cryptic membrane antigen: Possible explanation for neuraminidase-induced increase in cell immunogenicity. J. Natl. Cancer Inst., *52*: 1151–1155, 1974.

43. Rosenberg, S. A. and Rogentine, G. N., Jr. Natural human antibodies to "hidden" membrane components. Nature New Biol., *239*: 203–204, 1972.

44. Rogentine, G. N. and Plocinik, B. A. Carbohydrate inhibition studies of the naturally occuring human antibody to neuraminidase treated human lymphocytes. J. Immunol., *113*: 848–858, 1974.

Discussion of Paper of Drs. Simmons and Rios

DR. M. HOZUMI: Were the effects you observed with neuraminidase special to the *V. cholerae* variety? Also, have you investigated the effects of other enzymes, such as trypsin, on the facilitation of tumor regression?

DR. SIMMONS: The neuraminidases from both *Clostridium perfringens* and *V. cholerae* lyse 2-3, 2-6, and 2-8 glycosidic linkages, but the latter is available commercially in a purer form and was therefore utilized.

Trypsin had no effect in several studies we have performed, and we have screened a number of enzymes *in vitro* in the search for substances active on cell surface substrates which we can detect. Influenza virus neuraminidase has a substrate different from the bacterial varieties but, as it is different to secure, we are ignorant of its effects, if any, on the immunogenicity of tumor cells.

DR. M. HOZUMI: Is there any relationship between the membrane alterations produced by neuraminidase and by concanavalin A (con A)? Secondly, what was the valence of your con A preparation?

DR. SIMMONS: We worked only with tetravalent con A. The cell surface changes induced by these two substances are probably not the same. We have hypothesized that tumor cells treated with either VCN or con A are more easily processed by an animal, a common effect we expect might occur under a number of varying chemical circumstances.

DR. KOBAYASHI: What mode of inoculation of VCN-treated tumor cells offers the maximum effect? Have you examined various routes of administering BCG in the clinical situation?

DR. SIMMONS: In mice, intradermal (i.d.), subcutaneous, intraperitoneal, and intravenous administration all yield similar results. We have chosen to administer these cells i.d. and BCG intraepithelially directly over the VCN-treated tumor inoculum in order to avoid the local necrosis which accompanies i.d. BCG injection. We have not compared the route of BCG inoculation in our patients but have simply selected this one, which seems to least bother them.

DR. CASTRO: In your studies, 1 cm seems to be a critical diameter over which a positive effect with VCN treatment is not realized. Is this related to vascularization of the tumors you employed? Also, does neuraminidase lead to the re-expression of fetal antigens or phase specific antigens? Thirdly, the system in which you used C3H mice with a MTV-associated mammary carcinoma is the same ones in which Prehn noted immunostimulation of tumor growth. Have you observed a similar effect?

DR. SIMMONS: Most studies examining concomitant immunity as measured *in vitro* reveal disappearance of this phenomenon with tumor masses greater than 1 cm in diameter. This is also the size at which necrosis begins to occur. This diameter is, of course, not a sharp demarcation, but generally the smaller the initial neoplasm, the more completely they disappear in our system.

In one preliminary experiment, neuraminidase-treated fetal cells enhanced tumor growth whereas following irradiation they act like VCN-treated specific tumor cells.

We have not seen enhancement using the MTV-associated mammary tumor. There is less local recurrence in the VCN tumor cell inoculum groups, but the incidence at secondaries is the same for all groups when adjusted for individual survival times. Dr. Hosokawa from Hokkaido University is now working in our laboratory and, upon modifying our scheme to give 1×10^6 MCA-induced fibrosacorma cells followed by a VCN-modified tumor cell inoculum on the third day, he noted enhancement.

DR. Y. IKAWA: The majority of tumors which you examined was experimentally induced neoplasms of moderate to high antigenicity. Do you feel that your system is thus directly applicable to the clinical situation which involves many spontaneous epithelial neoplarms of low antigenicity?

DR. SIMMONS: The private tumor-specific antigen on our mammary carcinoma is extremely weak, and evidence for its existence is very difficult to glean *in vitro*, as it is not active in cytotoxicity and immunization systems. The private antigen is so weak that it must be inoculated and rejected two to three times in order to secure good immunization. Some of our other neoplasms are certainly stronger antigenically, but at present we're stuck for models. Some 5 years may be necessary before we can determine strict clinical correlations with the models we have chosen.

DR. KOBAYASHI: Why didn't VCN treatment increase the immunogenicity of MTV-associated antigens?

DR. SIMMONS: We are not sure, but it is possible that the MTV system involves sialic acid containing antigens which we are removing. With this unexpected exception, neuraminidase appears to increase the immunogenicity of almost every detectable cell surface antigen, weak histocompatability antigens, certain red cell antigens, antigens of *Schistosoma mansoni*, and glycoproteins of various types.

DR. HOBBS: Our Westminster group has an eight year experience treating 180 patients with malignant melanoma, and has noted an important difference from your animal model. Here irradiation is ineffective, as we have treated autologous tumor cells with 12,000 R, used them for immunization with and without BCG, and found no significant alteration of survival in 80 patients followed for 5 years. We have no experience with neuraminidase, however, and wish you luck.

Adrenocortical Function and Serum Properdin Level of Thymectomized and Sham-operated Rats Bearing Chemically Induced Tumors

J. Fachet,[*1] M. Zombory,[*2] K. Mihály,[*3] and G. Cseh[*4]

*Immunogenetic Labs., Inst. of Genetics, Biol. Res. Ctr., Hung. Acad. Sci. Szeged, 2nd Hungary,[*1] Inst. of Pathology, Univ. Med. School, Budapest, Hungary,[*2] Dept. of Pathophysiology, Inst. of Exptl. Medicine, Hung. Acad. Sci., Budapest, Hungary,[*3] and Pharmaceutical Res. Inst., Budapest, Hungary[*4]*

Abstract: Alteration of adrenocortical function and serum properdin level during chemical carcinogenesis was studied in young-adult thymectomized (ATx) and sham-operated (sham-op.) male Wistar rats.

The corticosterone level of peripheral blood and production of corticosterone by adrenals *in vitro* were found to be significantly higher in sham-op. than in ATx rats 120 days after 3,4-benzpyrene (BP) treatment.

Properdin level of the serum was found to be significantly lower in BP-treated sham-op. rats than in BP-treated ATx rats, being both significantly lower than the corresponding control.

The time of first appearance of tumors and the death of tumor-bearing rats occurred not sooner, but slightly later in ATx, than in sham-op. rats. Hypertrophy of adrenals and spleens was found in BP-treated sham-op. and ATx rats. The weight of thymus was less in BP-treated sham-op. rats than in untreated controls. The weight of tumors was less in BP-treated ATx, than in BP-treated sham-op. rats.

In ATx rats fed by yellow butter (YB, *p*-dimethylaminoazobenzene) for 14 months, there was a significant increase of the corticosterone level in the peripheral blood and a decrease of it in the sham-op. rats. Weights of adrenals and liver was most conspicuously increased in ATx, than in any other groups.

In summary, contrary to expectations, ATx rats treated with BP did not show higher incidence or accelerated development of tumors, but had slightly lower incidence and slower appearance of tumors and their death occurred slightly later than in sham-op. BP-treated rats.

Lower properdin levels and higher corticosterone concentrations were associated with early appearance and fast progress of chemically induced tumors. Properdin may be involved with non-specific immunological defense against cancer and the higher corticosterone levels may interfere with host's defense directly or through suppression of the immune system.

Numerous and repeated attempts have been made during the last centuries in order to explore the aetiology and to find effective treatment of neoplastic diseases.

Although it has been established that genesis and development of malignant diseases are pluricausal and the outcome is dependent mainly on the host's defense, regrettable enough, these works have not provided us with the necessary knowledge and means to prevent from or stop the fatal progress of neoplastic diseases.

The greatest progress has been made on the line of tumor immunology, since Foley (1), Prehn and Main (2), and Klein and his coworkers (3) demonstrated that chemically induced tumors might be immunogenic as syngeneic grafts and irradiated tumor cells may confer resistance to subsequent transplants of the same tumor. But further studies have revealed the variable importance of specific immune responses against tumors, according to their aetiology (viral, chemical, or spontaneous) and latent period. Tumors with a short latent period were more immunogenic than those growing over a longer time (4).

Furthermore, recent data seem to suggest that in case of spontaneous tumors, the immunological surveillance may be only a late acting and inefficient defense reaction of the host (5) among other regulatory processes called into play also in order to get these mutant cells under physiological control and stop this unwanted malignant proliferation, regrettable in most of the patients in vain.

Being aware of these difficulties, two approaches seem to be left for further trial; either to increase the specific and non-specific immune responses or to look for other defense reactions of the host against neoplastic cells to be strengthened in hope of finding a more efficient combined therapy.

The specific immune responses against transplanted tumors have been studied extensively in numerous laboratories, but their relevance to the naturally occurring tumors has not been elucidated. We have selected, therefore, a long-term and syngeneic tumor-host system for studying the non-specific reactions of the host to chemical carcinogens; (1) effects of young-adult thymectomy on incidence and development of chemically induced tumors, (2) alteration of adrenocortical function, and (3) serum properdin level in young-adult thymectomized (ATx) and sham-operated (sham-op.) rats bearing chemically induced tumors. We have performed our studies on three series of experiments:

1) In the first group, male Wistar rats of one month of age, body weight 110 ± 10 g, were thymectomized and sham-operated under ether anesthesia, according to our earlier method (6). Two days and nine days later 1 ml of 0.1% 3,4-benzpyrene (BP) in oleum helianthae (sunflower-seed oil) was injected subcutaneously into the thigh of left legs. Controls received the same volume of the vehiculum.

All animals were decapitated 120 days later and the plasma level of corticosterone and the *in vitro* production of corticosterone and aldosterone was determined according to our method as published earlier (6). Properdin content was determined as described by Fritsche *et al.* (7) based on the fact that properdin combines with zymosan to form a complex and inactivates C'3 (8). Weight of some organs and of the tumors was measured and chequed by histology (referred as BP-I exp.).

2)   In the second group, the animals were operated and treated as in group one, but all were left to die, while the first appearance of tumors and the survival time was recorded. At the time of their death, weight of body and organs was also measured and chequed by histology (referred as BP-II exp.).

3)   In the third group, the animals were operated as indicated earlier, but from the second day onwards they were fed by standard-diet pellets (like purina chow) which was moistured and mixed with 8 mg/day/rat of yellow butter (YB, p-dimethylaminoazobenzene) for 14 months. Controls received the same standard diet without YB for 14 months. All animals were then decapitated and the plasma corticosterone level and the production of corticosterone and aldosterone by *in vitro* adrenals were determined as in group one. The weight of some organs and tumors was measured and chequed by histology (referred as YB exp.).

Carcinogenesis in Thymectomized Animals

Since the thymus has an important role in the development of peripheral lymphoid organs and homograft immunity, the removal or disorders of thymus or thymus-dependent system is associated in most cases with a higher incidence of tumors in experimental animals and clinical patients as well (for a review, see Refs. *9–11*). Although this generalization may be valid for the consequences of neonatal thymectomy, it seems to be not valid equivocally for adult thymectomy (*4*).

We have selected some publications that are in some way arguing against a decisive role of the thymus-dependent system in immune surveillance mechanism.

According to Prehn (*12*) a weak immune response, rather than being inhibitory, may stimulate the growth of tumor cells. Furthermore, Custer and his coworkers (*13*) did not find more frequent incidence of spontaneous tumors in athymic nude mice, than in others. In accordance with these data, Stutman (*14*) reported more recently that athymic nude mice showed the same incidence and latency period of local sarcomas or lung adenomas 120 days after 3-methylcholanthrene treatment at birth, as the controls.

Fumarola and Giordano (*15*) have reported significantly lower incidence of fibrosarcoma and longer survival time in young-adult thymectomized rats, than in controls treated with BP. Prehn (*16*) also found a decreased incidence of fibro-sacoma in adult thymectomized animals after methylcholanthrene treatment, consonant with other data (*17*). Martinez (*18*) published further evidences that thymectomy at 6 days of age reduces the incidence of mammary tumor development in C3H/Bi female mice.

Since contradictory data were also published demonstrating that adult thymectomy may result in a higher incidence of tumors (*19, 20*) we have been prompted to reinvestigate the consequences of young-adult thymectomy on chemical carcinogenesis.

In the first group of our experiments, the percentage incidence of tumors

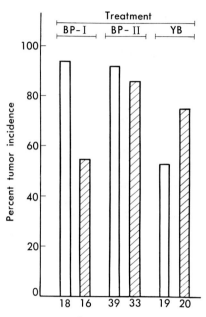

FIG. 1.   Percentage of tumor incidence induced by chemical carcinogens in young-adult ATx and in sham-op. rats. Numbers at bottom of columns indicate number of animals. ☐ sham-op.; ▨ ATx.

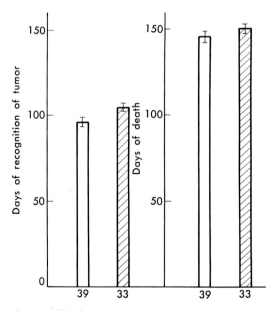

FIG. 2.   The first appearance of tumors and time of death of young-adult ATx and sham-op. rats, both having been treated with BP. Columns represent means ($\bar{x}$), bars indicate standard errors ($S\bar{x}$), and numbers at bottom of columns give number of animals. Footnote : This note for the means, standard errors and numbers applies to all other figures also. ☐ sham-op.+BP-II; ▨ ATx+BP-II.

induced by two consecutive injection of BP by day 120 was significantly lower in ATx rats than in sham-op. controls. In the second group, at the time of their death (Fig. 1), the incidence of tumors was still lower in ATx animals, but the difference

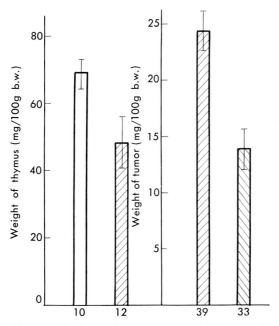

FIG. 3.   Weights of thymus and tumor of BP- treated rats at the time of their spontaneous death. □ sham-op.; ▨ sham-op.+BP-II; ▧ ATx+BP-II.

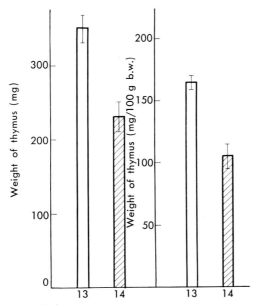

FIG. 4.   Effect of treatment on the weight of thymus 120 days after injection of carcinogen or vehiculum. □ sham-op.; ▨ sham-op.+BP-I.

was not significant. In case of the third group, we have considered those weight of livers pathologically enlarged which were over the highest values of the normal weights of control livers. According to this calculation, the pathological enlargement of livers was more frequent in ATx than in sham-op. rats, both group having been fed by YB (Fig. 1).

These results are in accordance with the later appearance of tumor in ATx

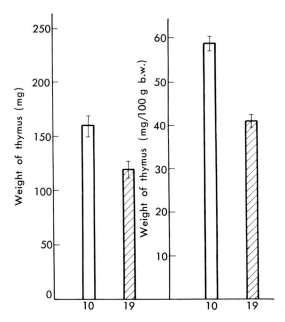

FIG. 5. Weight of thymuses of sham-op. rats kept on normal standard diet and of sham-op. rats fed by YB. ☐ sham-op.; ▨ sham-op.+YB.

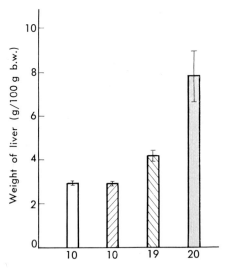

FIG. 6. Weight of livers of sham-op. rats kept on normal standard diet and of sham-op. rats fed by YB. ☐ sham-op.; ▨ ATx; ◨ sham-op.+YB; ▩ ATx+YB.

rats than in sham-op. controls ($P<0.05$), but their death occurred not significantly later (Fig. 2).

Furthermore, the weight of tumors at the time of their spontaneous death was considerable lower in ATx than in sham-op. controls, having been treated with BP (Fig. 3).

At the same time, the weight of thymus in all three groups treated by BP or

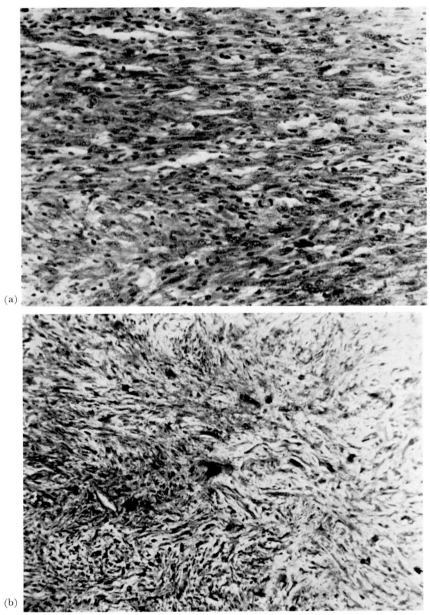

Fig. 7.   Fibrosarcoma (a) and fibrosarcoma with giant cells (b) 120 days after BP injection into the thigh of 1-month-old male Wistar rats. Haematoxylin and Eosin staining (H-E). × 158.

YB significantly decreased ($P<0.01$), comparable to the appropriate controls (Figs. 3, 4, and 5).

In the third group, the relative weight of the enlarged livers was significantly increased in both groups fed by YB, but considerably higher in ATx rats (Fig. 6).

Histological studies verified the type of tumors; as a result of BP treatment

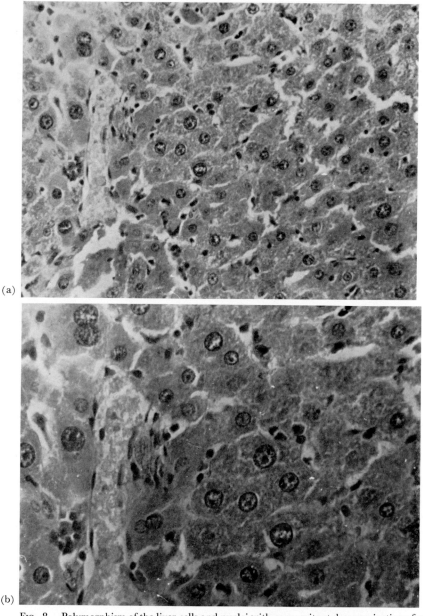

(a)

(b)

FIG. 8.   Polymorphism of the liver cells and nuclei with concomitant desorganization of normal hepatic structure and necrobiosis of rats fed by YB for 14 months. (a) H.-E. ×158. (b) H.-E. ×252.

at the site of injection fibrosarcoma or fibromyxosarcoma was detected, sometimes with giant cells.

In case of pathologically enlarged livers, histology revealed a high degree of polymorphism of liver cells and nuclei with desorganisation of the normal hepatic structure, that we have considered as indications of serious precancerous stage induced by chronic feeding with YB (Fig. 8 (a) and (b)).

Adrenocortical Function in Tumor-bearing Animals

The involution of thymus in tumor-bearing animals might be attributed to hypersecretion of adrenals, as a result of the stress caused by injection of toxic carcinogens, or transplantation of a large quantity of malignant cells (*21*). This view seems to be supported by earlier reports demonstrating hyperplasia of adrenals in rats with Walker carcinosarcoma 256 (*22*). Histological studies have revealed enlarged adrenal cortices and significant increase in zona reticularis (*23*), but secretion rate and type of corticosteroids produced by the adrenals remained to be determined. In guinea pigs transplantation of lymphoblastic leukemia resulted in a higher production of cortisol (*24*).

Furthermore, there are accumulating evidences that endocrine (mainly Cushing-syndrome) and metabolic complications in patients suffering from neoplastic disease may be attributed to hypersecretion of polypeptides, mainly with corticotropin-like hormone activity. This secondary Cushing's syndrome most frequently associated with carcinoma of bronchus, thymus or breast, since these

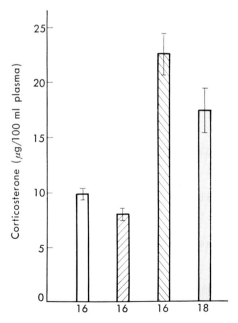

Fig. 9.   Corticosterone level of peripheral blood of sham-op. and young-adult ATx rats 120 days after BP treatment. □ sham-op. ; ▨ ATx ; ◩ sham-op.+BP-I. ; □ ATx+BP-I.

tumors might secrete considerable quantities of adrenocorticotrophic hormone (ACTH)-like polypeptides and complete remission can be observed after surgical removal of the tumor (25–29).

Nevertheless, there were some publications, reporting no adrenal abnormality due to carcinogen treatment in rats (30) and even a decrease of zona fasciculata with concomitant enlargement of zona reticularis associated with neoplasia in SJL/J mice (31).

The purpose of our studies was to reinvestigate the function of adrenals in chemically induced tumor-bearing animals in detail, therefore we determined the plasma level of corticosterone, and the production of corticosterone and aldosterone by adrenals in vitro and their responsiveness to ACTH.

We performed our studies on sham-op. and adult ATx rats also, since we expected different response to carcinogens, in respect of the incidence and development of tumors, which in turn may influence the function of adrenals.

In the first group, the weight of adrenals of sham-op. and ATx rats was found to be increased 120 days after BP treatment, but the difference to the untreated controls was not significant ($P < 0.05$). The corticosterone level in both BP-treated groups was considerably elevated ($P < 0.01$) and even more higher in sham-op. rats ($P > 0.05$) (Fig. 9).

These findings were supported by the observation, that production of corticosterone by adrenals was increased especially in presence of ACTH in vitro circumstances. (Fig. 10).

At the same time and under the same in vitro circumstances, the production of aldosterone was lower in both BP-treated groups (Fig. 11).

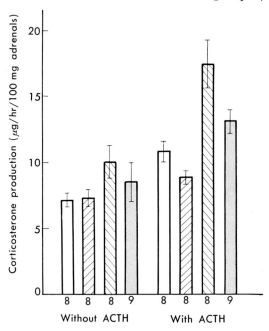

FIG. 10.   In vitro production of corticosterone by adrenals of sham-op. and ATx rats 120 days after BP treatment. □ sham-op.; ▨ ATx; ◨ sham-op.+BP-I; ▧ ATx+BP-I.

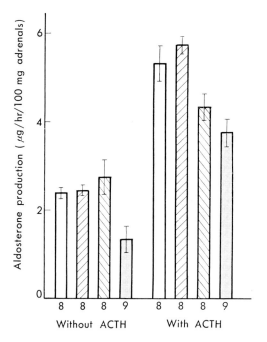

FIG. 11. *In vitro* production of aldosterone by adrenals of sham-op. and ATx rats 120 days after BP treatment. ☐ sham-op.; ▨ ATx; ▧ sham-op.+BP-I; ☐ ATx+BP-I.

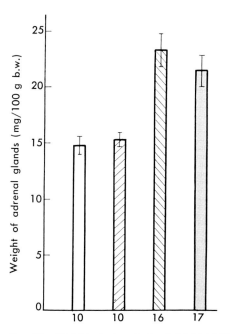

FIG. 12. Weight of adrenal glands (right+left) of sham-op. and ATx rats treated with BP at the time of their spontaneous death. ☐ sham-op.; ▨ ATx; ▧ sham-op.+BP-II; ☐ ATx+BP-II.

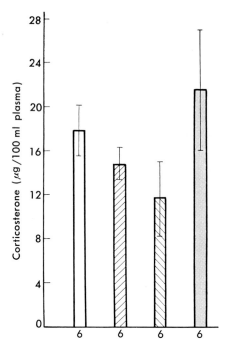

FIG. 13. Corticosterone level of peripheral blood of sham-op. and ATx rats fed by YB for 14 months. ☐ sham-op.; ▨ ATx; ▨ sham-op.+YB; ▨ ATx+YB.

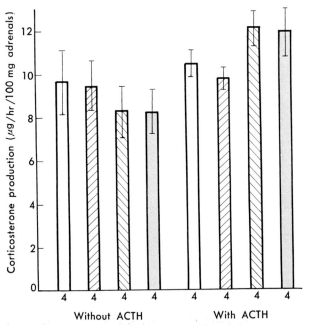

FIG. 14. *In vitro* production of corticosterone by adrenals of sham-op. and ATx rats fed by YB for 14 months. ☐ sham-op.; ▨ ATx; ▨ sham-op.+YB; ▨ ATx+YB.

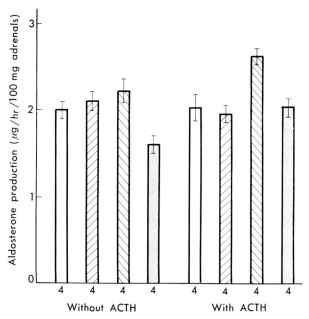

Fig. 15.   *In vitro* production of aldosterone by adrenals of sham-op. and ATx rats fed by YB for 14 months. □ sham-op.; ▨ ATx; ◩ sham-op.+YB; ▨ ATx+YB.

The weight of adrenals was increased significantly even at the time of their death in rats of both BP-treated groups, comparable to the appropriate controls ($P<0.01$) (Fig. 12).

In the third group, where the sham-op. and ATx animals were fed by YB for 14 months, the weight of adrenals only in ATx rats was increased significantly ($P<0.01$). The corticosterone level of the peripheral blood was considerably higher in ATx than in sham-op. rats, both having been fed by YB, but the difference was not significant due to the unusual high standard errors ($P>0.05$) (Fig. 13).

The spontaneous production of corticosterone by adrenals *in vitro* was lower, and their response to ACTH was higher in rats of both YB-fed groups, comparable to the untreated controls ($P>0.05$) (Fig. 14).

The production of aldosterone *in vitro* with and without ACTH was lower in ATx than in sham-op. rats fed by YB ($P<0.02$) (Fig. 15).

Histological studies revealed in case of enlarged adrenals widening of and hyperplasia in the zona fasciculata, without remarkable changes in zona glomerulosa and reticularis.

Serum Properdin Level in Tumor-bearing Animals

Pillemer and his coworkers (*32*) in 1954 demonstrated the existence of a new serum protein, properdin which acts only in conjunction with complement (C'3) and Mg^{2+}, and participates in destruction of bacteria, in lysis of certain red cells, and in neutralization of viruses (*32*). Subsequent studies have demonstrated that the serum level of properdin was lower in patients with carcinoma or other malignant diseases (*33–36*). Furthermore, Southam and Pillemer (*33*) found a close parallelism existing between the serum properdin levels of human patients and their ability to reject cancer cell homografts, although there was no evidence for a casual relationship.

Successful transplantation of tumors in experimental animals was also associated with a significant decrease of the properdin level in the serum (*37–39*) and it was higher in those rats which were more resistant to transplantation of Jensen sarcoma (*40*). At last Pensky and his coworkers (*41*) in 1968 isolated the human properdin and found it to be β-globulin with MW 223,000.

Since we found significantly higher levels of serum properdin in young-adult ATx rats, than in sham-op. controls (*42*), we supposed that lower incidence and slower development of tumors induced by BP in ATx rats might be associated with a relatively higher serum properdin level, than that of sham-op. BP-treated rats.

As it can be seen in Fig. 16 the properdin level in the serum is significantly higher in the untreated ATx than in sham-op. rats ($P<0.001$).

Furthermore, it shows that BP treatment resulted in a considerable decrease in the properdin level in the sham-op. and ATx animals as well, although in the latter group it is still significantly higher, than in the former one ($P<0.01$).

Since we do not know the precise mechanism responsible for the decrease of properdin level in the animals bearing chemically induced tumors, we might only suppose that polysaccharides on, or released from, the tumors might bind or inactivate the serum properdin and possibly exhaust its production.

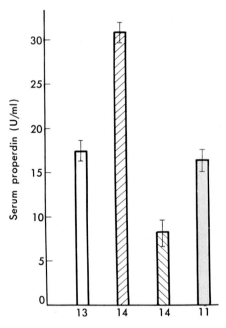

Fig. 16. Serum properdin level of sham-op. and ATx rats 120 days after BP treatment. □ sham-op.; ▨ ATx; ▨ sham-op.+BP-I; ▨ ATx+BP-I.

Our finding, that properdin level increases after young-adult thymectomy, has been strengthened by our more recent results (43) that properdin level is higher in neonatally ATx rats also. It seems that neither the thymus, nor the thymus-derived cells (T cells) have a share in the production of properdin; on the contrary, either of them may inhibit it to some extent.

The increases of serum properdin level after thymectomy may be a result of the release from the suppressor effect of T cells exerted on those cells involved in elaboration of properdin. This hypothesis might be in accord with the modern concept of suppressor T-cell's function (44, 45). The cells, responsible for the higher production of properdin after thymectomy might be among those cells of the reticulo-endothelial system which are proliferating not only in lymphoid organs, but even in the liver too (46, 47).

COMMENTS AND CONCLUSIONS

It has been assumed for a long time that fatal outcome of malignant diseases is pluricausal and dependent mainly on host's defense.

The specific immune responses against transplanted tumors have been studied extensively in numerous laboratories but their effectiveness against and their relevance to the naturally occurring tumors have been questioned also (5).

According to our results, thymectomy in young-adult rats did not increase the incidence and did not accelerate the development of chemically induced tumors, but produced a slightly opposite effect. In contrast to these findings there are numerous data demonstrating that especially neonatally ATx animals are more susceptible to the oncogenic effect of viruses and chemical carcinogens (4, 10, 11). The exact interpretation of this discrepancy cannot be done until more knowledge is gained concerning the regulatory role of the suppressor T-cells and the other non-immunological functions of the thymus (48), e.g., participation in the physiological regulation of the proliferative processes. (49–51).

In our experiments, the increase of corticosterone level in the peripheral blood and in vitro production of corticosterone was observed, but this was not associated with absence of thymus or carcinogen treatment, but rather with the tumorous state. It might be of importance that not the aldosterone with mineralocorticoid activity, but the corticosterone production was increased, which may exert considerable immunosuppression on the thymus-lymphatic system (52, 53) and interfere with the host's defense against malignancies. Hypersecretion of glycocorticoids might be even more dangerous resulting in "hormonal thymectomy" (54, 55).

There are accumulating other evidences demonstrating that not only the specific immune reactions, which develop in time, but other immediate defense reactions are also called into play against tumors (4, 5, 10, 11, 56). As one among them properdin might also contribute to the resistance against cancer as demonstrated in patients (33–36) and in experimental animals as well (37–40), since, most of the polysaccharides employed for immunopotentiation against tumors enhance properdin level also (42, 43, and review Ref. 57).

Of course, our studies should be extended to more detailed analysis of the genetic factors determining the effectiveness of the immune and non-specific defense reactions against induction and development of tumors.

REFERENCES

1. Foley, E. J. Antigenic properties of methyl-cholanthrene induced tumors in mice of the strain of origin. Cancer Res., *13*: 835–837, 1953.
2. Prehn, R. T. and Main, J. M. Immunity to methylcholanthrene-induced sarcomas. J. Natl. Cancer Inst., *18*: 769–778, 1957.
3. Klein, G., Sjögren, H. O., Klein, E., and Hellström, K. E. Demonstration of resistance against methylcholanthrene-induced sarcomas in the primary autochthonous host. Cancer Res., *20*: 1561–1572, 1960.
4. Weston, B. J. The thymus and immune surveillance. *In*; A.J.S. Davies and R. L. Carter (eds.), Contemporary Topics in Immunobiology, vol. 2, chap. 15, pp. 237–263, Plenum Press, New York / London, 1973.
5. Prehn, R. T. Cancer and the immune response. Proc. Inst. Med. Chicago, *29*: 1–7, 1973.
6. Fachet, J., Stark, E., Vallent, K., and Palkovits, M. Some observation on the functional interrelationship between the thymus and the adrenal cortex. Acta Med. Acad. Sci. Hung., *18*: 461–466, 1962.
7. Fritsche, W., Fischer, H., Schwick, G., and Schultze, H. E. Über die Bestimmung von Properdin und Komplementfraktion. Klin. Wochenschr., *36*: 100–105, 1958.
8. Pillemer, L., Blum, L., Lepow, L. H., Ross, C. A., Todd, E. W., and Wardlaw, A. C. The properdin system and immunity. I. Demonstration and isolation of a new serum protein, properdin and its role in immune phenomena. Science, *120*: 279–285, 1954.
9. Law, L. W. Studies of thymic function with emphasis on the role of the thymus in oncogenesis. Cancer Res., *26*: 551–574, 1966.
10. Metcalf, D. The Thymus, Recent Results in Cancer Research, vol. 5, Springer-Verlag, New York, 1966.
11. Miller, J.F.A.P. and Osoba, D. Current concepts of the immunological function of the thymus. Physiol. Rev., *47*: 437–520, 1967.
12. Prehn, R. T. The immune reaction as a stimulator of tumor growth. Science, *176*: 170–171, 1972.
13. Custer, R. P., Outzen, H. C., Eaton, G. J., and Prehn, R. T. Does the absence of immunologic surveillance affect the tumor incidence in "Nude" mice? First recorded spontaneous lymphoma in a nude mouse. J. Natl. Cancer Inst., *51*: 707–711, 1973.
14. Stutman, O. Tumor development after 3-methylcholanthrene in immunologically deficient athymic nude mice. Science, *183*: 534–536, 1974.
15. Fumarola, D. and Giordano, D. Influence of thymectomy and of thymic-extract treatment in the development and growth of 3, 4-benzpyrene induced sarcomas in the rat. Tumori, *48*: 5–12, 1962.
16. Prehn, R. T. Personal communication, 1964.
17. Fachet, J. Absence of tumor induction by repeated partial hepatectomy in thymectomized rats. Unpublished.
18. Martinez, C. Effect of early thymectomy on development of mammary tumours in mice. Nature, *203*: 1188, 1964.

19. Nishizuka, Y., Nakakuki, K., and Usui, N. Enhancing effect of thymectomy on hepatotumorigenesis in Swiss mice following neonatal injection of 20-methylcholanthrene. Nature, *205*: 1236–1238, 1965.

20. Linker-Israeli, M. and Trainin, N. Influence of adult thymectomy on growth of transplanted tumors in mice. J. Natl. Cancer Inst., *41*: 411–420, 1968.

21. Selye, H. Thymus and adrenals in the response of the organism to injuries and intoxications. Brit. J. Exp. Pathol., *17*: 234–239, 1936.

22. Ball, H. A. and Samuels, L. T. Adrenal weights in tumour-bearing rats. Proc. Soc. Exp. Biol. Med., *38*: 441–443, 1938.

23. Coombs, R.R.H., Castro, J. E., and Sellwood, R. A. Adrenal hyperplasia in rats with Walker carcinosarcoma 256. Brit. J. Surg., *61*: 136–140, 1974.

24. Burstein, S. and Nadel, E. M. Corticosteroid production rates in strain 2 guinea pigs following L2C/NB leukemia transplantation. Cancer Res., *27*: 2118–2122, 1967.

25. Hymes, A. C. and Doe, R. P. Adrenal function in cancer of the lung with and without Cushing's syndrome. Am. J. Med., *33*: 398–407, 1962.

26. Ross, E. J. Endocrine and metabolic consequences of carcinoma of the bronchus. Proc. Roy. Soc. Med., *58*: 485–487, 1965.

27. Ross, E. J. Endocrine syndromes of non-endocrine origin. Proc. Roy. Soc. Med., *59*: 335–338, 1966.

28. Miura, K., Sasaki, C., Katsushima, I., Ohtomo, I., Sato, S., Demura, H., Torikai, T., and Sasano, N. Pituitary-adrenocortical studies in a patient with Cushing's syndrome induced by thymoma. J. Clin. Endocrinol., *27*: 631–637, 1967.

29. Jones, J. E., Shane, S. R., Gilbert, E., and Flink, E. B. Cushing's syndrome induced by the ectopic production of ACTH by a bronchial carcinoid. J. Clin. Endocrinol., *29*: 1–5, 1969.

30. Hamilton, T. and Sneddon, A. Endocrine organ weight differences between rats bearing simple and malignant tumours. Brit. J. Surg., *54*: 230, 1967.

31. Pierapaoli, W., Haran-Ghera, N., Bianchi, E., Müller, J., Meshorer, A., and Bree, M. Endocrine disorders as a contributory factor to neoplasia in SJL/J mice. J. Natl. Cancer Inst., *53*: 731–744, 1974.

32. Pillemer, L., Blum, L., Lepow, I. H., Ross, O. A., Todd, E. W., and Wardlaw, A. C. Science, *120*: 279–285, 1954.

33. Southam, C. M. and Pillemer, L. Serum properdin levels and cancer cell homografts in man. Proc. Soc. Exp. Biol. Med., *96*: 596–601, 1957.

34. Rottino, A., Levy, A. L., and Conte, A. A study of the serum properdin levels of patients with malignant tumors. Cancer, *11*: 351–356, 1958.

35. Meyerburg, R. J. Levels of properdin in patients with carcinoma. Am. J. Clin. Pathol., *31*: 415–421, 1959.

36. Cron, J. A contribution to the role of properdin in anticancer defense of the organism. Neoplasma, *17*: 155–168, 1970.

37. Troeh, M. R., Slater, C. R., Larson, W. M., Jr., and McKee, R. W. Changes in serum properdin of mice during tumor growth and following immunization to Ehrlich ascites carcinoma. Proc. Soc. Exp. Biol. Med., *109*: 51–54, 1962.

38. Bradner, W. T. and Clarke, D. A. Serum properdin levels in mice with sarcoma 180. Proc. Am. Assoc. Cancer Res., *2*: 282–290, 1958.

39. Herbut, P. A., Kraemer, W. H., Pillemer, L., and Todd, E. W. Studies on the properdin system in rats bearing transplantable human carcinoma HR-132. Cancer Res., *18*: 1191–1195, 1958.

40. Pfordte, K. and Matthies, E. Tumorresistenz und Properdinspiegel. Naturwissenschaften, *53*: 135, 1960.

41. Pensky, J., Hinz, C. F., Jr., Todd, E. W., Wedgwood, R. J., Boyer, J. T., and Lepow, I. H. Properties of highly purified human properdin. J. Immunol., *100*: 142–158, 1968.

42. Fachet, J. and Cseh, G. Zusammenhänge zwischen Thymus und Nebennierenrindenhormonen bei der Beeinflussung des Serum-Properdinspiegels. Med. Exp., *10*: 39–44, 1964.

43. Fachet, J. and Szemere, G. Effects of endotoxin on the serum properdin content in neonatally thymectomized and splenectomized rats. 1975. Unpublished.

44. Kerbel, R. S. and Eidinger, D. Variable effects of anti-lymphocyte-serum on humoral antibody formation; role of thymus dependency of antigen. J. Immunol., *106*: 917–926, 1971.

45. Baker, P. J., Stashak, P. W., Amsbaugh, D. F., and Prescott, B. Regulation of the antibody response to type III. Pneumococcal polysaccharide. II. Mode of action of thymic-derived suppressor cells. J. Immunol., *112*: 404–409, 1974.

46. Fachet, J., Stark, E., Palkovits, M., and Mihály, K. Effect of neonatal thymectomy on endocrine and lymphatic organs, reticular elements and blood count. I. Findings in rats not suffering from wasting syndrome. Acta Med. Acad. Sci. Hung., *21*: 304–310, 1965.

47. Fachet, J., Palkovits, M., and Vallent, K. Effect of neonatal thymectomy on endocrine and lymphatic organs, reticular elements and blood counts. II. Findings in rats with wasting syndrome. Acta Med. Acad. Sci. Hung., *21*: 304–310, 1965.

48. Grant, G. A. and Miller, J.F.A.P. Effect of neonatal thymectomy on the induction of sarcomata in C57BL mice. Nature, *205*: 1124–1125, 1965.

49. Fachet, J., Stark, E., Palkovits, M., and Vallent, K. Der Einfluss der Thymektomie auf die Leberregeneration nach partieller Hepatektomie. Z. Zellforsch., *60*: 609–614, 1963.

50. Fachet, J., Vallent, K., Palkovits, M., and Ács, Zs. The role of the thymus in the hyperfunction of the adrenal cortex caused by experimental hyperthyroidism. Acta Med. Acad. Sci. Hung., *20*: 281–287, 1969.

51. Fachet, J., Palkovits, M., and Vallent, K. Über die Rolle des Thymus bei den durch Nebennierenrindenhormon—Thyroxin-und Heparin-behandlung herforgerufenen volumenveränderungen der Leberzellkerne. Acta Morphol. Acad. Sci. Hung., *15*: 15–21, 1967.

52. Fachet, J. and Parrott, D.M.V. Effect of corticosteroids and adult thymectomy on induction and recall of contact sensitivity in mice. Clin. Exp. Immunol., *10*: 661–672, 1972.

53. DeSousa, M. B. and Fachet, J. The cellular basis of the mechanism of action of cortisone acetate on contact sensitivity to oxazolone in the mouse. Clin. Exp. Immunol., *10*: 673–684, 1972.

54. Fachet, J., Palkovits, M., Vallent, K., and Stark, E. Effect of a single glycocorticoid injection on the first day of life in rats. Acta Endocrinol. (Kbh.), *51*: 71–76, 1966.

55. Fachet, J., Stark, E., and Palkovits, M. Effect of a single neonatal glycocorticoid injection on the thymus-lymphatic and endocrine system and on the growth of the rat and the dog. Acta Med. Acad. Sci. Hung., *25*: 395–407, 1968.

56. Keller, R. and Hess, M. W. Role of activated macrophages in the suppression of

tumour growth. *In*; W.-H. Wagner and H. Hahn (eds.), Activation of Macrophages, pp. 291–292, Excerpta Medica, Amsterdam, 1974.

57. G.E.W. Wolstenholme and J. Knight (eds.), Immunopotentiation (Ciba Foundation Symposium), vol. 18, Elsevier/Excerpta Medica/North Holland, Amsterdam/London /New York, 1973.

Discussion of Paper of Drs. Fachet et al.

DR. JANKOVIĆ: Did you search for mediastinal thymic remnants and extra thymic lobes in the region of the thyroid gland in your ATx rats? Frequently, such extra thymuses are overlooked when supposedly complete thymectomies were performed in rats and mice.

DR. FACHET: Yes, we checked these areas both macroscopically and microscopically and discarded those animals with signs of thymic tissue.

DR. NISHIOKA: How did you measure serum properdin levels? Did you record the protein itself or a mixture with factors B and D and C3?

DR. FACHET: We examined hemolytic activity in a sheep red blood cell system, measuring the consumption of C3 by a properdin-zymosan complex.

DR. M. KODAMA (Aichi Cancer Center Research Institute, Nagoya):   We recorded the results similar to yours in the mouse, as thymectomy prolonged the survival of polyoma virus infected animals (J. Natl. Cancer Inst., *30*: 225, 1963). However, this amelioration was observed only in AKR mice which have large immature thymuses, and not in C3H mice which have smaller and more mature thymus glands. Did you investigate the size of the thymus and its degree of histologic maturation at the time of thymectomy?

DR. FACHET: We followed the weight and histologic maturation of the thymus and other lymphoid organs in our rats and at the time of thymectomy the thymus was fully mature.

HOST DEFENSE AGAINST CANCER AND ITS POTENTIATION, D. MIZUNO ET AL. (EDS.),
UNIV. OF TOKYO PRESS, TOKYO / UNIV. PARK PRESS, BALTIMORE, PP. 265–279, 1975

Host Factors Influencing Mammary and Ovarian Tumorigenesis in Neonatally Thymectomized Mice*

Yasuaki Nishizuka and Teruyo Sakakura

Laboratory of Experimental Pathology, Aichi Cancer Center Research Institute, Nagoya, Japan

Abstract: In attempting to investigate the mechanism of reduced appearance of spontaneous mammary cancers in the mouse after neonatal thymectomy, endocrinologic and immunologic analyses were performed on (C3H/HeMs × 129/J)F_1 hybrid mice thymectomized at 3 days of age. The following conclusions were obtained:

1) Thymectomy at 2–4 days after birth resulted in a particular type of ovarian dysgenesis, which seemed to be a main cause of reduced mammary tumorigenesis. Poor development of the mammary gland and depressed appearance of hyperplastic alveolar nodules, morphologic precursors of cancers, were noticed also.

2) The ovarian dysgenesis thus induced is characterized by complete loss of oocytes and follicles, and hyperplasia of interstitial cells capable of producing androgenic steroids. Hence, profound disturbances in reproductive performance were recognized in thymectomized mice.

3) The initial change leading to anovular ovarian dysgenesis seemed to be lymphocyte infiltration giving a histological pattern of "lymphocyte oophoritis." The similar acute reaction probably of delayed type of hypersensitivity was evoked in syngenic ovaries grafted into thymectomized mice bearing the dysgenetic ovaries. These results may indicate possible autoimmune nature of the ovarian dysgenesis.

4) Ovarian tumors of tubular and granulosa cell types developed not infrequently from this anovular ovaries at older ages. Endocrinologic mechanism of ovarian tumorigenesis might be similar to that in X-ray irradiated mice. In both systems, high level of gonadotrophin secretion and production of androgenic steroids from the damaged ovaries were demonstrated.

5) Replacement of thymectomized mice either with thymus or spleen tissues or with injections of cell suspensions containing thymus-dependent cells was successfully performed and all the abnormalities in ovarian function and morphogenesis

* The work described in this paper was supported by Grant-in-Aid for Scientific Research from Japanese Ministry of Education, Science and Culture, National Cancer Institute (NIH, U.S.A.) Research Contract (NO1-CP-55650), and the Princess Takamatsu Cancer Research Fund.

disappeared. No ovarian tumor developed, and mammary tumorigenesis returned to normal, except for the fact that development of mammary cancers was still inhibited in reconstituted mice with spleen cell injections.

Since 1964, it has been reported that complete removal of the thymus at neonatal ages results in a significant decrease in the incidence and in a marked delay of the appearance of spontaneous mammary cancers in different mouse systems. This was proved in C3H mice (1, 2), (C3H/HeMs × 129/J)F$_1$ hybrids (3), BALB/c mice infected with mammary tumor virus (MTV) of C3H origin (4–6), and RIII mice (6).

Although Squartini et al. (6) emphasized that the inhibitory effect of thymectomy on MTV-induced mammary tumorigenesis is dependent, to a large extent, on the mouse strains used, there exist probably three possible mechanisms to explain the role of the thymus in such an experimental condition (7):

1)   The presence of the thymus is required to build up a proper hormonal stimulation in the host for mammary cancer development.

2)   The intact thymus is necessary for a "balanced" immunologic interaction between MTV or MTV-induced antigen(s) and host during the sequences of cancer development.

3)   The thymus may provide an indispensable and suitable site for MTV replication.

The last possibility seemed unlikely, because our bioassay with (C3H/HeMs × 129/J)F$_1$ mice indicated that the spleen of neonatally thymectomized 2- to 3-month-old female mice contained MTV in an amount sufficient enough to induce mammary cancer when its cell-free extracts were given through intraperitoneal route into intact MTV-free BALB/c mice as neonates. Heppner (5) also reported that no effect of thymectomy could be detected on the presence either of blood associated, or milk-borne MTV activity. Thus, our efforts had been mostly focused on investigating other possibilities. This communication deals with our experiments conducted to understand mechanism of reduced occurrence of mammary cancers from the endocrinologic and immunologic aspects mentioned above.

It has been reported also from our laboratory that neonatal thymectomy may cause "spontaneous" development of ovarian tumors of granulosa cell type and tubular adenoma type (8). Mechanism of ovarian tumorigenesis in this experimental condition will be briefly described.

Mechanism of Reduced Mammary Tumorigenesis after Neonatal Thymectomy

The experiments described herein were mainly concerned with thymectomized (C3H/HeMs × 129/J)F$_1$ hybrid mice unless otherwise mentioned. Thymectomy was performed at 3 days of age in almost all the experiments, because it became certain that this age is the earliest age for thymectomy after which the vast majority of the operated mice can be alive in healthy conditions for their life span, showing

TABLE 1.   Inhibitory Effect of Thymectomy on Mammary Tumor Development in (C3H/HeMs×129/J)F$_1$ Mice[a]

Experimental groups	Tumor incidence	HAN per gland
Control (virgin)	2/19 (11%)	1.6
Thymectomized (virgin)[b]	0/25	0.0
Control (breeder)	12/35 (34%)	1.7
Thymectomized (breeder)[b]	0/64	0.3

[a] Data at 12 months of age.   [b] Thymectomized at 3 days of age.

neither significant retardation of body growth nor higher susceptibility to common laboratory infections and wasting disease.

Table 1 indicates a set of experiments which clearly shows that thymectomy at this particular age reduces the incidence of mammary cancers accompanied with markedly depressed appearance of hyperplastic alveolar nodules (HAN), virus-induced morphologic precursors of mammary cancers in this hybrids. Such inhibitory effect of thymectomy was eventually observed in both virgin and breeding groups. Since it has been generally accepted that HANs appear most frequently in the normally developed mammary gland (9), a comparative study on the grade of morphologic mammogenesis was made between thymectomized and non-thymectomized mice with whole-mount preparations of the gland. To evaluate lubulo-alveolar development of the glands, they were divided into 5 grades: Grade 0 means the most poorly developed gland and Grade IV the most highly developed gland. As summarized in Table 2, many thymectomized mice had the mammary glands of Grade 0 or I, whereas, non-thymectomized controls the glands of Grade II or III. The similar tendency was obvious in (129/J×C3H/HeMs)F$_1$ mice where no MTV is transmitted through mother's milk. These results indicate that poor development of the mammary gland may be responsible for markedly decreased occurrence of HANs and conclusively for reduced development of cancers, because it is proved that HANs transform into cancers under a suitable hormonal condition (9).

At present, nothing is known about functional connection between the thymus and mammary gland. Chronologic studies with neonatally thymectomized mice were made to examine histologic abnormalities of various organs possibly related to mammary morphogenesis. Of interest was the fact that a drastic histologic

TABLE 2.   Grade of Mammary Gland Development after Neonatal Thymectomy in Mice (3)

Groups of mice	Thymectomy[a]	Grade of development[b]				
		0	I	II	III	IV
(C3H/HeMs×129/J)F$_1$	−	0	0	16	3	0
	+	1	8	2	0	0
(129/J×C3H/HeMs)F$_1$	−	0	3	32	2	0
	+	5	4	2	0	0

[a] Thymectomized at 3 days of age.   [b] Observed on whole-mount preparations at 12 months of age.

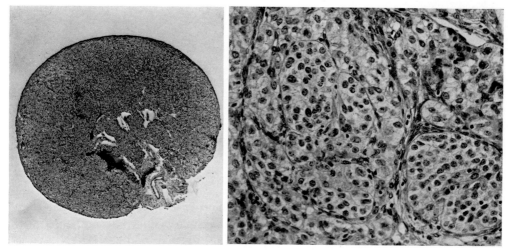

FIG. 1. Ovarian dysgenesis appearing in a neonatally thymectomized (C3H × 129)F$_1$ mouse aged 90 days. Note absence of oocyte, follicle, and corpus luteum. The ovary is covered by a layer of intact surface epithelium and entirely occupied by large interstitial cells arranged in masses partly mimicking luteinizing follicles. Hematoxylin and Eosin staining (H-E). Left × 32; right × 170.

change which could account for poor lubulo-alveolar development of the mammary gland was found only in the ovary (*10, 11*). The morphology of the ovarian change at the most florid stage is characterized by complete loss of oocytes, follicular elements and corpora lutea, and subsequent hyperplasia of interstitial cells is conspicuous (Fig. 1). This ovarian change was noticed clearly at 8–12 weeks of age in 60–70% of thymectomized (C3H × 129)F$_1$ mice. The interstitial cells are, in general, slightly hypertrophic and show typical morphology of steroid-producing cells. In electron micrographs they contain abundant mitochondriae with tubular cristae, numerous prominent lipid droplets, and apparent Golgi complex associated with remarkable development of both smooth and rough surfaced endoplasmic reticulum in tubular to vesicular form. It is interesting enough to note that evidences for secretion of androgenic steroids from these interstitial cells are obtained in both *in vivo* and *in vitro* studies (*11, 12*).

The majority of (C3H × 129)F$_1$ females with dysgenetic ovaries had slightly or moderately masculinized submandibular salivary gland which showed obviously larger intercalated tubules composed of taller cells with larger amounts of eosinophilic granules compared with those of control females (*11*). It was also demonstrated that, when ^{3}H-3-hydroxypregn-5-en-20-one, ^{14}C-progesterone, or ^{14}C-17-hydroxyprogesterone was incubated with ovarian homogenates, androstendione and testosterone were synthesized by the dysgenetic ovaries, while much less of these C$_{19}$-steroids were formed by homogenates of normal ovaries. Estimation of enzyme activities related to steroid conversion supported these biosynthetic data. Homogenates of dysgenetic ovaries contained very low activity of 20α-hydroxysteroid dehydrogenase and very high activities of 17-hydrolase and the lyase, but

TABLE 3. Effect of Neonatal Thymectomy on Reproductive Performance of (C3H/HeMs×129/J)F₁ Female Mice (13)

Experimental groups	Total sterility (No. sterile/ No. mice)	Averave age at 1st birth (weeks)	Number of litters in 10 months						Ovarian dysgenesis[a] (No. dysg./ No. mice)
			Distribution						
			1	2	3	4	5	6	
Control	0/31	11.5	0	0	0	2	9	20	0/31
Thymectomy[b]	11/55	9.5[c]	13	4	2	5	7	13	36/53[d]

[a] Ovarian dysgenesis was determind by histologic examination at 12 months of age.   [b] Thymectomy at 3 days of age.   [c] Average age of 44 parous mice.   [d] Two mice, histologically not examined, were excluded.

activity of 3β-hydroxysteroid dehydrogenase was at a similar level in dysgenetic and normal ovaries (12).

In accordance with these ovarian changes, irreversible irregularity of vaginal cycles and profound disturbances in fertility capacity of thymectomized mice were noticed with age (13). Approximately 20% of thymectomized (C3H×129)F₁ females were rendered completely sterile and 40–50% of the operated mice were relatively infertile at the age of 6 months and thereafter (Table 3).

It is likely, therefore, that poor development of the mammary gland after neonatal thymectomy is mostly due to hormonal disturbances evoked by ovarian dysfunction.

Mechanism of Occurrence of Ovarian Dysfunction after Neonatal Thymectomy

The ovarian dysgenesis after early thymectomy was observed in all the strains and F₁ hybrids tested, and even in random bred colonies such as ICR/Swiss mice, although there existed striking strain differences in incidence, ranging 10 to 90%, and in time course (14). Of a great significance was the fact that the strict critical age for effective thymectomy in terms of development of the ovarian dysgenesis

TABLE 4. Critical Age of Effective Thymectomy for Induction of Ovarian Dysgenesis in (C3H/HeMs× 129/J)F₁ Mice (14)

Age at thymectomy (days)	No. of mice tested	No. of mice with dysgenesis[a]	Incidence (%)	Effect
0		Death due to wasting disease		
2	10	6	(60.0)	+
3	39	25	(64.1)	+
4	17	11	(64.7)	+
5	17	1	(5.8)	±
6	12	1	(8.3)	±
7	20	0	(0)	−
20	25	0	(0)	−
40±0	22	0	(0)	−

Data of mice killed at 120 days of age.   [a] Ovarian dysgenesis was determined by histologic examination.

was clearly recognized; namely, thymectomy at 2, 3, and 4 days of age resulted in ovarian dysgenesis in many strains, while thymectomy at 7 days or later was no longer associated with postnatal ovarian morphogenesis. The data obtained in $(C3H \times 129)F_1$ mice are summarized in Table 4.

Histologic studies on ovaries at earlier ages after effective thymectomy revealed that the principal change leading to such an anovular ovary seemed to be very rapid and progressive decrease in the number of oocytes and growing follicles (15). Apparently, it is impossible to postulate however, that this anovular change is a

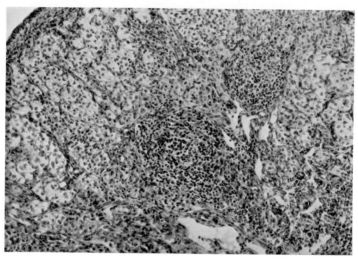

FIG. 2.   Lymphocyte infiltration detected in the ovary of a thymectomized $(C57BL/6J \times A/Jax)F_1$ mouse aged 8 weeks. Note lymphocyte accumulation around markedly degenerating follicles. H-E. $\times 145$.

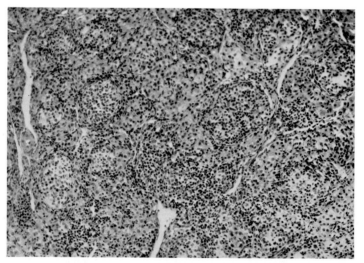

FIG. 3.   Severe lymphocyte oophoritis induced by human chorionic gonadotrophin, 72 hr after the last injection, 10 units per day for 3 successive days, in a thymectomized $(C3H \times 129)F_1$ mouse aged 8 weeks. H-E. $\times 125$.

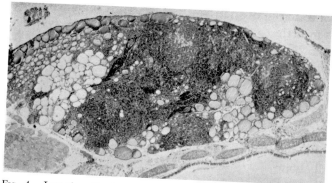

FIG. 4. Lymphocytic thyroiditis found in a thymectomized (BALB/c × 129/J)F₁ mouse aged 12 months. Note lymphatic follicles with germinal center. H-E. ×30.

simple acceleration of ageing process of the ovary, because, in some strains, lymphocyte infiltration in a greater or lesser degree was observable in the ovaries prior to the onset of apparent ovarian dysgenesis (Fig. 2). Thus, rapid and severe destruction of rather smaller growing follicles followed by or preceeded death to oocytes was taken place, and finally anovular dysgenetic ovaries appeared. This ovarian change could be referred to as "lymphocyte oophoritis" (11). The more intensive cellular infiltration was easily induced by injections of human chorionic gonadotrophin to thymectomized mice at 5–6 weeks of age, the age just before the appearance of typical dysgenesis. Two to three days after exogeneous gonadotrophin stimulation, abortive and imcomplete luteinization of growing follicles and drastic infiltration of lymphocytes, which often mixed with plasma cells and was pronounced around and within degenerating follicles, were observed (Fig. 3). Not infrequently, lymphocytic thyroiditis was detected in thymectomized animals with lymphocyte oophoritis (Fig. 4, Ref. 16). Higher titers of antibodies against mouse-thyroid globulin were detected in sera of thymectomized mice with thyroiditis (17).

Occurrence of the ovarian damage in thymectomized mice can be completely prevented either by grafting of thymus or spleen or by injections of cell suspensions containing thymus-independent (T) cells prepared from syngenic tissues (18). A summary of the experments along this line is given in Table 5. Sufficient numbers

TABLE 5. Procedures Tested for Prevention of Ovarian Dysgenesis in Thymectomized Mice

Effective :
1) Grafting of syngenic thymus or spleen tissues
2) Injection (i.p.[a]) of syngenic thymus or spleen cells

Non-effective :
1) Injection (i.p.) of bone marrow cells
2) Injection (i.p.) of spleen cells taken from thymectomized mice
3) Injection (i.p.) of spleen cells taken from syngenic mice pretreated with anti-thymocyte rabbit serum
4) Grafting and injection (i.p.) of allogenic thymus or spleen tissues or cells
5) Insertion (i.p.) of Millipore chamber containing syngenic spleen or thymus cells

[a] Intraperitoneal.

of T cel
but not
Conger
show r
ovariar
numbe
hetero:
results
is a T
upon i

It
kidney
follicle
adult
of ov:
of all
grafte
comp
Proba
conn
The
orgai
react

concluded that lower incidence of mammary cancer in thymectomized mice was caused by endocrine impairment of the ovary due to an autoimmune oophoritis after ablation of T-cell population after the critical early postnatal age.

TABLE 7. Mammary Tumorigenesis after Neonatal Thymectomy in (C3H/HeMs×129/J)F$_1$ Hybrid Mice

Experimental groups	Tumor incidence	HAN per gland[a]	Development of mammary gland	Morphology of ovary
Control	12/35 (34%)	1.7	Normal	Normal
Thymectomy[b]	0/64	0.3	Poor	Dysgenesis
Thymectomy+ thymus grafting[c]	6/28 (17%)	4.3	Normal	Normal
Thymectomy+ spleen cell injection[c]	0/29	0.5	Normal	Normal

Data at 12 months of age. [a] HAN: hyperplastic alveolar nodule in the right thoracical mammary gland. [b] Thymectomy at 3 days of age. [c] Thymus grafting (1-day-old whole thymus) and spleen cell injection (10^7 cells) at 7 days of age.

Connecting with this conclusion, preliminary and rather descriptive data given in Table 7 may suggest another possible role of immune reaction contributing to the development and establishment of mammary cancers in the mouse system. Table 7 shows that thymectomized mice replaced with thymus grafts restore both endocrine function of the ovary and mammary cancer susceptibility; in contrast, thymectomized mice which had received injections of spleen cells from adult syngenic mice showed normal ovarian and mammary gland morphogenesis, but cancer susceptibility is still highly inhibited.

Ovarian Tumorigenesis in Neonatally Thymectomized Mice

Induction of ovarian tumors in the mouse has been reported by different procedures such as X-ray irradiation (21), application of chemical carcinogen (22), and intrasplenic transplantation of autochthonous or syngenic ovaries in gonadectomized hosts (23, 24). The concept has been proposed that the most basic and common event caused by these different techniques, which is essentially responsible for later development of ovarian tumors, may be disappearance of oocytes at early young adult ages (25). This was supported by spontaneous appearance of bilateral ovarian tubular ademona complex in mutant sterile mice, such as (C57BL/6J × C3H/HeJ)F$_1$-W^x/W^v hybrids in which no oocyte was found at 13 weeks of age because of very rapid exponential deletion of oocytes at postnatal ages (26).

Morphology of the post-thymectomy ovarian dysgenesis resembles that of the ovary of mice exposed to whole-body X-ray irradiation at young adulthood (15). It is well documented that growing oocytes in developing follicles are extremely sensitive to irradiation and destroyed. Ovarian tumors arise very frequently at older age in these anovular ovaries (27). Since the dysgenetic ovary after thymectomy does not contain oocyte, appearance of the tumors from these ovaries is

TABLE 8.   Ovarian Tumorigenesis in Thymectomized Mice

Animals	Thymectomy[a]	Total No. of mice	Ovarian tumors	Mammary cancers
(C3H/HeMs × 129/J)F$_1$	−	29	0	19
	+	20	7 (35%)	3
(C57BL/6J × A/Jax)F$_1$	−	29	0	0
	+	24	8 (33%)	0

Data on virgin mice survived over 15 months.   [a] Thymectomized at 3 days of age.

conceivably expected. This was proved in the two hybrid systems examined as illustrated in Table 8. Approximately 35% of the thymectomized mice that had survived over 15 months had ovarian tumors with histology of tubular adenoma, luteoma or granulosa cell tumor, and of their mixtures (8). Metastasis mostly to the liver was detected in granulosa cell tumors in a few occasions.

Comparative studies on thymectomized and X-ray irradiated mice revealed that histogenetic sequences to ovarian tumorigenesis and changes in the anterior pituitary at varying ages prior to tumor development were quite analogous (15). In brief, at 8–10 months of age and afterwards, progressive downgrowth proliferation of the surface epithelium was prominent and finally formed tubular adenoma, often accompanied with patchy and nodular hyperplasia of luteinized stroma cells. In some areas, nodular luteomas were detected. At 12 months or later, small or large foci composed of undifferentiated granulosa cells appeared, not always closely connected with the proliferative surface epithelium, and developed into tumors. Tumor cells were usually arranged in follicular or nodular patterns, although areas of undifferentiated growth were found as well. Electron micrographs of these tumor cells had a striking resemblance to normal granulosa cells. Many mitotic figures suggested that the tissue was growing rapidly. Signs of estrogenic stimulation in the uterine endometrium were recognized in many cases of granulosa cell tumors in thymectomized animals. In the pituitary, increased numbers of hypertrophic FSH cells, and LH cells in a lesser degree, were clearly recognized by electronmicroscopic studies at 6–12 months of age. Continuous production of androgenic steroids in large quantities from changed ovaries was demonstrated by in vivo and in vitro analyses in the two systems. These findings may indicate that the similar hormonal imbalance involves tumorigenesis in the ovary of both thymectomized and irradiated mice. Thymectomized mice replaced either with thymus grafts or with spleen cells had normal hormonal balance, ovarian morphology, and fertility capacity. No ovarian tumor developed in these reconstituted mice.

In summary, the experiments presented here suggest that an immunologic alteration, induced by thymectomy at the critical neonatal age, contributes to modulation of spontaneous tumorigenesis in the mouse through different ways: one is concerned with inhibitory effect as seen in mammary tumorigenesis, and the other is to furnish a basis for tumor occurrence in the ovary. It is of interest that abnormal hormonal balances may result in divergent modulation of tumorigenesis in this system.

REFERENCES

1. Martinez, C. Effect of early thymectomy on development of mammary tumors in mice. Nature, *203*: 1188, 1964.
2. Law, L. W. Studies on thymic function with emphasis on the role of the thymus in oncogenesis. Cancer Res., *26*: 551–574, 1966.
3. Sakakura, T. and Nishizuka, Y. Effect of thymectomy on mammary tumorigenesis, noduligenesis, and mammogenesis in the mouse. Gann, *58*: 441–450, 1967.
4. Heppner, G. H., Wood, P. C., and Weiss, D. W. Studies on the role of the thymus in viral tumorigenesis. I. Effect of thymectomy on induction of hyperplastic alveolar nodules and mammary tumors in BALB/cfC3H mice. Israel J. Med. Sci., *4*: 1195–1203, 1968.
5. Heppner, G. H. Neonatal thymectomy and mouse mammary tumorigenesis. *In;* L. Severi (ed.), Immunity and Tolerance in Oncogenesis, pp. 503–524, Division of Cancer Research, Perugia, Italy, 1970.
6. Squartini, F., Olivi, M., and Bolis, G. B. Mouse strain and breeding stimulation as factors influencing the effect of thymectomy on mammary tumorigenesis. Cancer Res., *30*: 2069–2072, 1970.
7. Yunis, E. J., Martinez, C., Smith, J., Stutman, O., and Good, R. A. Spontaneous mammary adenocarcinoma in mice: Influence of thymectomy and reconstitution with thymus grafts or spleen cells. Cancer Res., *29*: 174–178, 1969.
8. Nishizuka, Y., Tanaka, Y., Sakakura, T., and Kojima, A. Frequent development of ovarian tumors from dysgenetic ovaries of neonatally thymectomized mice. Gann, *63*: 139–140, 1972.
9. Bern, H. A. and Nandi, S. Recent studies of the hormonal influence in mouse mammary tumorigenesis. *In;* F. Homberger (ed.), Progress in Experimental Tumor Research, vol. 2, pp. 90–144, S. Karger AG, Basel, 1961.
10. Nishizuka, Y. and Sakakura, T. Thymus and reproduction: Sex-linked dysgenesis of the gonad after neonatal thymectomy in mice. Science, *166*: 753–755, 1969.
11. Nishizuka, Y. and Sakakura, T. Ovarian dysgenesis induced by neonatal thymectomy in the mouse. Endocrinology, *89*: 886–893, 1971.
12. Nishizuka, Y., Sakakura, T., Tsujimura, T., and Matsumoto, K. Steroid biosynthesis *in vitro* by dysgenetic ovaries induced by neonatal thymectomy in mice. Endocrinology, *93*: 786–792, 1973.
13. Kojima, A., Sakakura, T., Tanaka, Y., and Nishizuka, Y. Sterility in neonatally thymectomized mice: Its nature and prevention by the injection of spleen cells. Biol. Reprod., *8*: 356–361, 1973.
14. Nishizuka, Y., Sakakura, T., Tanaka, Y., and Kojima, A. Disturbance in female reproductive function in neonatally thymectomized mice. *In;* H. Peters (ed.), The Development and Maturation of the Ovary and Its Functions, pp. 171–180, Excerpta Medica, Amsterdam, 1973.
15. Nishizuka, Y. An experimental pathobiological study on thymus function. Transact. Soc. Pathol. Japan, *62*: 41–67, 1973 (in Japanese).
16. Nishizuka, Y., Tanaka, Y., Sakakura, T., and Kojima, A. Murine thyroiditis induced by neonatal thymectomy. Experientia, *29*: 1396–1398, 1973.
17. Kojima, A., Kojima-Tanaka, Y., Sakakura, T., and Nishizuka, Y. Experimental autoimmune thyroiditis induced in thymectomized mice. Unpublished.

18. Sakakura, T. and Nishizuka, Y. Thymic control mechanism in ovarian development: Reconstitution of ovarian dysgenesis in thymectomized mice by replacement with thymus and other lymphoid tissues. Endocrinology, *90*: 431–437, 1972.

19. Kojima, A. and Nishizuka, Y. Unpublished.

20. Sakakura, T., Hiai, H., Taguchi, O., and Nishizuka, Y. Experimental autoimmune oophoritis. I. Acute reaction to the ovarian isograft in thymectomized mice. Unpublished.

21. Furth, J. and Butterworth, J. S. Neoplastic diseases occurring among mice subjected to general irradiation with X-rays. Am. J. Cancer, *28*: 66–95, 1936.

22. Howell, J. S., Marchant, J., and Orr, J. W. The induction of ovarian tumours in mice with 9: 10-dimethyl-1: 2-benzanthracene. Brit. J. Cancer, *8*: 635–646, 1954.

23. Furth, J. and Sobel, H. Neoplastic transformation of granulosa cells in grafts of normal ovaries into spleen of gonadectomized mice. J. Natl. Cancer Inst., *8*: 7–16, 1947.

24. Li, M. H. and Gardner, W. U. Tumors in intrasplenic ovarian transplants in castrated mice. Science, *105*: 13–15, 1947.

25. Krarup, T. Oocyte destruction and ovarian tumorigenesis after direct application of of chemical carcinogen (9: 10-dimethyl-1: 2-benzanthracene) to the mouse ovary. Int. J. Cancer, *4*: 61–75, 1969.

26. Murphy, E. D. Hyperplastic and early neoplastic changes in the ovaries of mice after genic deletion of germ cells. J. Natl. Cancer Inst., *48*: 1283–1295, 1972.

27. Peters, H. The effect of radiation in early life on the morphology and reproductive function of the mouse ovary. *In;* A. McLaren (ed.), Advances in Reproductive Physiology, vol. 4, pp. 149–185, Logos Press Limited, London, 1969.

Discussion of Paper of Drs. Nishizuka and Sakakura

DR. ALEXANDER: What is the basis for your preference of an immunological interpretation of the mammary and ovarian tumorigenesis observed following thymectomy rather than simple stimulation of the hypophysis? The thymus is under the
control of the anterior pituitary, and it is not unreasonable to postulate that a
feedback mechanism is operative so that thymectomy results in hormonal stimulation equivalent to that produced by, for example, bilateral adrenalectomy. In this
regard, does adrenalectomy in a strain with a high incidence of mammary tumors
effect the tumor incidence? The ovarian changes you observed could be a direct
consequence of an over production of hypophyseal hormones.

DR. NISHIZUKA: We are examining the pituitary glands from thymectomized mice
and neonatally cortisone-treated animals electronmicroscopically, but have no conclusive data as yet. We have observed no changes in the adrenals or other endocrine
glands which might be expected to accompany an increased secretion of hypophyseal
hormones. No significant and direct changes in hypophyseal ovarian feedback
control actually realized upon thymectomy, I think. I do not know whether adrenalectomy affects tumor incidence in mice at high risk for mammary carcinoma.

DR. FACHET: We did not note significant changes in adrenocortical or thyroid
function in adult and neonatally thymectomized rats. The weights and detailed
histologies of the testes, ovaries, and hypophyses in these animals were examined
along with a quantitative determination of the various hypophyseal cell types,
again without significant alteration, except in those animals near death from
runting disease. Thus, in agreement with Dr. Nishizuka's experience, thymectomy
did not substantially change the feedback mechanisms of these hormones.

DR. DUKOR: Female Nude mice are unable to nurse their babies as they have
atrophic mammary glands, although this may not be directly correlated with the
absence of thymus glands in these animals. Have you compared the histological
picture of the underdeveloped mammary glands in your thymectomized mice with
those of Nude mice?

Secondly, do you think it likely that you will find a viral basis as responsible
for the oophoritis and ovarian dysgenesis observed in thymectomized mice?

DR. NISHIZUKA: It is true that the ovary of Nude mice shows the normal morphology except for frequent absence of corpora lutea. This may mean that complete loss of T cells is not a simple cause of development of oophoritis and subsequent ovarian dysgenesis. Dr. Kojima *et al.* in our laboratory (unpublished) demonstrated that, when Nu/Nu BALB/c mice were injected intraperitoneally with a small number of spleen or thymus cells taken from Nu/+ and/or +/+ BALB/c mice, at 7 days of age, typical dysgenetic changes with lymphocyte infiltration arised in the ovaries of athymic recipients.

So far as our electronmicroscopic studies on the ovaries with dysgenesis and its acute reaction, and bioassays with cell-free filtrates from dysgenetic ovaries and other tissues of thymectomized mice are concerned, no positive evidence indicating possible participation of viral agents is available to date.

Dr. Hobbs: We find antibody in the plasma of patients with Hashimoto's thyroiditis and autoimmune adrenalitis that will attract lymphocytes to thyroid and adrenal gland tissue, respectively. We believe that both diseases are the result of excess B-cell activity due to a deficiency of suppressor T-cells. Organs from these patients are infiltrated by small round cells which we believe are K cells attracted by antibody. You noted a lymphocytic oophoritis with some plasma cell infiltration prior to ovarian dysgenesis after thymectomy. Have you determined the nature of these lymphocytes? I assume they can't be T cells because the animals were thymectomized.

Dr. Nishizuka: We have not yet classified the type of lymphocyte infiltrate in the ovary. Some T cell may be present in thymectomized hosts for at least 6–8 weeks after thymectomy, when ovarian changes begin appearing. The population of T cells in the spleen at this age is about 1/3 of the normal T-cell population. We can assume that the ovarian alterations may indeed be the result of a probable over activity of B cells in the host in which a relative deficiency of T-cell control may exist.

HOST DEFENSE AGAINST CANCER AND ITS POTENTIATION, D. MIZUNO ET AL. (EDS.),
UNIV. OF TOKYO PRESS, TOKYO / UNIV. PARK PRESS, BALTIMORE, PP. 281–301, 1975

The Role of the Neuroendocrine System in Murine Mammary Tumorigenesis*

Clifford W. Welsch

Department of Anatomy, Michigan State University, East Lansing, Michigan, U.S.A.

Abstract: One of the first groups to investigate the role of the central nervous system on the genesis of murine mammary tumors was that of Lacassagne and Duplan, who showed that the administration of the tranquilizer reserpine hastened the development of mammary tumors in mice. Subsequently, we demonstrated that the administration of the tranquilizer to rats bearing carcinogen-induced mammary carcinomas resulted in a prompt increase in growth of these tumors. Mechanical alterations of discrete areas of the central nervous system also has a significant influence on this process. Median eminence-hypothalamic electrolytic lesions placed in rats bearing carcinogen-induced mammary carcinomas results in a sharp increase in growth of the tumors and also markedly increase the incidence of spontaneous mammary tumors in female rats. Such surgical procedures, as well as the administration of tranquilizing drugs, invariably result in an altered endocrine system characterized by an enhanced secretion of pituitary prolactin and frequently a reduced secretion of all other anterior pituitary hormones.

Certain ergot alkaloids and ergoline derivatives appear to mimic the activity of the hypothalamic-prolactin release-inhibiting factor, *i.e.*, they appear to be relatively specific for prolactin and are efficacious inhibitors of the secretion of this hormone. The administration of these drugs to rats bearing carcinogen-induced mammary carcinomas results in a prompt regression of these tumors closely mimicking the mammary oncolytic benefits of hypophysectomy. Furthermore, chronic treatment of a high-mammary cancer strain of mice with these drugs virtually *prevents* the subsequent development of spontaneous mammary carcinomas. Thus there appears to be little doubt, from the results of these studies, and others, that prolactin is a key hormone in murine mammary tumorigenesis and that the central nervous system, by virtue of its influence on pituitary gland activity, is a significant overseer in this oncogenic process.

* U.S.P.H.S. (NCI) Research Career Development Awardee, CA-35027. This research was supported in part by research grants from the U.S. National Science Foundation (GB-17034), the American Cancer Society (ET-59) and the U.S. National Institutes of Health (NCI) (CA-13777).

281

Perhaps the most significant advance in endocrinology during the past 25 years has been the recognition that the endocrine system is extensively regulated by the central nervous system, creating an area of study currently referred to as neuroendocrinology. Hormones associated with normal and cancerous mammary development are among those which appear to be significantly affected by changes in central nervous system activity. The hormone which efficaciously binds the central nervous system-mammary tumorigenesis relationship is prolactin, an anterior pituitary peptide whose singular existence has long been recognized in lower animals but only recently verified in humans. Thus, the purpose of this treatise is to provide evidence demonstrating: (1) a significant central nervous system-mammary tumorigenesis relationship in rodents and, (2) that prolactin may be the primary hormonal mediator in this tumorigenic process.

Central Nervous System-Murine Mammary Tumorigenesis Relationship

Sufficient evidence is available to support the existence of a central nervous system-mammary tumorigenesis relationship in experimental animals as well as in man. Murine mammary tumor development and growth have been reported to be significantly influenced by a variety of factors that affect central nervous system activity, *e.g.*, stress (*1*), androgenization (*2*), hypothalamic implant of estrogen (*3*) and constant light (*4*). A variety of psychological factors have also been reported to have a direct bearing on the incidence and progression of mammary cancer in man (*5*).

Perhaps the first group to investigate the effect of tranquilizers on the genesis of murine mammary tumors was Lacassagne and Duplan (*6*). They reported that reserpine, a Rauwolfia tranquilizer, hastened the development of mammary tumors in C3H mice. Mice treated with reserpine developed mammary tumors in the 8th to the 15th month of life, in contrast to the controls, which developed mammary tumors in the 11th to the 17th month. In accord, Welsch and Meites (*7*) administered reserpine to female rats bearing 7,12-dimethylbenzanthracene (DMBA)-induced mammary tumors and observed a marked stimulation of mammary tumor growth. Tumor-bearing rats treated with 100 μg reserpine/100 g body weight for 10 and 25 days showed 58 and 115% increases in tumor growth, in contrast to 18 and 61% increases in the saline-treated controls. Reserpine, however, could not reactivate growth of regressing mammary tumors in ovariectomized rats. Similarly, Pearson *et al.* (*8*) administered perphenazine, a phenothiazine tranquilizer, to DMBA-treated rats to determine whether or not this drug would influence the development of mammary tumors. After 5 months of treatment, 100% of the perphenazine-treated animals developed mammary tumors, in contrast to 70% of the saline-treated controls. The number and size of the tumors in the perphenazine-treated group exceeded that of the control group by a factor of two. Perphenazine was also administered to DMBA-treated, tumor-bearing rats following ovariectomy and adrenalectomy. After 5 months of treatment with the drug, 15 rats had a total of 15 mammary tumors, in contrast to none in the 11 saline-treated controls. These studies are particularly relevant in view of three very recent independent epidemiological studies demonstrating a positive correlation between the use of reserpine in humans and breast cancerigenesis. A comparison of newly diagnosed cases of breast cancer and matched controls indicated that the risk of breast cancer is over threefold in women using reserpine compared with women not exposed to the tranquilizer (9–11). It has been well established that the administration of either Rauwolfia (e.g., reserpine) or phenothiazine (e.g., perphenazine) tranquilizers to either rodents (7, 8) or humans (12) causes a prompt increase in pituitary prolactin secretion. It remains to be determined, particularly in humans, whether or not tranquilizer-induced increased prolactin secretion is the sole mechanism by which these drugs influence mammary tumorigenesis. In rodents at least, the evidence strongly suggests that the primary means by which these tranquilizers increase development and growth of mammary tumors is via an increased secretion of this hormone, presumably caused by depletion of central nervous system stores of catecholamines.

Numerous studies have indicated that hypothalamic catecholamines influence the secretion of all anterior pituitary hormones, but in particular prolactin. In general, an adrenergic tonus is believed to inhibit prolactin release and a reduction of hypothalamic catecholamines to promote prolactin secretion. Iproniazid, a monoamine oxidase inhibitor, is an effective inhibitor of prolactin secretion (13), presumably by interfering with the catabolism of catecholamines and thereby increasing their concentration in the hypothalamus. Nagasawa and Meites (14) investigated the effects of iproniazid on growth of DMBA-induced mammary tumors in female Sprague-Dawley rats. After these tumors reached approximately one centimeter in diameter, the rats were injected daily for 25 days with the drug. Iproniazid markedly suppressed mammary tumor growth and prevented development of new tumors, whereas in the controls growth of the initial tumors increased about 100%. Similarly, pargyline and levodopa (L-dopa), drugs which also increase catecholamines, thus suppressing pituitary prolactin secretion (13), significantly inhibited DMBA-induced mammary tumor growth (15). The results of these studies have provided impetus for the use of catecholamines in the treatment of disseminated breast cancer in humans. L-dopa therapy has been reported recently to provide alleviation of bone pain in women with advanced metastatic carcinoma of the breast (16). Murray et al. (17) reported improvement in 2/7 patients with metastatic breast carcinoma following L-dopa therapy. In another study, L-dopa was ineffective alone, but in combination with estrogen was effective in causing regression of the disease (18).

Experimentally, a more direct approach in evaluating the central nervous system-mammary tumorigenesis interrelationship is to manipulate the brain using stereotaxic procedures and subsequently evaluate the effects of these procedures on the development and growth of mammary tumors. In one of the earliest attempts to directly establish this relationship, Liebelt (19) induced hypothalamic damage in R111 × CBA virgin female mice by a single injection of goldthioglucose. All mice were treated at 70–80 days of age and developed a persistent obesity. Even though irregularities could not be detected in the estrous cycle, these animals were incapable of reproduction. Mammary tumors developed in 100% of the goldthioglucose-treated mice in contrast to 85% tumor incidence in the untreated virgins. Time of mammary tumor appearance was accelerated in the mice with hypothalamic drugs, with 50% developing tumors by 240 days as compared with 350 days in controls. Mammary tumors per animal averaged 3.2 in the goldthioglucose-treated mice, in contrast to 1.9 in the controls. Liebelt concluded that enhancement of mammary tumorigenesis in the mice bearing hypothalamic damage was associated with a hormonal imbalance initiated by an altered neuroendocrine mechanism.

One of the first studies designed to evaluate discrete areas of the central nervous system on growth of mammary tumors was that of Welsch et al. (20). Female Sprague-Dawley rats, 55 days of age, were treated with DMBA. Seventy to 90 days after carcinogen treatment, when all rats had at least one palpable mammary tumor, they were divided into groups and treated as follows: (1) intact controls, sham-operated; (2) intact and lesions placed in the median eminence area of the hypothalamus; (3) ovariectomized controls, sham-operated; (4) ovariectomized and lesions placed in the median eminence. At 0, 10, and 25 days after placement of the lesions, all rats were examined for number of palpable mammary tumors. Intact rats bearing mammary tumors responded to 10 and 25 days after lesions were placed in the median eminence with 138 and 200% increases, respectively, in number of palpable mammary tumors/rat, in contrast to increases of only 23 and 27%, respectively, in the intact controls. A significant increase in mean mammary tumor diameter also was observed in the intact median eminence-lesioned rats. Rats with lesions placed in the median eminence and ovariectomized immediately thereafter responded 10 days later with 25% increase, and 25 days later with 35% decrease in number of palpable mammary tumors/rat in contrast to 40 and 58% decreases at 10 and 25 days, respectively, in the ovariectomized controls. By contrast when ovariectomy preceded the median eminence lesions by 10 days, no significant effect of the lesion was observed in the number of mammary tumors/rat or mean tumor diameter. These results were confirmed by Klaiber et al. (21), who reported that median eminence-hypothalamic lesions accelerated growth of established carcinogen-induced rat mammary tumors, and ovariectomy reduced this enhancing effect. In their study, the number of tumors/rat 21 days after placement of lesions was 9.1 in contrast to 5.5 in the controls. When ovariectomy and median eminence lesions were combined, 5.4 mammary tumors/rat were observed as compared to 3.2 in the ovariectomized controls.

The effects of median eminence-hypothalamic lesions on pituitary function are, in many respects, qualitatively similar to those seen after stalk section or transplantation of pituitary, i.e., increased secretion of prolactin and significantly reduced secretion of all other anterior pituitary hormones (22, 23). Welsch et al. (24) reported that placement of median eminence lesions in Sprague-Dawley female rats resulted in a 10-fold increase in serum prolactin levels just 30 min after the lesion. Serum prolactin levels remained significantly higher than control levels for a period of at least 5 months (Fig. 1). The persistence of the increased serum prolactin levels constitutes further evidence that the predominant influence of the hypothalamus on prolactin release is inhibitory. Lesions in the median eminence are be-

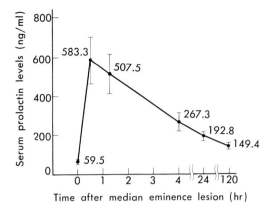

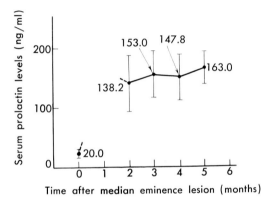

FIG. 1.   Effects of median eminence-hypothalamic lesions on serum prolactin levels of female rats at 1/2, 1, 2, 4, 24, and 120 hr after lesion placement (top).   At 2, 3, 4, and 5 months after lesion placement (bottom). (From Ref. 24)

lieved to act, at least in part, by disrupting the hypothalamic-pituitary portal system, the final common vascular pathway from the hypothalamus to the pituitary, thereby preventing the prolactin release-inhibiting factor (PIF) from reaching the pituitary gland.

Few investigations have been initiated to evaluate the role of sites other than the median eminence area of the hypothalamus in tumorigenesis. Welsch et al. (20) placed bilateral electrolytic lesions in the preoptic area of the hypothalamus or amygdaloid complex of female Sprague-Dawley rats bearing the DMBA-induced mammary tumors. Rats with lesions in the preoptic area showed significant tumor regression for up to 25 days, as indicated by a decrease in the number of mammary tumors/rat and a marked decrease in the mean tumor diameter. The mean tumor diameter in rats bearing amygdaloid lesions was also significantly decreased 25 days after lesion placement, but this treatment had no effect on the number of mammary tumors/rat. Unfortunately, an insufficient number of studies have been conducted to adequately analyze the precise hormonal alterations produced as a result of lesions in these areas.

The effect of median eminence-hypothalamic lesions on development of spon-

taneous mammary tumors was investigated by Welsch *et al.* (*25*). Mature mul-
tiparous, female Sprague-Dawley rats, free of palpable mammary tumors, were
divided into 2 groups: one group was given bilateral electrolytic lesions in the
median eminence, the other group served as sham-lesioned controls. Twenty-five
weeks after placement of the lesions all rats were sacrificed, blood was withdrawn
and assayed for prolactin and number of mammary tumors in each group was
determined. Mammary tumor incidence in the median eminence-lesioned rats was
52% in contrast to 19% in the sham-lesioned controls. Blood prolactin levels were
more than 3 times greater in the rats bearing the hypothalamic lesions (179.8
ng/ml) than in the controls (50.9 ng/ml). It is clear from this study that an endocrine
imbalance, consisting of elevated prolactin secretion and reduced secretion of all
other anterior pituitary hormones can be tumorigenic in the rat.

Bruni and Montemurro (*26*) place electrolytic lesions in the anterior, medial
or posterior hypothalamus of nulliparous C302 F female mice. They observed
that anterior and medial hypothalamic lesions significantly altered pituitary function to the extent that a number of mice in each of these groups were rendered
permanently sterile. Concomitantly, these lesions increased the incidence of spontaneous mammary tumors and reduced the latency period when compared to
controls. Lesions placed in the posterior hypothalamus, as well as those in the
anterior and medial hypothalamus that did not cause sterility, were essentially
ineffective in influencing tumor incidence. Thus it appears that electrolytic lesions
placed in the central nervous system not only have a profound effect on growth of
established mammary tumors but also markedly influence the genesis of these
neoplasms. These results strongly support our hypothesis that certain alterations
in function of the central nervous system may be one of the key etiological factors in
the development and progression of tumors of the mammary gland. That prolactin
is the "key" hormonal mediator in this complex tumorigenic process, in rodents,
is persuasively suggested by these studies.

Prolactin and Murine Mammary Tumorigenesis

Strains of rats that are normally highly susceptible to spontaneous mammary
tumorigenesis do not ordinarily develop mammary tumors if hypophysectomized
(*27*). On the other hand, administration of pituitary hormones to these animals
markedly increases the incidence of mammary tumors. For example, transplantation of multiple pituitaries (*28–30*) (Fig. 2) or pituitary tumors (*31*) to mice or rats
significantly increases the incidence and decreases the latency period for development of spontaneous and carcinogen-induced mammary tumors. Numerous neuro-
endocrine studies have demonstrated that the transplanted pituitary secretes large
amounts of prolactin and greatly reduced amounts of all other pituitary hormones
(*22*), thus further implicating prolactin as the principal pituitary hormone in
development of murine mammary tumors. This concept is considerably strengthened by a report by Boot *et al.* (*32*) of increased mammary tumor incidence in mice
chronically injected with prolactin.

Pituitary hormones have also emerged as important hormones in maintaining

Sprague-Dawley female rats (nulliparous)

8% mammary tumor incidence   75% mammary tumor incidence

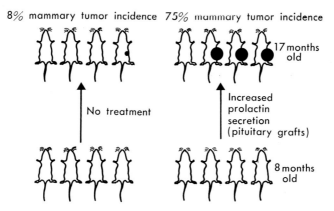

FIG. 2.   Effects of multiple pituitary homografts on mammary tumor incidence 9 months after grafting (30).

growth of carcinogen-induced rat mammary tumors. Growth of these tumors can be easily enhanced in intact (20, 21) or even in ovariectomized rats by grafting prolactin and growth hormone-secreting pituitary tumors (33) or by the concurrent administration of prolactin and growth hormone (34). That prolactin is the principal pituitary hormone in this growth-promoting process is further indicated by more recent studies demonstrating enhanced growth of mammary tumors in ovariecto-mized-adrenalectomized rats injected daily with prolactin (8, 35). Administration of growth hormone alone was without any stimulatory effect.

The interaction of pituitary and ovarian hormones in murine mammary tumorigenesis has long been and is currently an obscure relationship. It is known that administered estrogens markedly increase prolactin secretion whereas ovari-ectomy decreases the secretion of this hormone (36, 37), an observation which has led to the well-known hypothesis that estrogens are mammary oncogenic primarily because of their stimulatory effect on prolactin secretion (33). This concept is supported by studies such as those demonstrating the inability of estrogen to re-activate or even maintain tumor growth in mammary tumor-bearing, hypoph-ysectomized rats (38) and a lack of detectable growth stimulatory effect of the steroid on growth of mammary tumor tissue in vitro (39, 40). It is doubtful, however, that the mechanism of action of estrogen in the genesis and maintenance of mammary tumors is solely indirect, i.e., via the pituitary. For example, although a striking increase in mammary tumor growth after median eminence-hypothalamic lesions provides substantial evidence that prolactin is the principal pituitary hor-mone in this growth process, ovarian hormones also appear to be critical (41, 42), as diminished growth response of the mammary tumors is eventually observed in ovariectomized, median eminence-lesioned rats (20). This concept is further sup-ported by Sinha et al. (43) who reported that growth of carcinogen-induced mam-mary tumors could be reactivated in ovariectomized, median eminence-lesioned rats by ovarian grafts. They also reported that mammary tumors initially grew quite progressively, but eventually regressed in *ovariectomized* median eminence-lesioned rats despite the presence of high levels of blood prolactin in these animals, results which were also observed in our laboratory (*44*). Although previous reports demonstrated increased growth of carcinogen-induced mammary tumors in ovariectomized-adrenalectomized rats injected daily with prolactin (*8, 35*), these treatments were only given for a limited duration and the effects observed may not have persisted over a long period of time. There is evidence that estrogen can act directly on mammary tumor tissue increasing specific activity of certain enzyme systems (*45*).

Although moderate dose levels of estrogen are stimulatory to mammary tumor development and growth *in vitro*, large doses of the steroid inhibit growth of established mammary tumors in experimental animals as well as in man (*46–48*). It has been suggested that large doses of estrogen inhibit mammary tumor growth by reducing prolactin secretion below normal levels (*49*). However, more recent evidence (*50*) is to the contrary, as a wide range of doses of estrogen, when administered to rats, have been found to elevate blood prolactin levels. Moderate doses (5 μg) and high doses (500 μg) increase blood prolactin levels from 10–20 times greater than that observed in the non-treated controls.

Recent studies have provided evidence that the inhibitory effect of large doses of estrogen on mammary tumor growth may be primarily a result of direct action of the steroid on the tumor, directly interfering with the stimulatory effects of prolactin on cellular proliferation and perhaps also interfering with cellular metabolic processes. Meites *et al.* (*51*) provide *in vivo* evidence that large doses of estrogen directly inhibit prolactin stimulation of carcinogen-induced mammary tumor growth. They demonstrated that large doses of prolactin could overcome the inhibitory effects of administered estrogen, suggesting that the steroid interfered with the peripheral action of prolactin on the tumor tissue. Welsch and Rivera (*40*) reported the results of a study designed to determine and compare the capacity of estrogen and prolactin to promote DNA synthesis in organ cultures of carcinogen-induced rat mammary tumors. The results of this study demonstrated that: prolactin stimulates DNA synthesis in organ cultures of rat mammary tumors (Fig. 3), and

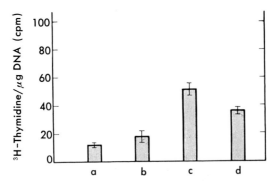

Fig. 3. Effect of estrogen and prolactin on ^{3}H-thymidine incorporation into DNA of organ cultures of DMBA-induced rat mammary carcinoma (*40*). a, controls; b, estrogen 0.01 μg/ml; c, prolactin 5.0 μg/ml; d, estrogen 0.01 μg/ml+prolactin 5.0 μg/ml.

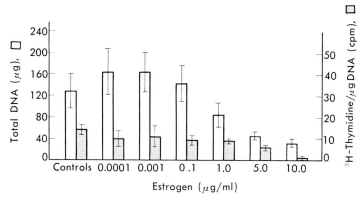

Fig. 4. Effect of varying levels of estrogen on DNA synthesis of organ cultures of DMBA-induced rat mammary carcinoma (40).

estrogen at moderate dose levels was without effect and at high dose levels was inhibitory to DNA synthesis (Fig. 4). Estrogen also suppressed prolactin-induced DNA synthesis (Fig. 3). Evidence, therefore, for an interaction of the steroid with the tumor either by directly interfering with DNA synthesis and/or by suppressing the prolactin stimulating effect is provided in this study. In accord, Turkington and Hilf (39) have reported an estrogen-induced inhibition of DNA synthesis of cultured C3H mouse mammary tumor. The observed stimulatory effect of prolactin on DNA synthesis (40) provides *in vitro* evidence that prolactin is an important hormone in promoting growth of rat mammary tumors, and the total lack of a stimulatory effect of estrogen *in vitro* lends credence to the hypothesis that estrogens are mammary oncogenic, at least in part, as a result of their ability to influence prolactin secretion.

The regulation of mammary tumorigenesis by use of drugs which suppress prolactin secretion is receiving increased attention. Prolactin secretion can be significantly suppressed by the administration of certain ergot alkaloids and ergoline derivatives in rats and mice as well as in man (14, 52–55). Investigations pertaining to the mechanism of action of these ergots indicate that at least one ergot drug, ergocornine, suppresses pituitary prolactin secretion by acting on the pituitary, thus mimicking the hypothalamic PIF (24, 56), and also by acting at the hypothalamic level as well (57).

Because of the marked suppressing activities of these ergots on prolactin secretion, their effects on murine mammary tumor development and growth have been investigated. Ergocornine, or 2-bromo-α-ergocryptine (CB-154), administered to carcinogen-induced mammary tumor-bearing rats (14, 53, 58), or to old rats bearing spontaneous mammary tumors (59) caused significant regression of these tumors (Fig. 5). Ergocornine-induced tumor regression was found to be nearly comparable to that observed after hypophysectomy (53). When treatment with the ergots was withdrawn, prompt resumption of tumor growth was observed. Ergocornine-induced tumor regression paralleled that observed following ovariectomy and was more effective than CB-154 treatment in these rats (58). Over 50% of the palpable mammary tumors regressed so that they were no longer pal-

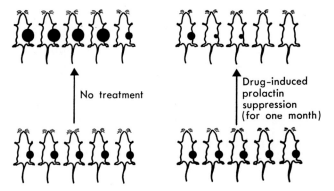

FIG. 5. Effect of the administration of ergocornine for one month, on growth of DMBA-induced rat mammary carcinoma (*53*). Dark circles denote mammary carcinomas. The size of the circle represents both number and size of the carcinoma.

pable after ergocornine treatment, whereas only 10% of these tumors failed to be affected by this drug. The rats continued to have a normal estrous cycle, suggesting specificity of the drug for prolactin. Treatment with the drugs at the doses given had no adverse effects on body weights.

In view of the marked oncolytic effect of the ergots on rat mammary tumors, the effect of these drugs on growth of spontaneous mouse mammary tumors was recently evaluated. Treatment of C3H/HeJ tumor-bearing mice with maximally tolerated doses of CB-154 failed to cause regression of these tumors (*60*). The lack of a significant effect of the ergots on established mouse mammary tumors is not surprising, as these tumors in their advanced state of development generally acquire

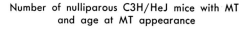

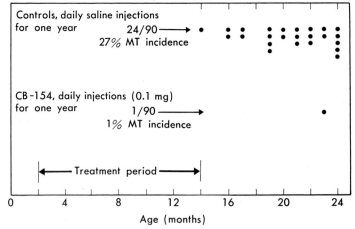

FIG. 6. Effect of CB-154 treatment on incidence of spontaneous mammary carcinomas (MT) in young nulliparous C3H/HeJ mice and age at mammary carcinoma appearance (*60*).

hormone independence (61, 62). However, it has been acknowledged by several investigators that the early developmental phases of spontaneous mouse mammary tumorigenesis are markedly hormone responsive (61–63). It was of interest, therefore, to determine whether or not treatment of mice with CB-154 could: (1) reduce the incidence and/or promote the regression of mammary hyperplastic alveolar nodules, as these hyperplasias have been reported to antedate the tumor (62), and (2) as a consequence, suppress or prevent the appearance of palpable mammary carcinomas. To test this, ninety 2-month-old nulliparous mice were given subcutaneous (s.c.) injections (daily for one year) of 0.1 mg CB-154 suspended in saline. A 2nd group of ninety 2-month-old mice, given s.c. injections of saline only (daily for one year), served as controls. A small number of the mice were sacrificed after one year of treatment, the majority of the mice were observed for an additional 10-month treatment, i.e., until the age of 2 years, during which time they received no treatment. Results (60) demonstrate that daily treatment of these mice with CB-154 for one year significantly reduced by greater than 50% the number of mammary hyperplastic alveolar nodules and, most important, virtually prevented the appearance of mammary carcinomas in these animals. Mammary tumor incidence was 27% in the controls (24/90) and 1% in ergot-treated mice (1/90) (Fig. 6).

Although blood prolactin has not yet been analyzed by radioimmunoassay in these ergot-treated mice, due to a lack of such an assay for this species, all other mammals thus far treated with CB-154 have shown highly significant suppression of blood prolactin levels by radioimmunoassay. CB-154-treated C3H female mice, however, have pituitary prolactin concentrations considerably less than those of untreated controls, measured by disc electrophoresis on polyacrylamide gel (64). There is no evidence to suggest that CB-154 directly interferes with other hormonal processes, that is, it appears to be relatively specific for prolactin. Mice or rats chronically treated with the ergot have normal estrous cycles, suggesting that the drug has no marked inhibitory effect on gonadotrophin secretion (60). Furthermore, growth hormone content of pituitaries of mice treated with CB-154 differs insignificantly from controls (64). In our study (60), the mice treated with the ergot had pituitary, ovarian, uterine, and adrenal weights differing insignificantly from the controls and had normal estrous cycles. Only the mammary gland showed marked disparity between controls and experimental animals. This is particularly significant since it suggests that mammary tumorigenesis can be blocked *even in animals with normal ovarian activity*, as long as prolactin secretion is minimal. CB-154 at the dose levels and schedules used in this study did not interfere with normal body weight gains. More recently we have observed that the administration of CB-154 to female mice profoundly suppresses the development of estrogen-induced mammary dysplasia (65). Mammary tumor incidence as well as mammary hyperplasias were significantly reduced in the CB-154-estrogen treated mice in comparison to the control mice treated with the steroid alone. We also have observed that normal C3H/HeJ female mice chronically treated with CB-154 would only infrequently become pregnant when mated with males of the same strain, but upon drug withdrawal, normal fecundity was immediately reestablished (66). Suppression of fecundity in the ergot-treated mice is probably due to the inhibition of prolactin-induced luteal maintenance.

Considerably fewer studies have involved the utilization of ergoline derivatives in either the prophylactic or chemotherapeutic control of murine mammary tumorigenesis. 6-Methyl-8-β-ergolineacetonitrile (MEA), an efficacious inhibitor of prolactin secretion in rodents (55), and apparently less toxic than some of the ergot alkaloids, has also been reported to suppress the development of mammary hyperplastic alveolar nodules (63) and spontaneous mammary carcinoma (67) in C3H/HeJ female mice. These studies involving prophylaxis of spontaneously developing mammary carcinomas are in accord with the reports of Yanai and Nagasawa (52) and Clemens and Shaar (68), demonstrating that chronic suppression of prolactin secretion inhibits development of *induced* mammary tumors in mice bearing pituitary isografts (52) and rats treated with DMBA (68). These results suggest that prolactin is extremely important, *perhaps essential,* in the early development phases of both induced and spontaneous murine mammary tumorigenesis.

Although the evidence for a key role for prolactin in murine mammary tumorigenesis is striking, whether or not this hormone is significantly influential in the development and growth of human breast tumors remains to be determined. It is not surprising that we know so little about this hormone in humans, since its singular existence in primates has only recently been verified (69), although it has been known to exist as a single entity in lower animals for many years. A number of *in vivo* studies have been initiated to evaluate the role of prolactin in growth of human breast carcinoma (9–11, 16, 17, 70–72). The results of these studies, however, do not provide a basis for a definitive conclusion regarding this question. Women with metastatic breast carcinoma have been reported to have higher mean basal serum levels of prolactin than patients without the disease (17). On the other hand, Boyns *et al.* (70) reported a lack of correlation between serum prolactin levels and the presence or absence of breast carcinoma. CB-154 has been reported to promote regression of metastatic breast carcinoma in a limited number of patients (71), whereas in another study (72), the ergot was found to be essentially ineffective in controlling the advanced stages of this disease. In addition, pituitary stalk section, a treatment known to increase prolactin secretion, does not appear to excite growth of existing metastatic breast carcinoma (73). It was previously mentioned that prolactin suppression by L-dopa therapy has benefited patients with the disease (16, 17) and chronic use of the tranquilizer, reserpine (a potent stimulator of prolactin secretion), may excite the development of breast carcinoma (9–11).

To my knowledge there are only three reported *in vitro* studies (74–76) that attempted to evaluate the potential of prolactin as a growth stimulant for human breast carcinoma. Mioduszewska *et al.* (74) reported that ovine prolactin-treated cell cultures or organ cultures of human breast carcinomas responded with a significant increase in cellular proliferation. They found that 21/37 of the carcinomas grown in cell cultures and 13/20 of those grown in organ cultures responded to the hormone. Furthermore, a positive response to prolactin *in vitro* was correlated with a favorable clinical prognosis. Salih *et al.* (75) recently reported that 16/50 human breast carcinomas, grown in organ culture for 24 hr, responded positively to the

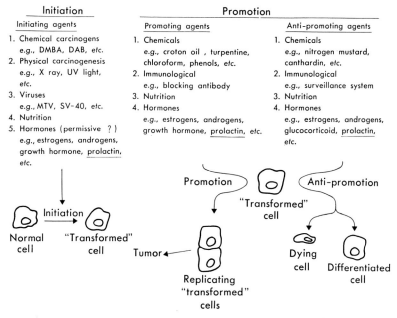

FIG. 7. Berenblum hypothesis (two-stage mechanism). The Berenblum hypothesis (77) is a well-known theoretical model of cancerigenesis depicting this oncogenic process as a two-step mechanism, *i.e.*, initiation and promotion. According to this model, prolactin probably participates in both the initiation and promotion steps of mammary tumorigenesis. In the initiation phase, variations in prolactin levels appear to influence the metabolism of the mammary epithelium, so that the epithelium would be either more receptive to or refractory to an initiating agent (*e.g.*, chemical carcinogens, physical carcinogens, *etc.*), *i.e.*, a "permissive" action. In the promotion phase, prolactin may act as either a promoter or an anti-promoter of the "transformed" cells. In promotion, the hormone may, either directly or indirectly (*via* the ovary), stimulate mitotic activity of the "transformed" cells. In anti-promotion the hormone, in the presence of requisite hormones (*e.g.*, glucocorticoids), may synergistically induce differentiation (*i.e.*, lactation) in the "transformed" cells. A tumor would be induced in the former (promotion) but not in the latter (anti-promotion) case.

stimulatory effects of prolactin by increased pentose shunt activity. They used a histochemical determination for dehydrogenase activity as an assessment of the total activity of this pathway, a metabolic cycle very important in providing 5-carbon sugars for nucleotide biosynthesis. More recently, we observed an increase in the incorporation of ^{3}H-thymidine into DNA in a significant fraction of prolactin-treated organ cultures of human breast carcinoma biopsy specimens (76).

It should be emphasized that the lack of a demonstration of an effect of prolactin on growth of human breast carcinoma does not necessarily imply that the hormone was not critically involved in its development. Bear in mind that the advanced spontaneous mouse mammary carcinoma is clearly not responsive to this hormone, but in the earlier development stages the hormone appears to be prerequisite for subsequent neoplastic development (60). Thus, it seems clear that prolactin markedly influences the development (transformation?), perhaps *via* a permissive mechanism, and/or growth (direct or indirect *via* the ovary) of the commonly investigated rodent mammary tumor models (Fig. 7). There is a pressing need to define the relationship of prolactin, as well as ovarian hormones, to development and growth of normal, hyperplastic and neoplastic mammae in humans. Once these hormonal requirements are known, prophylaxis or control of the disease may be possible by appropriate drug-mediated hormone suppression.

REFERENCES

1. Andervont, H. B. Influence of environment on mammary cancer in mice. J. Natl. Cancer Inst., *4*: 579–585, 1944.
2. Kovacs, K. Effect of androgenisation on the development of mammary tumors in rats induced by the oral administration of 9, 10-dimethyl-1, 2-benzanthracene. Brit. J. Cancer, *19*: 531–537, 1965.
3. Nagasawa, H. and Meites, J. Effects of hypothalamic estrogen implant on growth of carcinogen-induced mammary tumors in rats. Cancer Res., *30*: 1327–1329, 1970.
4. Jull, J. W. The effect of infection, hormonal environment, and genetic constitution in mammary tumor induction in rats by 7, 12-dimethylbenzanthracene. Cancer Res., *26*: 2368–2373, 1966.
5. LeShan, L. Psychological states as factors in the development of malignant disease: A critical review. J. Natl. Cancer Inst., *22*: 1–18, 1959.
6. Lacassagne, A. and Duplan, A. F. LeMécanisme de la cancerisation de la mamelle chez la souris, consideré d'après les résultats d'expériences au moyen de la reserpine. Compt. Rend. Acad. Sci., *249*: 810–812, 1959.
7. Welsch, C. W. and Meites, J. Effects of reserpine on development of 7, 12-dimethyl-benzanthracene induced mammary tumors in female rats. Experientia, *26*: 1133–1134, 1970.
8. Pearson, O. H., Llerna, O., Llerna, L., Molina, A., and Butler, T. Prolactin dependent rat mammary cancer: A model for man? Trans. Assoc. Am. Phys., *82*: 225–238, 1969.
9. Jick, H. Reserpine and breast cancer. Lancet, *2*: 669–671, 1974.
10. Armstrong, B., Stevens, N., and Doll, R. Retrospective study of the association between use of rauwolfia derivatives and breast cancer in English women. Lancet, *2*: 672–675, 1974.
11. Heinonen, O. P., Shapiro, S., Tuominen, L., and Turunen, M. I. Reserpine use in relation to breast cancer. Lancet, *2*: 675–677, 1974.
12. Frantz, A. G., Kleinberg, D. L., and Noel, G. L. Studies of prolactin in man. Rec. Prog. Hormone Res., *28*: 527–590, 1972.
13. Lu, K. H. and Meites, J. Inhibition of L-dopa and monoamine oxidase inhibitors of pituitary prolactin release; stimulation of methyldopa and *d*-amphetamine. Proc. Soc. Exp. Biol. Med., *137*: 480–483, 1972.
14. Nagasawa, H. and Meites, J. Suppression by ergocornine and iproniazid of carcinogen-induced mammary tumors in rats: Effects on serum and pituitary prolactin levels. Proc. Soc. Exp. Biol. Med., *135*: 469–472, 1970.
15. Meites, J., Lu, K. H., Wuttke, W., Welsch, C. W., Nagasawa, H., and Quadri, S. K. Recent studies on functions and control of prolactin secretion in rats. Rec. Prog. Hormone Res., *28*: 471–526, 1972.
16. Dickey, R. P. and Minton J. P. Levodopa relief of bone pain from breast cancer. New Engl. J. Med., *286*: 843, 1972.

17. Murray, R.M.L., Mozaffarian, G., and Pearson, O. H. Prolactin levels with L-dopa treatment in metastatic breast carcinoma. *In;* A. R. Boyns and K. Griffiths (eds.), Prolactin and Carcinogenesis, pp. 158–161, Alpha Omega Alpha Publ., Cardiff, Wales, U. K., 1972.

18. Stoll, B. A. Brain catecholamines and breast cancer. A hypothesis. Lancet, *1*: 431, 1972.

19. Liebelt, R. A. Effects of gold-thioglucose-induced hypothalamic lesions in mammary tumorigenesis in RIII × CBA mice. Proc. Am. Assoc. Cancer Res., *3*: 37, 1959.

20. Welsch, C. W., Clemens, J. A., and Meites, J. Effects of hypothalamic and amygdaloids lesions on development and growth of carcinogen-induced mammary tumors in the female rat. Cancer Res., *29*: 1541–1549, 1969.

21. Klaiber, M. S., Gruenstein, M., Meranze, D. R., and Shimkin, M. B. Influence of hypothalamic lesions on induction and growth of mammary cancers in Sprague-Dawley rats receiving 7, 12-dimethylbenzanthracene. Cancer Res., *29*: 999–1001, 1969.

22. Welsch, C. W., Negro-Vilar, A., and Meites, J. Effects of pituitary homografts on host pituitary prolactin and hypothalamic PIF levels. Neuroendocrinology, *3*: 238–245, 1968.

23. Welsch, C. W., Jenkins, T., Amenomori, Y., and Meites, J. Tumorous development of *in situ* and grafted anterior pituitaries in female rats treated with diethylstilbestrol. Experientia, *27*: 1350–1352, 1971.

24. Welsch, C. W., Squiers, M. D., Cassell, E., Chen, C. L., and Meites, J. Median eminence lesions and serum prolactin: Influence of ovariectomy and ergocornine. Am. J. Physiol., *221*: 1714–1717, 1971.

25. Welsch, C. W., Nagasawa, H., and Meites, J. Increased incidence of spontaneous mammary tumors in female rats with induced hypothalamic lesions. Cancer Res., *30*: 2310–2313, 1970.

26. Bruni, J. E. and Montemurro, D. G. Effect of hypothalamic lesions on the genesis of spontaneous mammary gland tumors in the mouse. Cancer Res., *31*: 854–863, 1971.

27. Moon, H. D., Simpson, M. E., Li, C. H., and Evans, H. M. Neoplasms in rats treated with pituitary growth hormone. V. Absence of neoplasms in hypophysectomized rats. Cancer Res., *11*: 535–539, 1951.

28. Mühlbock, O. and Boot, L. M. Induction of mammary cancer in mice without the mammary tumor agent by isografts of hypophyses. Cancer Res., *19*: 402–412, 1959.

29. Welsch, C. W., Clemens, J. A., and Meites, J. Effects of multiple pituitary homografts or progesterone on 7, 12-dimethylbenzanthracene induced mammary tumors in rats. J. Natl. Cancer Inst., *41*: 465–471, 1968.

30. Welsch, C. W., Jenkins, T. W., and Meites, J. Increased incidence of mammary tumors in the female rat grafted with multiple pituitaries. Cancer Res., *30*: 1024–1029, 1970.

31. Haran-Ghera, N. The role of mammotrophin in mammary tumor induction in mice. Cancer Res., *21*: 790–795, 1961.

32. Boot, L. M., Mühlbock, O., and Ropche, G. Prolactin and the induction of mammary tumors in mice. Gen. Comp. Endrocrinol., *2*: 601–603, 1962.

33. Kim, U. and Furth, J. Relation of mammary tumors to mammotropes. II. Hormone responsiveness of 3-methylcholanthrene induced mammary carcinomas. Proc. Soc. Exp. Biol. Med., *103*: 643–645, 1960.

34. Talwalker, P. K., Meites, J., and Mizuno, H. Mammary tumor induction by estrogen or anterior pituitary hormones in ovariectomized rats given 7,12-dimethylbenzanthracene. Proc. Soc. Exp. Biol. Med., *116*: 531–534, 1964.

35. Nagasawa, H. and Yanai, R. Effects of prolactin or growth hormone on growth of carcinogen-induced mammary tumors of adreno-ovariectomized rats. Int. J. Cancer, *6*: 488–495, 1970.

36. Meites, J. and Nicoll, C. S. Adenohypophysis: Prolactin. Annu. Rev. Physiol., *28*: 57–88, 1966.

37. Welsch, C. W., Sar, M., Clemens, J. A., and Meites, J. Effects of estrogen on pituitary prolactin levels of female rats bearing median eminence implants of prolactin. Proc. Soc. Exp. Biol. Med., *129*: 817–820, 1968.

38. Sterental, A., Dominquez, J. M., Weissman, C., and Pearson, O. H. Pituitary role in the estrogen dependency of experimental mammary cancer. Cancer Res., *23*: 481–484, 1963.

39. Turkington, R. W. and Hilf, R. Hormonal dependence of DNA synthesis in mammary carcinoma cells *in vitro*. Science, *160*: 1457–1460, 1968.

40. Welsch, C. W. and Rivera, E. M. Differential effects of estrogen and prolactin on DNA synthesis in organ cultures of DMBA-induced rat mammary carcinoma. Proc. Soc. Exp. Biol. Med., *139*: 623–626, 1972.

41. Dao, T. L. Studies on mechanism of carcinogenesis in the mammary gland. Prog. Exp. Tumor Res., *11*: 235–261, 1969.

42. Welsch, C. W. Growth inhibition of rat mammary carcinoma induced by *cis*-platinum diaminodichloride-II. J. Natl. Cancer Inst., *47*: 1071–1078, 1971.

43. Sinha, D., Cooper, D., and Dao, T. L. The nature of estrogen and prolactin effect on mammary tumorigenesis. Cancer Res., *33*: 411–414, 1973.

44. Welsch, C. W. Effect of brain lesions on mammary tumorigenesis. *In;* T. L. Dao (ed.), Estrogen Target Tissue and Neoplasia, pp. 317–331, Univ. of Chicago Press, Chicago, Ill., 1972.

45. Hollander, V. P., Jonas, H., and Smith, D. E. Estradiol-sensitive isocitric dehydrogenase in non-cancerous and cancerous human breast tissue. Cancer, *11*: 803–809, 1958.

46. Huggins, C., Moon, R. C., and Morii, S. Extinction of experimental mammary cancer. I. Estradiol-17β and progesterone. Proc. Natl. Acad. Sci. U.S., *48*: 379–386, 1962.

47. Welsch, C. W. and Meites, J. Effects of norethynodrel-mestranol combination (Enovid) on development and growth of carcinogen-induced mammary tumors in female rats. Cancer, *23*: 601–607, 1969.

48. Stoll, B. A. Tumor regression following ovarian steroid therapy. *In;* B. A. Stoll (ed.), Mammary Cancer and Neuroendocrine Therapy, pp. 57–81, Butterworth, London, 1974.

49. Kim, U. Pituitary function and hormonal therapy of experimental breast cancer. Cancer Res., *25*: 1146–1161, 1965.

50. Chen, C. L. and Meites, J. Effects of estrogen and progesterone on serum and pituitary prolactin levels in ovariectomized rats. Endocrinology, *86*: 503–505, 1970.

51. Meites, J., Cassell, E., and Clark, J. Estrogen inhibition of mammary tumor growth in rats; counteraction by prolactin. Proc. Soc. Exp. Biol. Med., *137*; 1225–1227, 1971.

52. Yanai, R. and Nagasawa, H. Inhibition by ergocornine and 2-Br-α-ergocryptin of spontaneous mammary tumor appearance in mice. Experientia, *27*: 934, 1971.

53. Welsch, C. W., Iturri, G., and Meites, J. Comparative effects of hypophysectomy, ergocornine and ergocornine-reserpine treatments on rat mammary carcinoma. Int. J. Cancer, *12*: 205–212, 1973.

54. Lutterbeck, P. M., Pryor, J. S., Varga, L., and Wenner, R. Treatment of nonpuerperal galactorrhea with an ergot alkaloid. Brit. Med. J., *3*: 228–229, 1971.

55. Brooks, C. L. and Welsch, C. W. Reduction of serum prolactin in rats by 2 ergot alkaloids and 2 ergoline derivatives: A comparison. Proc. Soc. Exp. Biol. Med., *146*: 863–867, 1974.

56. Lu, K. H., Koch, Y., and Meites, J. Direct inhibition by ergocornine of pituitary prolactin release. Endocrinology, *89*: 229–233, 1970.

57. Wuttke, W., Cassel, E., and Meites, J. Effects of ergocornine on serum prolactin and LH and on hypothalamic content of PIF and LRF. Endocrinology, *88*: 737–741, 1971.

58. Cassell, E. E., Meites, J., and Welsch, C. W. Effects of ergocornine and ergocryptine on growth of 7,12-dimethylbenzanthracene-induced mammary tumors in rats. Cancer Res., *31*: 1051–1053, 1971.

59. Quadri, S. K. and Meites, J. Regression of spontaneous mammary tumors in rats by ergot drugs. Proc. Soc. Exp. Biol. Med., *138*: 999–1001, 1971.

60. Welsch, C. W. and Gribler, C. Prophylaxis of spontaneously developing mammary carcinoma in C3H/HeJ female mice by suppression of prolactin. Cancer Res., *33*: 2939–2946, 1973.

61. Dux, A. and Mühlbock, O. Enhancement by hypophyseal hormones on the malignant transformation of transplanted hyperplastic nodules of the mouse mammary gland. Eur. J. Cancer, *5*: 191–194, 1969.

62. DeOme, K. B., Faulkin, L. J., Bern, H. A., and Blair, P. B. Development of Mammary tumors from hyperplastic alveolar nodules transplanted into gland-free mammary fat pads of female C3H mice. Cancer Res., *19*: 515–520, 1959.

63. Welsch, C. W. and Clemens, J. A. 6-Methyl-8-β-ergoline-acetonitrile-induced inhibition of mammary hyperplastic alveolar nodular development and growth in C3H/HeJ female mice. Proc. Soc. Exp. Biol. Med., *142*: 1067–1071, 1973.

64. Yanai, R. and Nagasawa, H. Suppression of mammary hyperplastic nodule formation and pituitary prolactin secretion in mice induced by ergocornine or 2-bromo-α-ergocryptine. J. Natl. Cancer Inst., *45*: 1105–1112, 1970.

65. Brooks, C. L. and Welsch, C. W. Inhibition of mammary dysplasia in estrogen-treated C3H/HeJ female mice by treatment with 2-bromo-α-ergocryptine. Proc. Soc. Exp. Biol. Med., *145*: 484–487, 1974.

66. Welsch, C. W. and Morford, L. K. Influence of chronic treatment with 2-bromo-α-ergocryptine (CB-154) on the reproductive and lactational performance of the C3H/HeJ female mouse. Experientia, *30*: 1353–1355, 1974.

67. Welsch, C. W., Gribler, C., and Clemens, J. A. 6-Methyl-8-β-ergoline-acetonitrile (MEA)-induced suppression of mammary tumorigenesis in C3H/HeJ female mice. Eur. J. Cancer, *10*: 595–600, 1974.

68. Clemens, J. A. and Shaar, C. J. Inhibition by ergocornine of initiation and growth of 7,12-dimethylbenzanthracene-induced mammary tumors in rats: Effect of tumor size. Proc. Soc. Exp. Biol. Med., *139*: 659–662, 1972.

69. Friesen, H. G. Human placental lactogen and human pituitary prolactin. Clin. Obstet. Gynecol., *14*: 669–684, 1971.

70. Boyns, A. R., Cole, E. N., Griffiths, K., Roberts, M. M., Buchan, R., Wilson, R. G.,

and Forrest, A.P.M. Plasma prolactin in breast cancer. Eur. J. Cancer, *9*: 99–102, 1973.

71. Schultz, J. D. Czygan, P. J., del Pozo, E., and Frieser, H. Varying response of human metastasizing breast cancer to the treatment with 2-Br-alpha-ergocryptine (CB-154): Case report. *In;* J. L. Pasteels and C. Robyn (eds.), International Symposium of Human Prolactin (International Congress Series, No. 368), pp. 268–271, Excerpta Medica, Amsterdam, 1973.

72. Heuson, J. C., Coune, A., and Staquet, M. Clinical trial of 2-Br-α-ergocryptine (CB-154) in advanced breast cancer. Eur. J. Cancer, *8*: 155–156, 1972.

73. Antony, G. J., VanWyk, J. J., French, F. S., Weaver, R. P., Dugger, G. S., Timmons, R. L., and Newsome, J. F. Influence of pituitary stalk section on growth hormone insulin and TSH secretion in women with metastatic breast cancer. J. Clin. Endocrinol. Metabol., *29*: 1238–1250, 1969.

74. Mioduszewska, O., Kawzarowski, T., and Gorski, C. The influence of hormones on breast cancer *in vitro* in relation to the clinical course of the disease. *In;* A.P.M. Forrest and P. B. Kunkler (eds.), Prognostic Factors in Breast Cancer, pp. 347–360, The Williams and Williams Co., Baltimore, 1968.

75. Salih, H., Flax, H., Brander, W., and Hobbs, J. R. Prolactin dependence in human breast cancer. Lancet, *2*: 1103–1105, 1972.

76. Welsch, C. W. Effect of prolactin on the *in vitro* incorporation of H^3-thymidine into DNA of human breast malignancies. Abstr. Papers 11th Int. Cancer Congr., Florence, Italy, pp. 122, 1974.

77. Berenblum, I. Carcinogenesis and tumor pathogenesis. Adv. Cancer Res., *2*: 129–175, 1954.

Discussion of Paper of Dr. Welsch

Dr. J. C. Laurence (University of Chicago Pritzker School of Medicine, Chicago, Illinois, and Institute for Cancer Research, Osaka University Medical School, Osaka): Some interesting clinical data bearing on a possible relationship between human mammary carcinogenesis and elevated serum prolactin levels appeared in a series of papers in a September, 1974, issue of the Lancet. Three groups, representing Boston (Jick, H. *et al.*, Lancet. *2*: 669, 1974), Oxford (Armstrong, B., Stevens, N., and Doll, R., Lancet, *2*: 672, 1974), and Helsinki (Heinonen, O. P. *et al.*, Lancet, *2*: 673, 1974), incited by preliminary findings from the Boston collaborative Drug Surveillance Program in its routine scanning of information gleaned from a survey of hospital patients, recorded significant retrospective associations between the use of reserpine or other Rauwolfia derivatives, such as methoserpidine, and breast cancer incidence in females. Reserpine was here employed as a therapeutic for individuals suffering from mild to moderate hypertension, and controls were matched for age, personal habits, prior drug history, and degree of hypertension either untreated or being managed with alternative regimens. A simple explanation based solely on acute stimulation of prolactin is untenable, as no association between the use of α-methyldopa, an anti-hypertensive which can also enhance prolactin release, and breast cancer was realized, but the suggestive evidence is provocative. Would you care to comment?

Dr. Welsch: In these independent analyses, women being treated with the tranquilizer reserpine appeared to be in a 2–3 fold higher risk group for the development of breast cancer. The actual number of cases involved is low, however, and E. Wynder in N.Y.C. is presently conducting more extensive investigations along similar lines. One must retain great caution in interpreting these data, as a number of very potent prolactin stimulators, including other types of tranquilizers, such as the phenothiazines, did not yield comparable associations. I would, of course, be extremely excited if a causal relationship for prolactin is confirmed in these studies, because of all the anterior pituitary hormones it is the one hormone which, at present, can be most effectively controlled with drugs.

Dr. J. C. Laurence: With this concern, is it possible to employ the hypothalamic prolactin inhibitory factor in the specific depression of prolactin release in man, rather than the ergot alkaloids and ergoline derivatives which you have investigated?

DR. WELSCH: While we are confident that a prolactin inhibitory activity exists in the hypothalamus, PIF as yet remains a hypothetical moiety, never having been isolated. It would certainly be a tremendous asset should it ever become available. However, the ergot preparations we employed mimic PIF activity to a significant degree, and at least in lower mammals, appear to be relatively specific for prolactin, not markedly influencing the secretion of the other hypophyseal peptides in mice and rats.

DR. Y. IKAWA: The majority of rodent mammary carcinomas present well dif-ferentiated histologies, which might be expected to be sensitive to hormonal manip-ulation. Are the transplantable Huggins rat carcinomas, which are more variable histologically, as susceptible to prolactin stimulation? Also, is there a relationship between the degree of differentiation of human breast carcinomas and their prolactin responsiveness?

DR. WELSCH: Transplantable rat mammary neoplasms exhibit great diversity in their response to prolactin, most being stimulated by the hormone while others are actually inhibited by the peptide. Prolactin appears to induce secretory activity in a number of these latter types of tumors. We have not observed a good correla-tion between the histological characteristics of either a rodent or human tumor and the responsiveness of that tumor to prolactin.

DR. NISHIZUKA: Have you noted a relationship between the degree of *in vitro* responsiveness of a tumor to prolactin and the time of its appearance following DMBA induction?

DR. WELSCH: Those tumors which arise quickly following DMBA treatment are generally much more sensitive to prolactin in our *in vitro* system. Only approximately 2/3 of those tumors taking very prolonged periods to appear respond at all to this hormone. Of those tumors which respond, there is also a marked variation in the percent incorporation of ^{3}H-thymidine *in vitro*, with a range of 75–250%. We have yet to correlate this difference with *in vivo* tumor growth.

DR. NAUTS: Has anyone examined blood prolactin levels of women at potentially greater risks for the development of breast cancers because of a putative genetic association?

DR. WELSCH: Pearson and his colleagues in the U.S.A. have noted a positive correlation between blood prolactin levels and the incidence of breast cancers in women, but a group in Europe (Boyns *et al.*) did not confirm these findings.

DR. HALPERN: Have attempts been made to suppress prolactin secretion by means of an anti-prolactin antiserum?

DR. WELSCH: In 1971 Butler and Pearson obtained regression of an existing carcinogen-induced rat mammary neoplasm with such an antiserum.

DR. HOBBS: Does the chronic suppression of prolactin beginning early in life prevent normal pubertal breast development?

Secondly, just as you've noted that prolactin sometimes inhibits tumor growth, I suspect that increased secretion of this hormone may explain the rare patients whose tumors have regressed following infundibular section.

DR. WELSCH: Prolactin suppressed animals retain a normal sized mamma but the epithelial elements are very atrophic.

Pituitary stalk section leading to breast carcinoma regression in humans was first reported by Eckles in 1959. High secretory activity was observed both in the residual breast tissue and in the neoplasm, so that the regression appeared to be associated with a lactational response, *i.e.*, a differentiation rather than increased mitogenic activity. We believe this is also true in the rodent system, *i.e.*, prolactin may inhibit tumor growth as it promotes differentiation and secretory function.

DR. ALEXANDER: Was prolonged prolactin suppression the equivalent of mastectomy, in that an irreversible change was induced so that on resumption of prolactin secretion the breast no longer responded to it?

DR. WELSCH: Within two weeks after a 10–12 month period of prolactin withdrawal, during which time the mammary gland epithelium is extremely atrophic, the induced changes were fully reversible, yielding normal lobular-alveolar development in response to prolactin treatment. It is not truly a medical mastectomy as the ductal elements persist during the period of chronic prolactin suppression, remaining simply in a quiescent state as they lack the complete hormonal stimulus required for induction of cell division.

DR. JANKOVIĆ: It is known that hypothalamic lesion and reserpine treatment induce tremendous alterations in the cellular structure of the thymus. Did you examine the thymus during the course of your experiments?

DR. WELSCH: No, but we may in the future. However, reserpine does not affect advanced, spontaneous hormone-insensitive mouse mammary carcinomas, suggesting that an immunologic phenomenon is not playing a key role in the processes we have described.

Brown Adipose Tissue: Relationship to Cell-mediated Immunity

Branislav D. Janković

Immunology Research Center, Belgrade, Yugoslavia

Abstract: The role of the brown adipose tissue (BAT) in humoral and cellular immunity was investigated in normal rats treated with saline extract of the tissue, and in rats from which the interscapular BAT was removed at birth (partially adipectomized rats). Repeated injections of allogeneic tissue extract did not affect the formation of antibody, but markedly suppressed the Arthus reactivity and delayed skin sensitivity to bovine serum albumin.

In adipectomized rats, the production of antibody and the number of plaque-forming cells to sheep erythrocytes seemed to remain normal. However, adipectomy caused a general potentiation of cell-mediated immunity, as shown by the increased delayed skin hypersensitivity, more pronounced clinical and histopathological signs of allergic encephalomyelitis, enhanced enlargement of the popliteal lymph nodes in a host-*versus*-graft reaction, and accelerated rejection of thyroid allograft implanted under the kidney capsule. So far as the development and expression of experimental allergic encephalomyelitis is concerned, it seems that BAT and the thymus are natural antagonists in the domain of cellular immunity.

The growth of primary sarcoma transplants was studied in mice adipectomized at 6 weeks of age. In allogeneic combinations, adipectomized mice rejected tumor in an accelerated manner. In the isogeneic combination, an exciting finding was that adipectomized mice survived much longer the inoculation of tumor cells than sham-adipectomized controls.

Although these results suggest a thymus-dependent cell (T cell) orientation of the immunopotentiation induced by adipectomy, the relevance of BAT to T lymphocytes still remains to be elucidated. It seems that this tissue influences the function of lymphocytes rather than the proliferation of lymphocytes. The immune role of this tissue probably is dependent on the capacity of the BAT microenvironment to synthesize and release biologically active substances (noradrenaline? unsaturated fatty acids?), and on the functional relationship between BAT and other tissues.

The structure and function of the immune system cannot be studied in isolation from other systems of the body. It is now clear that the field of immunological activities is triangular, with three systems for its sides: the immune system, nervous system, and endocrine system. It is in this context that the development, morphology and physiology of lymphocytes and their associates should be considered and studied. Consequently, the nonlymphoid cells, such as reticular cells and neurons, and neurohumoral, hormonal, and lymphochemical agents should be regarded as normal constituents of the dynamic immune microenvironment (1). The present report introduces a nonlymphoid tissue, the brown adipose tissue (BAT), into cell-mediated immunity.

General Features of BAT

The BAT (brown fat, hibernating gland, embryonal fat, *etc.*) is the subject of several comprehensive reviews (2–5). I shall confine myself here to some basic information relevant to the purpose of this report.

The BAT was first identified in the marmot by Gesner (6). It occurs in appreciable amounts only in certain newborn nonhibernators (man, monkey, cat, sheep, rabbit, rat, mouse, *etc.*), in hibernators (marmot, hedgehog, ground squirrel, *etc.*), and in cold-acclimated animals. The topography of this tissue in adult rats is described by Hammar (7), the largest portion being situated between the blade shoulders. In the rat, the amount of BAT decreases with age (8).

Morphologically, the most outstanding features are its lobulated nature, dense capillary networks surrounding the cells (9), and abundance of intercellular sympathetic nerve endings (10). BAT contains numerous mitochondria, large amounts of unsaturated fatty acids (11) and noradrenaline (12), and several steroids which are not present in white fat (13). Functionally, the tissue possesses an extraordinarily metabolic potential (5). In the past, BAT was regarded as part of the thymus, an endocrine gland, or a reservoire for food substances (14, 15), but it is now widely recognized as the principal source of nonshivering thermogenesis. Its calorigenic function and its postulated endocrine function are controlled by the sympathetic nerve system, most probably *via* stimulation of adenyl cyclase and acceleration of lipolysis by catecholamines (5).

A variety of stress factors and hormones affect the morphology and physiology of BAT in both hibernators and nonhibernators (3, 16). The tissue may serve as a reservoire for encephalitis, rabies and Coxsackie viruses (17). Hypertrophy of BAT has been observed in humans with pheochromocytoma (18).

The current interest of biologists in BAT is focused on its role in the regulation of metabolic processes, and its function in nonshivering production of heat. This tissue has remained, however, little known to immunologists. Since earlier studies have shown that deep hibernation and artificially induced hypothermia suppress the formation of antibody (17, 19–22), and since BAT is the most important heat-producing organ in hibernating animals, the first experiments to discover the role of the tissue in immunity were directly concerned with its thermogenic function, and were performed on the cultured explants of tissue of hibernating animals (23, 24).

The experiments that will be described here differ conceptually and methodologically from the above-mentioned reports. Our studies were motivated by the extraordinary and heterogeneous metabolic activities of BAT, and its relation to the sympathetic nervous system and hormones. Moreover, the immune function of the tissue was investigated *in vivo*, in nonhibernators and at normal body temperature.

Influences of BAT Extract on Antibody Production, Arthus Reactivity, and Delayed Sensitivity

Our first studies were concerned with the effect of BAT extract on immune reactions in the rat (25, 26). The saline extract was prepared from lyophilized interscapular BAT of 1-day-old rats, and used for the treatment of normal 8-week-old rats of the same strain. Control rats received multiple injections of saline extract of white fat or of saline alone. Bearing in mind the high concentration of noradrenaline in the tissue (12), and in an attempt to find out the possible role of catecholamines in immune reactions, adult rats were given injections of 12 μg of noradrenaline, an amount which is higher than that found in a single dose of BAT extract. Rats of all groups were challenged with bovine serum albumin (BSA) in complete Freund's adjuvant.

The results summarized in Table 1 indicate that rats treated with BAT extract produced circulating anti-BSA antibody at a level similar to that of controls. On the other hand, there was a striking diminution of Arthus reactivity and delayed skin hypersensitivity in rats treated with BAT extract. These results indicate that BAT may be involved in reactions of cell-mediated type.

The failure of BAT extract, taken from nonhibernating animals and injected into animals which do not normally experience seasonal hibernation, to exert an effect on antibody production, is not in accordance with observations on hibernating animals. Namely, it has been reported that brown fat extract from hibernating ground squirrels can inhibit antibody production *in vitro* (23, 24), and that the chloroform extract of brown fat of hibernating ground squirrels, cold-acclimated

TABLE 1. Antibody Production, Arthus Reactivity, and Delayed Skin Hypersensitivity to BSA in Rats Treated with BAT Extract

Rats treated with[a]	Mean antibody titer ($\log_2$)		Mean Arthus reaction (mm)		Mean delayed reaction (mm)	
	10 days	20 days	10 days	20 days	10 days	20 days
BAT extract	1.8	5.1	0	6.1	0.8	11.2
WAT extract	2.5	6.0	5.2	15.7	10.4	18.2
Noradrenaline	2.2	5.8	5.6	16.1	9.5	17.0
Saline	2.4	6.2	6.0	17.8	8.5	11.6

WAT: white adipose tissue.   [a] Eight rats in each group.

deer mice, brown bats and newborn rabbits exert an immunosuppressive effect on antibody production by fragments of the hamster's spleen cultured with sheep red cells (27). The use of nonhibernators in the *in vivo* studies, the manner of preparing the extract, and the amount of extract employed for the treatment may account for this discrepancy between the results of our group and those of Dr. Sidky's group. A number of other circumstances are mentioned elsewhere (28). At the present state of our knowledge, the role of BAT in humoral immunity of non-hibernators must be regarded as unresolved.

Although the influence that the sympathetic nervous system exerts on BAT (10) would imply that noradrenaline may be a factor responsible for the immune function of BAT, the rats given multiple injections of noradrenaline for a period of 26 days did not exhibit apparent immunological abnormalities. These negative results may be ascribed to the rapid decomposition of injected noradrenaline (29, 30). The possibility still remains, therefore, that this agent is capable of interfering with immune processes under experimental conditions differing from those described here (31).

Effect of Neonatal Adipectomy on Hemolysin-forming Cells, Antibody Production and Delayed Skin Hypersensitivity

Most of experiments to be reported here were performed on rats from which the interscapular BAT was surgically extirpated at birth (adipectomy). Such an adipectomy should be considered as incomplete one since it leaves intact 40–50% of the newborn rat BAT. As a rule, sham-adipectomized animals served as controls.

Table 2 illustrates the number of hemolysin-forming cells to sheep erythrocytes, and antibody production and delayed skin reactions to BSA in sham-adipectomized and adipectomized rats challenged at the age of 8 weeks. Hemolytic plaque assays with spleen cells revealed a statistically insignificant difference between the number of direct plaque-forming cells (PFC) in control and adipectomized rats. The amounts of anti-BSA antibody, as determined by a passive microhemagglutination reaction, were also quite similar in both groups of rats. These findings are in substantial agreement with observations on antibody formation in rats treated with BAT extract (25, 26).

As for delayed skin hypersensitivity, the neonatal ablation of BAT induced a

TABLE 2. IgM PFC to Sheep Erythrocytes, and Antibody Production and Delayed Skin Hypersensitivity to BSA in Sham-adipectomized and Adipectomized Rats

Group	Mean number of PFC per 10^6 spleen cells[a]	Mean antibody titer $(\log_2)$[b]		Mean diameter (mm) of skin reaction[b]	
		10 days	20 days	10 days	20 days
Sham-adipectomized	3,013	2.1	5.9	7.2	16.3
Adipectomized	2,672	2.2	5.6	19.8	21.8

[a] Five rats in group; PFC were detected 5 days after intravenous immunization with 7×10^8 sheep red cells. [b] Twelve rats in group; tests were performed 10 and 20 days after immunization with BSA in complete Freund's adjuvant.

marked potentiation of skin reactions to BSA (*28*), this being particularly clear in rats skin-tested 10 days after immunization (Table 2). Undoubtedly, these results supplement those showing the immunosuppressive influence of the tissue extract on delayed sensitivity (*25, 26*).

Essential Features of the Adipectomy Effect on Experimental Allergic Encephalomyelitis, and the Antagonistic Influences of Thymectomy and Adipectomy on Cell-mediated Immunity

The most striking immunopotentiating effect of neonatal adipectomy was observed in rats which were sensitized with allogeneic spinal cord in complete Freund's adjuvant in order to induce allergic encephalomyelitis (Fig. 1). Neonatally thymectomized, and thymectomized-adipectomized animals were also included in this experiment. The incidence and severity of clinical and histopathological signs of the disease reached the highest level in adipectomized rats. On the other hand, none of thymectomized and thymo-adipectomized rats developed paralysis, and only a small number of thymectomized animals exhibited mild histological lesions in the brain and spinal cord. The intensity and distribution of lesions were quite similar in control sham-adipectomized and thymectomized-adipectomized rats (*28, 32*).

On the basis of these observations, it may be concluded that rats lacking BAT exhibit a higher capacity to develop allergic encephalomyelitis whereas thymectomized rats show markedly less propensity to develop this disease (*33*). In other words, BAT acts as an antagonist of the thymus in cell-mediated immunity. This view is supported by the fact that thymectomized-adipectomized rats possessed a normal capacity to respond to encephalitogenic stimulus, *i.e.*, the suppressive effect of neonatal thymectomy on encephalomyelitis is neutralized by the potentiating effect of neonatal adipectomy, and *vice versa*.

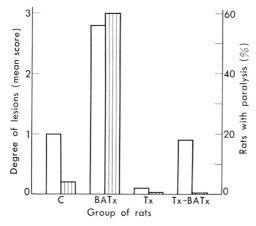

FIG. 1. Severity of allergic encephalomyelitis lesions (open bars) and incidence of paralysis (striped bars) in sham-adipectomized (C), adipectomized (BATx), thymectomized (Tx), and thymectomized-adipectomized (Tx-BATx) rats. Histological lesions were graded as follows: negative, 0; +, 1; ++, 2; and +++, 3. The arithmetic score reflecting an overall response was calculated for each group.

Enhancement of Popliteal Lymph Node Enlargement (LNE) in a Host-versus-Graft Reaction by Neonatal Adipectomy

The enlargement of the rat popliteal lymph nodes following the injection of parental cells into the footpad proved to be a sensitive measure of graft-*versus*-host reaction (*34*). On the other hand, the current methods of evaluating a host-*versus*-graft reaction *in vivo* are still qualitative and subjective (*35*). Recently, a quantitative lymph node weight assay for allogeneic interactions in the rat has been described (*36*), in which the interference of graft-*versus*-host component was excluded by exposing donor cells to Mitomycin-C prior to their injection into the footpad of the recipient rat.

In order to avoid participation of donor immunocompetent cells in the LNE assay, we have employed the thyroid, which is poor in lymphocytes, as allogeneic graft (Janković, Janežić, and Popesković, manuscript in preparation). For this purpose, the thyroid of Lewis rats was implanted in the immediate vicinity of the popliteal lymph nodes of Wistar rats. The ipsilateral lymph nodes were extirpated 6 days after transplantation, accurately weighed and examined histologically. The contralateral popliteal lymph nodes served as controls. This kind of LNE assay provided objective and quantitative parameters for the evaluation of local lymph node response to allograft.

The results summarized in Table 3 indicate that the magnitude of allograft response at 6 days was significantly greater in rats adipectomized at birth than in sham-adipectomized and neonatally thymectomized animals. These findings point to the relationship between the function of BAT and sensitization to allo-antigens.

TABLE 3. LNE in a Host-*versus*-Graft Reaction 6 Days after Implantation of Thyroid Allograft in the Immediate Vicinity of the Recipient's Popliteal Lymph Node

Group	No. of rats	LNE index[a]
Sham-adipectomized	8	1.42 ± 0.40
Adipectomized	6	2.95 ± 1.30[b]
Thymectomized	6	1.29 ± 0.55[c]

[a] LNE index $= \dfrac{\text{weight of ipsilateral lymph node (mg)}}{\text{weight of contralateral lymph node (mg)}}$. Student's *t* test was employed. Values are means $\pm$ standard errors. [b] $P < 0.02$. [c] $P > 0.05$.

Potentiation of Thyroid Allograft Rejection by Neonatal Adipectomy

Transplantation immunity was further ascertained by studying the kinetics of rejection of thyroid grafts taken from Lewis rats and implanted under the kidney capsule of Wistar rats (*28*). Several circumstances justified the use of that transplantation model: (a) since adipectomized rats were supposed to reject the allograft in an accelerated manner, it was expected that the characteristic cellular makeup of the thyroid would make it much easier to recognize the incipient signs of rejection, (b) the implantation of the thyroid under the kidney capsule is less harmful for the graft itself (*37*), and prevents postoperative injury of the graft, (c) the

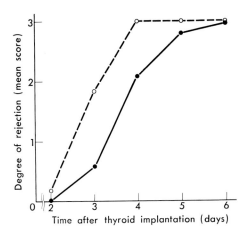

FIG. 2. Rejection of allogeneic thyroid graft implanted under the kidney capsule of sham-adipectomized (●) and adipectomized (○) rats. The degree of rejection was graded from 0 to 3. For calculation of mean score see the legend for Fig. 1. Mean score 3 means complete rejection.

traumatic component of the operation does not greatly affect the bed of the graft, and (d) the evaluation of rejection is based on histological inspection at different levels of the graft and thus is semi-quantitative.

The rejection of the thyroid allograft (Fig. 2) is enhanced in adipectomized rats. As early as 2 days after implantation, the host mononuclear cells form groups in the graft, and at 4 days, the normal cellular architecture of the thyroid is completely replaced by a mass of lymphoid cells. However, 4 days after transplantation there were several unchanged thyroid follicles in the graft in sham-adipectomized animals.

Growth of Primary Allogeneic and Isogeneic Sarcoma Transplants in Adipectomized Mice

Sarcoma I (SaI) tumor, which is regarded as almost insensitive to the action of antibodies (*38, 39*), was used in the study of tumor growth and rejection in normal and adipectomized mice (Janković, Vujanović, and Popesković, manuscript in preparation). The interscapular BAT was removed from 6-week-old inbred CBA, C57BL/6, and A/JAX mice, and 7 days later CBA and C57BL/6 animals were inoculated subcutaneously with 10^7, and A/JAX mice with 2×10^3 viable SaI cells. Sarcoma development was assessed by measuring the diameters of solid tumors. Those mice that died were autopsied to confirm the presence of a tumor.

The growth of sarcomas in allogeneic combinations (Fig. 3) was characterized by accelerated rejection of the tumor both in CBA and C57BL/6 mice lacking the interscapular BAT. The most striking finding was revealed in the isogeneic combination (Fig. 4). Sham-adipectomized A/JAX mice did not survive the 60th day after inoculation of SaI cells. On the other hand, adipectomized A/JAX mice showed a higher survival rate since about 25% of those animals were still alive on day 60.

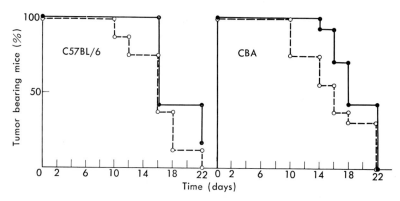

FIG. 3. Rejection of SaI tumor in C57BL/6 and CBA sham-adipectomized (●) and adipectomized (○) mice.

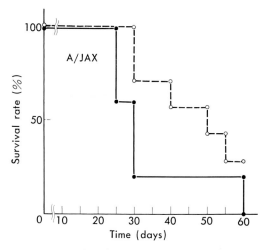

FIG. 4. Percentage survival of A/JAX sham-adipectomized (●) and adipectomized (○) mice
inoculated with syngeneic SaI tumor cells.

These results strongly suggest that BAT played a role in the immunity of CBA
and C57BL/6 mice to SaI tumor. Besides, the observations made in the isogeneic
combination would imply that the prolonged survival of adipectomized A/JAX
mice was due to the occurrence of cell-mediated immunity, *i.e.*, the extirpation of
the interscapular BAT resulted in a general increase of the cell-mediated immune
potential which enabled the recognition of even discrete histocompatibility differences between the SaI tumor and A/JAX mice.

DISCUSSION

The study of the role of BAT in the development and expression of cell-mediated immunity is in its initial phase so that the risk of generalization and over-
simplification cannot be avoided when theorizing about this subject. The first

question that naturally arises concerns the extent to which neonatal adipectomy affects the architecture of lymphoid tissues. Interestingly, histological examination of the thymus, spleen, lymph nodes, and Peyer's patches of sham-adipectomized and adipectomized rats did not reveal apparent differences (28). It seems that the effect of BAT is not mediated through stimulation of the proliferation of antigen-sensitive cells, as has been proposed for the immunopotentiating action of adjuvants (40). This view is supported by the observations that neonatally thymectomized-adipectomized rats exhibited a normal cellular immune response, as judged by their ability to develop allergic encephalomyelitis (28), in spite of the persistence of characteristic depletion of lymphocytes in thymus-dependent areas of the spleen and lymph nodes (41). Accordingly, the compromised cellular immunity due to neonatal thymectomy (33) can be repaired by adipectomy through mechanisms which concern primarily the humoral activity of BAT and the function of lymphocytes. In other words, some substances produced in the tissue take part, directly or indirectly, in the regulation of immune response, assuming that the function of lymphocytes can be influenced by immediate and remote surroundings and agents.

Because of the rich network of sympathetic nerve supply (10) and high concentration of noradrenaline (12) in BAT, the noradrenaline may be the suspect biologically active substance. To test such an assumption it would be appropriate to study the immune capacity of animals which are immunologically or chemically sympathectomized (42). Experiments of that kind are in progress in our laboratory.

Unsaturated fatty acids may be another substance by which BAT influences the immune machinery of the body. Indeed, triglycerides comprise 75–90%, oleate 30–70%, and linoleic acid 10–30% of the total lipid content of the tissue (43). Considerable attention has been recently paid to reports that unsaturated fatty acids (oleic acid, linoleic acid, etc.) interfere with lymphocyte-antigen interactions and thus exert an immunosuppressive or immunoregulatory effect (44, 45). It is reasonable to suppose that the lymphocyte immune response is influenced by fatty acids from BAT, and from other sites of the body which are functionally connected with this tissue (5). Viewed in this way, the extirpation of the interscapular BAT is followed by a marked decrease in fatty acids and thus by potentiation of immune responses. Some other diffusable agents related to the postulated endocrine function of BAT (5) should also be taken into consideration. Further analysis will show whether these effects were due to BAT alone or to its association with tissues which synthesize and release biologically active substances.

No matter which explanation may prove to be correct, the potentiated reactions of cell-mediated type in the rat have a common denominator: the lack of the interscapular BAT (partial adipectomy). It seems that the outlined results, although not yet conclusive, provide a sound basis for a number of further experiments pertaining to the role of BAT in immunity.

ACKNOWLEDGMENTS

I wish to acknowledge the collaboration of Drs. Lj. Popesković, A. Janežić, M. L. Lukić, and N. L. Vujanović in the performance of many of the experiments described here, and for permission to quote unpublished results. I am grateful to Dr. B.G.W. Arnason for stimulating discussions.

This work was supported by grants from the Republic Fund for Research of Serbia, Belgrade.

REFERENCES

1. Janković, B. D. Structural correlates of immune microenvironment. *In;* B. D. Janković and K. Isaković (eds.), Microenvironmental Aspects of Immunity, pp. 1–4, Plenum Press, New York, 1973.
2. Smalley, R. L. and Dryer, R. L. Brown fat in hibernation. *In;* K. C. Fisher, A. R. Dawe, C. P. Lyman, E. Schönbaum, and F. E. South (eds.), Mammalian Hibernation, vol. III, pp. 325–345, Oliver and Boyd, Edinburgh, 1967.
3. Smith, R. E. and Horwitz, B. A. Brown fat and thermogenesis. Physiol. Rev., *49*: 330–425, 1969.
4. Lindberg, O. (ed.). Brown Adipose Tissue. American Elsevier, New York, 1970.
5. Himms-Haggen, J. Effects of catecholamines on metabolism. *In;* H. Blaschko and E. Muscholl (eds.), Catecholamines, pp. 363–462, Springer Verlag, Berlin, 1972.
6. Gesner, C. Medici Tirugini Historiae Animalium Liber. II. Qui est de Quadrupedibus Ouiparis (de Mure Alpino). pp. 840–843, 1551.
7. Hammar, J. A. Zur Kenntnis des Fettgewebes. Arch. mikrosk. Anat. Entw. Mech., *45*: 512–547, 1895.
8. Hausberger, F. X. and Gujot, O. Über die Veränderungen des Gehaltes an Fett-, Wasser-, Glykogene-, und Trockensubstanz im wachsenden Fettgewebe junger Ratten. Arch. Exp. Pathol. Pharmacol., *187*: 647–654, 1937.
9. Hirzel, H. and Frey, H. Einiges über den Bau der sogenannten Winterschlafdrüssen. Z. Wiss. Zool., *12*: 165–174, 1863.
10. Cottle, W. H. The inervation of brown adipose tissue. *In;* O. Lindberg (ed.), Brown Adipose Tissue, pp. 155–178, American Elsevier, New York, 1970.
11. Chalvardjian, A. M. Fatty acids of brown and yellow fat in rats. Biochem. J., *90*: 518–521, 1964.
12. Sidman, R. L., Perkins, M., and Weiner, N. Noradrenaline and adrenaline content of adipose tissues. Nature, *193*: 36–37, 1962.
13. Zizine, J. Sur la présence de corticostéroids dans la graisse brune interscapulaire du rat. C. R. Acad. Sci., *242*: 681–684, 1856.
14. Rasmussen, A. T. The so-called hibernating gland. J. Morphol., *38*: 147–205, 1923–1924.
15. Johansson, B. Brown fat: A review. Metabolism, *8*: 221–239, 1959.
16. Selye, H. and Timiras, P. S. Participation of "brown fat" tissue in the alarm reaction. Nature, *164*: 745–746, 1949.
17. Schmidt, J. P. Response of hibernating mammals to physical, parasitic and infectious agents. *In;* K. C. Fischer, A. R. Dawe, C. P. Lyman, E. Schönbaum, and F. E. South (eds.), Mammalian Hibernation, vol. III, pp. 421–438, Oliver and Boyd, Edinburgh, 1967.
18. Melicow, M. M. Hibernating fat and pheochromocytoma. Am. Med. Assoc. Arch. Pathol., *63*: 367–372, 1957.
19. Petrik, J. Contribution à la sérologie des mammifères hibernants. Publ. Fac. Med. Brno R.C.S., *1(3)*: 3–15, 1922 (in Czech with French summary).

20. Kopeloff, L. M. and Stanton, A. H. The effect of body temperature upon hemolysin production in the rat. J. Immunol., *44*: 247–250, 1942.

21. Andjus, R. K. and Matic, O. Hibernation and immunological reactivity. Pflügers Arch. ges. Physiol., *270*: 55–56, 1959.

22. Jaroslaw, B. N. and Smith, D. E. Antigen disappearance in hibernating ground squirrels. Science, *134*: 734–735, 1961.

23. Sidky, Y. A., Daggett, L. R., and Auerbach, R. Brown fat: Its possible role in immunosuppression during hibernation. Proc. Soc. Exp. Biol. Med., *132*: 760–763, 1969.

24. Sidky, Y. A. and Hayward, J. S. Immunosuppression by extracts of brown fat. Fed. Proc., *31*: 800, 1972.

25. Janković, B. D., Popesković, Lj., Janežić, A., and Lukić, M. L. Immune reactions in rats treated with allogeneic brown adipose tissue and rats adipectomized at birth. Proc. Yugoslav. Immunol. Soc., *3*: 122–124, 1974.

26. Janković, B. D., Popesković, Lj., Janežić, A., and Lukić, M. L. Brown adipose tissue: Effect on immune reactions in the rat. Naturwissenschaften, *61*: 36, 1974.

27. Sidky, Y. A., Hayward, J. S., and Ruth, R. F. Personal communication.

28. Janković, B. D., Janežić, A., and Popesković, Lj. Brown adipose tissue and immunity. Effect of neonatal adipectomy on humoral and cellular immune reactions in the rat. Immunology, *28*: 597–609, 1975.

29. Ganong, W. F. and Lorenzen, L. Brain neurohumors and endocrine function. *In;* L. Martini and W. F. Ganong (eds.), Neuroendocrinology, vol. 2, pp. 583–640, Academic Press, New York, 1967.

30. Kopin, I. J. The adrenergic synapse. *In;* G. C. Quarton, T. Melnechuk, and F. O. Schmitt (eds.), The Neurosciences, pp. 427–432, Rockefeller Univ. Press, New York, 1967.

31. Janković, B. D. and Isaković, K. Neuro-endocrine correlates of immune response. I. Effects of brain lesions on antibody production, Arthus reactivity and delayed hypersensitivity in the rat. Int. Arch. Allergy Appl. Immunol., *45*: 360–372, 1973.

32. Janković, B. D. Janežić, A., and Popesković, Lj. Brown adipose tissue: Potentiation of delayed skin hypersensitivity and experimental allergic encephalomyelitis in adipectomized rats. Fed. Proc., *33*: 804, 1974.

33. Arnason, B. G., Janković, B. D., Waksman, B. H., and Wennersten, C. Role of the thymus in immune reactions in rats. II. Suppressive effect of thymectomy at birth on reactions of delayed (cellular) hypersensitivity and the circulating small lymphocytes. J. Exp. Med., *116*: 177–186, 1962.

34. Ford, W. L., Burr, W., and Simonsen, M. A lymph node weight assays for the graft-*versus*-host activity of rat lymphoid cells. Transplantation, *10*: 258–266, 1970.

35. Najarian, J. S. and Feldman, J. D. Quantitation of transplantation immunity. I. Method. J. Exp. Med., *121*: 521–531, 1965.

36. Dorsch, S. E. and Roser, B. A quantitative lymph node weight assay for allogeneic interactions in the rat. Aust. J. Exp. Biol. Med. Sci., *52*: 253–264, 1974.

37. Gibbs, J. E. and Field, E. O. Thyroid transplantation. An alternative to skin grafting. Transplantation, *12*: 490–492, 1971.

38. Kaliss, N. Induced alteration of the normal host-graft relationships in homotransplantation of mouse tumors. Ann. N. Y. Acad. Sci., *59*: 385–393, 1954.

39. Gorer, P. A. The value of ascites tumors in problems of tumor immunity. Ann. N. Y. Acad. Sci., *63*: 882–892, 1956.

40.   Dresser, D. W. The immune response: Circumvention and suppression. Proc. 4th Int. Congr. Pharmacol., *4*: 192–202, 1970.

41.   Waksman, B. H., Arnason, B. G., and Janković, B. D. Role of the thymus in immune reactions in rats. III. Changes in the lymphoid organs of thymectomized rats. J. Exp. Med., *116*: 187–206, 1962.

42.   Steiner, G. and Schönbaum, E. (eds.). Immunosympathectomy. Elsevier, Amsterdam, 1972.

43.   Prusiner, S., Sannon, B., and Lindberg, O. Mechanisms controlling oxidative metabolism in brown adipose tissue. *In;* O. Lindberg (ed.), Brown Adipose Tissue, pp. 283–318, American Elsevier, New York, 1970.

44.   Mertin, J., Shenton, B. K., and Field, E. J. Unsaturated fatty acids in multiple sclerosis. Brit. Med. J., *2*: 777–778, 1973.

45.   Offner, H. and Clausen, J. Inhibition of lymphocyte response to stimulants induced by unsaturated fatty acids and prostaglandins. Lancet, *ii*: 400–401, 1974.

Discussion of Paper of Dr. Janković

DR. CASTRO: Do your adipectomized animals suffer an alteration in body temperature?

DR. JANKOVIĆ: Rats do not. The body temperature remained normal even in rats cold-acclimated at 10°C.

DR. DUKOR: Does the adipectomy have to be performed neonatally in order to reveal an immunostimulatory effect?

DR. JANKOVIĆ: A lower degree of immunopotentiation was obtained when adipectomy was performed on 2-week-old rats. In mice, however, we did not succeed with neonatal adipectomy because of a very high mortality rate. Nevertheless, adipectomy performed on 1- to 2-month-old mice was quite effective in inducing immunopotentiation.

DR. AMOS: Have you attempted to manipulate the amount of BAT by alteration of diet, as dietary factors, especially those altering its lipid content, have an effect on lymphocyte reactivity?

DR. JANKOVIĆ: No, all animals were kept on a standard laboratory diet. With respect to the lipids, it is possible that the extirpation of BAT removes also a large amount of unsaturated fatty acids. It has been recently shown that fatty acids may exert an immunosuppressive effect on the multiple sclerosis (Mertin, J. *et al.*, Brit. Med. J., *2*: 777–778, 1973; Offner, H. *et al.*, Lancet, *ii*: 400–401, 1974).

DR. DRESSER: In your sham-operated controls, did you remove the BAT and then replace it, or simply form an incision and close it?

DR. JANKOVIĆ: The BAT was left *in situ* in those controls. In another experiments (Naturwissenschaften, *61*: 36, 1974) we have repeatedly injected normal rats with an extract prepared from the rat BAT, and this treatment produced an immunosuppressive effect. Thus, these results complement those described in this symposium.

DR. FACHET: Has the immune response of animals which exhibit a normal seasonal hibernation been examined during and outside of periods of hibernation? Also, are there any data bearing on the immune capacity of animals which do not normally hibernate but are placed in a state of deep hypothermia?

DR. JANKOVIĆ: In 1922 Dr. J. Petrik described a suppression of antibody formation in animals which were in deep hibernation. Similar results were obtained later on by several investigators who also used animals with artificially lowered body temperature. It is well known that hypothermia is followed by a decrease in metabolic rate including the synthesis of immunoglobulins. Therefore, the experiments performed on animals in hypothermia should not be confused with the experiments presented here.

DR. CASTRO: Have you examined macrophage responses in your adipectomized animals?

DR. JANKOVIĆ: We have not examined macrophages as yet, but we plan to do that both *in vivo* and *in vitro*.

DR. FROST: Does BAT produce prostaglandins? Secondly, what happens to BAT during tumor growth?

DR. JANKOVIĆ: BAT is certainly connected with the endocrine system, but I do not know any data showing a direct relationship between BAT and prostaglandins. We have not examined BAT during the tumor growth.

DR. FROST: We have preliminary data suggesting that prostaglandins cause a chemical thymectomy. This result may pertain to your system.

HOST DEFENSE AGAINST CANCER AND ITS POTENTIATION, D. MIZUNO ET AL. (EDS.), UNIV. OF TOKYO PRESS, TOKYO / UNIV. PARK PRESS, BALTIMORE, PP. 317-335, 1975

Chalones and Cancer

William S. Bullough

Mitosis Research Laboratory, Birkbeck College, University of London, London, U.K.

Abstract: The normal mitotic control mechanism of adult mammalian tissues is described. It depends basically on the conflicting actions of a tissue-specific mitotic inhibitor, the chalone, which permeates the tissue, and a non-tissue-specific mitotic promotor, the mesenchymal factor, which acts only in those cells that are in connective tissue contact. Thus "basal" cells tend to be mitotic while "distal" cells are forced by the high ambient chalone concentration to become post-mitotic and so to age and die. The basal cells are displaced distally by mitotic pressure and thus a perfect balance is maintained between cell gain and cell loss.

The evidence is that this mechanism breaks to allow tumour growth when the chalone concentration falls so low that the distal cells also tend to remain mitotic; this is caused by an abnormality of the cell membrane. Tumour cells continue to respond to the chalone of their tissue of origin so that when the chalone concentration rises, naturally or artificially, tumour growth ceases. With continued chalone treatment a tumour may disappear permanently evidently because, with the mitotic potential reduced, such destructive influences as the immune response predominate.

From the beginning of cancer research one thing has been self-evident: that no adequate understanding of the problem can be expected until the nature of the normal mitotic control mechanism itself is understood. It is not the many and diverse causes of cancer that are of primary significance: it is the particular form of damage that they all induce within the affected cells. This damage produces only one important effect: whereas in a normal tissue the rate of cell gain exactly matches the rate of cell loss, in a growing tumour. The rate of cell gain exceeds the rate of cell loss (*1, 2*). This is the kernel of the problem.

The present paper therefore considers, first, the outlines of mitotic control as they are now known in adult mammalian tissues, and second, the new light that this knowledge has thrown on the nature of cancer.

Mitotic Control

There are two major tissue types in an adult mammal: the mitosis-dependent tissue and the stem-cell-dependent tissue (see p. 322). The first consists partly of mitotic-cycle cells, from which new cells are formed, and partly of post-mitotic cells, which are the functional cells and which have only a limited life span. Both the mitotic rate and the post-mitotic life span are tissue-specific (1, 2).

There are two variations on this theme. First, there are the target tissues that become hyperplastic in the presence of a specific hormone (3). Second, there are the non-mitotic tissues, including nervous tissue and skeletal and heart muscles (3, 4); in the young animal these are normal mitotic tissues, but in the adult their mitotic genes are silenced (3, 5).

The most intensively studied mitotic tissue is the epidermis. Since epidermal thickness (epidermal mass) normally remains constant, the theoretical conclusion has been drawn that mitotic activity must be controlled by a feedback mechanism (6–8); the discovery of the tissue-specific antimitotic chalones provided the necessary messenger molecules; a chalone has been found in every tissue in which it has been sought (2, 9–12). The theory then grew that when a tissue grows to its appropriate mass the chalone concentration is adequate to prevent the production of any more cells; when tissue is lost or destroyed the chalone concentration falls, the mitotic rate rises, and regeneration occurs. This simple theory has now proved to be inadequate (1, 2).

1. Tissue mass

The mitosis-dependent tissues vary widely in their characteristics. In general, mitotic activity is high in the surface epithelia and low in the protected internal tissues. The mass of a tissue depends on two factors: the rate of new cell production and the rate at which the post-mitotic cells age and die. The tissue chalone inhibits both these processes in equal degree so that:

rate of mitosis : rate of post-mitotic ageing $= K$, a constant, which implies that

number of mitotic cells : number of post-mitotic cells $= K'$, another constant (1, 2). This alone disposes of the simple negative feedback theory.

In any tissue the specific mitotic rate and the specific post-mitotic life span fix the value of K, which in turn fixes the tissue mass. The lower the value of K the larger the tissue will be.

2. Tissue regeneration

When, after any form of tissue damage, the chalone concentration falls (13, 14), the mitotic rate rises and the newly forming post-mitotic cells then have a reduced life expectancy: in hyperplastic epidermis the post-mitotic life span may fall from the normal 14–21 days to only 4–5 days (15), while in regenerating liver it may fall from ca. 200–450 days to only ca. 26 days (16). The newly formed cells are not, however, lost since the damage is usually fully repaired within the reduced time limit; with the chalone concentration and the mitotic rate then reverting to normal, the post-mitotic life span follows suit.

If the damage persists and the raised mitotic rate becomes chronic, then the shortened post-mitotic life span ensures that the hyperplastic tissue mass does not become too large. The tissue mass plateaus, as for instance when constantly irritated epidermis thickens or when a cirrhotic liver enlarges.

Two main problems emerge: the first concerns the mechanism that ensures the perfect balance between cell gain and cell loss both in normal and in hyperplastic conditions; the second concerns the manner in which cell gain temporarily exceeds cell loss when a tissue is passing from a normal to a hyperplastic condition.

3. The dichophase ratio

The decision whether a mitotic daughter cell remains mitotic or whether instead it becomes post-mitotic is made in the dichophase which is part of the intermitotic interval. This dichophase decision is determined by the chalone concentration: below a critical chalone level the cell proceeds again to mitosis while above this critical chalone level the cell becomes post-mitotic. These are evidently alternative gene programmes activated or inhibited in response to the concentration of a messenger molecule (3).

In stable conditions, whether hypoplastic, normal, or hyperplastic, the average "dichophase decision ratio" is exactly 1 mitotic daughter cell: 1 post-mitotic daughter cell; in *changing* conditions, with an increasing mitotic rate, the dichophase ratio is temporarily distorted to >1 mitotic daughter cell: <1 post-mitotic daughter cell, which increases the cell number; with a decreasing mitotic rate the distortion is in the opposite direction.

Clearly in a normal tissue the 1: 1 dichophase ratio cannot be ensured by the chalone concentration alone since any change in that concentration would so destroy the balance that any chronic hyperplasia, such as epidermal psoriasis, would automatically lead to tumour formation. Since this does not happen the curious conclusion emerges that although the chalone concentration determines the dichophase decision, the dichophase ratio remains normal irrespective of the chalone concentration.

4. The mesenchymal factor

Evidently the mitotic control mechanism must contain at least one other controlling factor in addition to the chalone. Recently evidence has been reviewed (2) to suggest that this is the mesenchymal factor, a chemical messenger produced by connective tissue cells to counteract the chalone inhibition in the immediately adjacent epithelial tissue cells. The existence of this factor is indicated by an extensive literature: experimental evidence from both embryonic and adult tissues comes from salivary gland and pancreas (17), parotid gland (18), lung (19), mammary gland (20), gizzard (21), and prostate (22).

However, once again the best evidence comes from epidermis (23–28). When epidermis is separated from dermis *in vitro*, basal mitotic activity slows to a halt and all the cells ultimately die. In chick epidermis such death may involve keratinisation down to and including the basal cells, the implication being that, in the absence of the dermis, the chalone is so dominant as to force the whole epidermis into post-mitosis with keratinisation and death. When the separated epidermis is replaced on to the dermis, basal mitosis is again stimulated and the tissue remains normal. For this purpose the dermis may be inverted, other types of connective tissue may be substituted, fibroblast culture medium may be used as also may fresh serum or embryo extract. The conclusion is that the mesenchymal factor is not tissue-specific in its action.

5. The positional control of mitosis

Cellular homeostasis in the epidermis evidently depends on the interaction of the chalone with the mesenchymal factor. The whole tissue is permeated by a chalone concentration that is so high (even when reduced in hyperplasia) that, without the mesenchymal factor, all the cells would be directed to post-mitosis, keratin synthesis, and death; the chalone acts in a strictly tissue-specific way so that when it escapes into the adjacent tissues and the blood it has no action on these tissues; the dermal fibrocytes release the non-specific mesenchymal factor (or alternatively it reaches the dermis from the blood serum), which acts to neutralise the chalone action in those epidermal cells that are in dermal contact (this neutralisation may extend to higher cell layers when the chalone concentration is reduced in hyperplasia); the reason for the short range of action of the mesenchymal factor is not known; the possible relationship between the mesenchymal factor and the well-known serum factor (29) has not yet been adequately investigated.

The result is that the basal epidermal cells remain mitotic because the chalone effectiveness (chalone concentration *minus* mesenchymal factor concentration) is so low that the dichophase decision is for re-entry into mitosis; the distal cells are post-mitotic because in them the chalone effectiveness (chalone concentration alone) is high, even when it is reduced in hyperplasia. The precision of the dichophase ratio in all stable conditions from hypo- to hyperplasia is now explained; a cell is mitotic or post-mitotic according to its position within the tissue; as mitotic activity causes basal layer pressure, cells are forced distally, when they immediately become post-mitotic; thus the dichophase ratio must always remain precisely 1 new basal mitotic cell: 1 new distal post-mitotic cell.

This rule evidently applies to mitotic tissues in general. It is well known that in the various tissues of the skin, mitosis is always dermis-adjacent: this is seen in intra-epidermal melanocytes, in sebaceous glands and eccrine gland ducts, and in the hair root in which mitotic activity is related to the dermal papilla, which evidently contains an especially high mesenchymal factor concentration (2). In other tissues the "basal" cells are those that are connective-tissue-adjacent while the "distal" cells are those that are not. In some cases (especially the various epithelia) the "basal" cells are obviously the mitotic cells; in other cases (such as the liver) the permeating connective tissue network is so complex that the relationship is more difficult to establish.

6. The number of basal cells

The second question concerns the manner in which, when the mitotic rate is *changing*, the number of basal epidermal mitotic-cycle cells also changes, which can only mean that during this time the dichophase ratio is temporarily distorted. After epidermal damage it is observed that the increasing mitotic rate is accompanied by an increasing number of basal mitotic-cycle cells per unit area of skin, which leads to the recovery of the lost tissue or, if no tissue has been lost, to an epidermal hyperplasia. This hyperplasia results from the K ratio; with an increase in the number of basal cells per unit skin area there must be an equivalent increase in the number of distal cells, even though these distal cells are ageing and dying more quickly (1).

The details of this reaction are complex and are not yet adequately understood, but briefly the sequence of events is as follows. Damaged epidermal cells suffer a fall in their chalone concentration (about 50%, see Ref. 13) which is evidently due to excessive chalone loss across the damaged cell membranes; the mitotic rate therefore increases. The mitotic rate (number of mitoses per hundred cells per unit time) has two components: the speed of the mitotic cycle and the number of cells that are involved in this cycle. The first response to chalone loss is an increase in cycle speed: the dichophase shortens drastically and the dichophase cells are released *en masse* to enter the mitotic cycle in the form of a wave (30). In normal epidermis the pressure generated by each mitosis is relieved by the extrusion distally of a neighbouring dichophase cell, but when a wave of cells complete mitosis together the number of cells remaining in the dichophase is inadequate. Since the mitotic cells themselves are not usually extruded the pressure within the basal layer rises abnormally (31).

The cells then re-enter the dichophase in a wave and large numbers of them are forced distally (30). However, with the continuing low chalone concentration those cells that remain basal pass so quickly through the dichophase that the excess cells are not all lost. The increased pressure is not fully relieved. Thus the number of basal mitotic-cycle cells is increased; it is increased still further as the cells pass, still in the form of a wave, through their second mitosis (2).

The dichophase ratio returns to normal and so stabilises the system in one of two ways. On the one hand, the damage may heal and the chalone concentration return to normal, when the dichophase again lengthens and cell loss distally is adequate to relieve the basal pressure; the number of basal mitotic-cycle cells returns to normal.

On the other hand, the damage may be chronic. In this case the wave of cells passing round the cycle begins to flatten until the cell flow is again almost uniform. Once this occurs there is evidently an adequate number of dichophase cells always available to be forced distally to offset the pressure of each new mitosis. However, there is a continuing excess of cells in the basal layer and the consequent excess pressure leads to the folding or doubling of this layer (1, 2). A hyperplasia has been created which is stable since the dichophase ratio is again normal.

These responses need to be analysed in more detail; in particular it is necessary to learn more about dermoepidermal adhesion and about the method and timing of basal cell displacement (31).

7. Compensatory hypertrophy

The response to massive damage leading to large scale tissue loss may involve compensatory hypertrophy. This differs from wound healing in that it appears to depend on a simple chalone negative feedback mechanism (3, 4), although the mitosis-promoting mesenchymal or serum factor also plays its usual cooperative role (32).

When a tissue is large in relation to the general body space (*e.g.*, hepatocytes, granulocytes, or erythrocytes) the supply of its chalone is so great that enough escapes to create a significant concentration in the body, notably in the blood. If the liver is wounded the mitotic response is only local, but when the tissue loss exceeds 10% the mitotic response becomes general throughout the surviving cell mass (33, 34); beyond that point the mitotic rate of developing is in direct relation to the percentage of tissue lost; the response is also seen in similar tissue implanted at a distance or in the same tissue in a parabiotic twin (35, 36). The sequence of events, for instance after partial hepatectomy or the removal of one kidney, evidently begins with a proportional fall in the systemic chalone concentration and leads *via* a steeper diffusion gradient to a similarly proportional fall in the tissue chalone concentration.

In a tissue of small mass this cannot occur because, with so little chalone produced, the systemic concentration approximates to zero. Any reduction is then too slight to induce a response in the tissue remnant.

In compensatory hypertrophy, as in the liver, the cells that become mitotically active were previously post-mitotic and functional; they had been maintained in their post-mitotic state by the high chalone concentration. Their mitotic activity has the same consequences as that in normal healing; the cell numbers increase rapidly towards normality; and then, with both the systemic and tissue chalone concentrations rising, the mitotic activity dies down before any of the newly formed post-mitotic cells can pass to an early death.

Chronic general hyperplasia, as in liver cirrhosis, is similar except that it rises from the baseline of the normal tissue mass. The mass increases rapidly but it plateaus when the increased mitotic rate begins to be matched by the increased rate of post-mitotic cell ageing.

8. Stem-cell-dependent tissues

Uncommitted pluripotent stem cells, such as those in the bone marrow that give rise to the blood tissues (37), are self-maintaining in the manner of any ordinary mitotic tissue. Some cells remain mitotic; others undergo a terminal differentiation into one or other of the dependent tissues. The faster cells are withdrawn from the system the faster they are produced within it by typical compensatory hypertrophy; evidently the stem cell population has its own specific chalone system.

The recruitment of cells into a stem-cell-dependent tissue, such as the erythrocytic or granulocytic tissues, is a complex process (37, 38) but essentially it involves two steps. The first step is when a stem cell is induced to undergo a terminal differentiation into, for instance, a proerythrocyte; this change is irreversible. The second step is when this proerythrocyte passes through a sequence of mitoses to create a cell clone within the bone marrow. All these cells then become post-mitotic, synthesise haemoglobin, lose their nuclei, and pass into the blood, where as mature erythrocytes they survive for only a limited period. Thus each proery-throcyte gives rise only to dying cells, which is why constant cell recruitment from the stem cell reserve is essential.

When there is a sudden shortage of erythrocytes, as after haemorrhage, the response is twofold: a greater number of stem cells are induced to become pro-erythrocytes (this mechanism is imperfectly understood), and with a fall in the systemic erythrocytic chalone concentration each proerythrocyte clone passes through 1 or 2 extra mitoses before maturing and entering the circulation. This second response is a form of compensatory hypertrophy, similar to liver regeneration (*38, 39*).

The question why this curious system should exist at all has not previously been considered; there is no obvious reason why the mitotic activity of, for instance, the proerythrocytes should not be adequate to maintain the tissue in the normal manner. The answer could be that any dispersed cell tissue that is not connective-tissue-based must inevitably die and disappear, exactly as does isolated epidermis *in vitro* (*2*). Another range of tissues that present a peculiar problem are the connective tissues themselves; it is probable that they too are recruited from a stem cell population (*40–42*).

The Breakdown of Mitotic Control

It is self-evident that cancer must be caused by a local breakdown in the mitotic control mechanism; what is less evident is that a tumour grows not with a wild lack of control but according to a pattern that closely resembles that of compensatory hypertrophy (*2, 43*).

The only adequate definition of a growing tumour is that it is a group of cells in which the average outcome of each mitosis is >1 mitotic daughter cell: <1 post-mitotic daughter cell; the dichophase ratio is distorted. This is exactly the situation seen in a regenerating tissue and in a developing hyperplasia, and it contains the essence of the cancer problem.

Both compensatory hypertrophy and hyperplasia are dependent on a fall in the chalone concentration and therefore the chalone relations of tumours must be considered. It may be noted that the influence of the mesenchymal factor can be disregarded: should its concentration fall to zero the tissue would disappear for lack of mitosis; should the concentration rise abnormally a hyperplasia would develop but with the distal chalone concentration remaining normal the post-mitotic cells would continue to die at their normal rate.

A tumour will appear if a group of tissue cells fails to synthesise its chalone, or if it fails to respond normally to this chalone, or if the chalone produced is lost at too high a rate across damaged cell membranes. The available evidence (see below) all points to the last of these possibilities and indicates that the common, if not universal, condition of tumour cells is a low intracellular chalone concentration. In this a tumour closely resembles a hyperplasia. However, in a hyperplasia, stability is ensured because those cells that are forced distally enter a chalone concentration which, although reduced, is adequate to ensure post-mitosis; in a growing tumour the distal chalone concentration is so low that cells entering it do not necessarily become post-mitotic.

1. The chalone mechanism in tumours

The evidence in support of these conclusions is already extensive. The first two tumours studied were a rabbit epidermal carcinoma (44) and a rat granulocytic leukaemia (45–47). In both cases the results obtained were the same: the chalone content of the tumour cells was 10% or less of normal; the missing chalone was present in the body fluids which therefore had an abnormally high chalone concentration; this high systemic concentration greatly reduced the mitotic activity of the tissue of origin of the tumour; the basic damage was to the cell membrane which consequently allowed so much chalone to be lost; and the tumour cells still responded by mitotic inhibition when the chalone concentration was artificially raised to a higher level.

Supporting evidence has now come from 12 diverse tumours in 5 mammalian species including man: epidermal carcinomata from rabbit (44), hamster (48, 49), and mouse (50); melanomata from mouse and hamster (51, 52); granulocytic (myeloid) leukaemia from rat and man (45–47); lymphocytic leukaemia from mouse and man (53–55); cervix uterus from man (56); mammary carcinoma and plasmacytoma from mouse (57–60).

These tumours are so diverse and the results obtained are so uniform that it begins to appear that the common characteristic of any tumour is a severely reduced chalone concentration, while the common characteristic of any tumour-bearing animal is an abnormally high systemic chalone concentration and an abnormally low mitotic rate in the tumour's parent tissue.

2. The tumour cell membrane

The conclusion that the basic damage suffered by a neoplastic cell is to the cell membrane is not unexpected. There is a wide literature indicating that cell surface abnormalities are responsible for such well-known tumour cell characteristics as loss of contact inhibition, metastasis, and the induction of an immune response.

What is not yet clear is the way in which cell membrane damage impinges on the chalone mechanism. The view expressed here, that it leads to excessive chalone loss into the body, is based mainly on the observation that the chalone missing from the tumour cells can be found in the body fluids (45, 50). The alternative view put forward by Houck (61), that the chalone molecules act by occupying specific sites on the outer membrane surface, is based mainly on the observation that chalone washes more readily from leukaemic lymphocytes in which the sites are believed to be damaged. Either or both views may be correct but this does not alter the present argument.

3. The pattern of tumour growth

If a tumour continues to synthesise the chalone of its tissue of origin and then to lose it excessively into the body fluids, it should follow that the larger the tumour becomes the higher will be the systemic chalone concentration. That this indeed happens has been demonstrated, for instance, by Bullough and Deol (*50*), who found that a growing epidermal carcinoma causes a progressive fall in the mitotic rate of the epidermis but not of other tissues; other examples such as the suppression of normal granulocyte production by a developing granulocytic leukaemia are well known.

With further tumour growth and a higher systemic chalone concentration the growth of the tumour itself should be inhibited. It is this that evidently produces the well-known tumour sigmoid growth curve (*62–65*).

The slowing of tumour growth with increasing mass has long been known but it has commonly been explained in terms of a "major drain on the metabolic resources of the host" or of "vascular accidents that lead to total necrosis" as the newly forming capillaries "fail to keep up with the volume increase" (*66*). Central necrosis is a common feature of large tumours and has been widely held to be due to central vascular failure (*67*) perhaps leading to hypoxia (*68*). Certainly such factors do play some role (*43*), but it has been repeatedly emphasised that the slowing of tumour growth cannot be due to nutritional problems. Also it cannot be due to a developing immune response, since it occurs equally in tumours that are believed to be only slightly or non-antigenic.

From one of the earliest analyses of tumour growth dynamics, Laird (*62, 63*) reached the important conclusions that "the growth of nearly all tumours reported in the literature is characterised by a continuous deceleration from the earliest period of observation," and that "the retardation of growth . . . appears to be an actively increasing depression of the specific growth rate, rather than a passive limitation imposed by the exhaustion of available growth-supporting factors in the environment." Burns (*65*) concluded that a tumour may regulate its own growth "as normal and non-neoplastic tissues do by the production of a homologous specific mitotic inhibitor"; Bullough and Deol (*43*) added further evidence in support of the same conclusion; and Bichel (*60*) from a mathematical analysis of a series of tumours suggested "that tumour growth may be described as an exponential process limited by an exponential retardation, which can be explained by . . . the increasing concentration of an inhibitor produced by an increasing number of cells."

Thus there is a pattern in tumour growth that closely resembles that seen in compensatory hypertrophy, although it is often obscured by the distortions caused by the inadequacy of the available space, the breakdown of the blood supply, and the damage done by clinical treatment.

4. Tumour growth and compensatory hypertrophy

The close similarity of tumour growth to compensatory hypertrophy is most obvious in a chronic tumour, which reaches a stable mass, or plateau, before the host animal is killed. Theoretically, a lethal tumour is the same except that the host dies before the plateau is reached.

The experimental evidence includes that of Goodman (*69*), who found that at death the mass of tumour tissue is the same whether the tumour is single or double, and that if one of a pair of tumours is removed the growth rate of the other increases; of Trotter (70), who showed that partial hepatectomy encourages the growth of small adenomatous hepatic nodules; of Schatten (71) and Lewis and Cole (72), who found that the amputation of a large primary tumour may result in the rapid development of metastases that would not otherwise have appeared, which recalls the well-known clinical problem of metastatic growth after the excision of a primary tumour; of Burns (65), who found that in an old Ehrlich ascites tumour in which growth has slowed, mitotic activity begins again after most of the tumour cells have been washed from the body cavity; and of Brown (73), who showed that when two tumours of different tissue origins are present in one animal they grow independently of each other and that each reaches its usual plateau as if the other was not present, thus neatly disproving the suggestion that growth ceases because of nutrient exhaustion or of toxic metabolic products.

These results have been confirmed and enlarged upon by Bichel (57, 58, 74) using three different chronic ascites tumours of the mouse. He found that the reduction of the tumour mass from the plateau level induces immediate growth back to that level; that a large ascites mass in one mouse inhibits the growth of a small ascites mass in a parabiotic twin; that cell-free ascites fluid from the plateau phase, when injected into mice containing the rapid growth phase, causes this growth to be inhibited; and that, as the growth rate decreases, the mitotic cycle length increases. Bichel (59, 60) then studied the simultaneous growth of two different ascites tumours in the same animal: he confirmed that each reaches its plateau as if the other were not present, and showed that the injection of the cell-free ascites fluid from the plateau phase of one tumour type inhibited only the growth of that same tumour, leaving the other to grow without interruption. He concluded that each tumour continues to produce and to respond to a tumour-(and tissue-) specific growth regulator with the characteristics of a chalone.

Thus tumour growth and compensatory hypertrophy (e.g., of liver) have the same characteristic that they both stop their increase in mass when the systemic chalone concentration rises to an inhibiting level. The only difference between them is that a regenerating tissue is inhibited by a normal systemic chalone concentration, while a tumour is inhibited only by a higher-than-normal systemic chalone concentration. In the case of a lethal tumour the animal dies before an inhibiting chalone concentration can be reached.

The plateau phase of a chronic tumour is well known to be unstable. If any of its cells suffer further damage this can lead to further and perhaps lethal growth. This is termed "progression" (75) and it occurs in abrupt and irreversible steps. Thus the point of balance of any chronic tumour may become a receding goal as the chalone mechanism suffers more and more damage.

5. Chalone treatment of tumours

Such evidence provides the rationale for testing the effects of chalones on tumour growth. The extensive evidence, reviewed above, has all shown that the chalone of a tumour's tissue of origin inhibits the mitotic activity of the tumour cells, and that the tumour response to the chalone is as tissue-specific as is the response of the tissue of origin. This was even true in an anaplastic epidermal carcinoma that had been maintained by transplantation at 1- to 2-week intervals for more than 30 years (44).

However, most of this evidence derives from short-term experiments and what is now urgently needed is more information on the effects of long-term treatment. So far only two types of tumour have been treated for a long enough period to provide an indication of the results that might be obtained, the main difficulty being that of producing large enough supplies of chalone.

All the tumours tested were fast-growing, malignant and lethal, and all the results were strikingly similar. The first experiments were those of Mohr et al. (51) using mice with Harding-Passey melanomata and hamsters with Green-Fortner amelanotic melanomata. For 5 consecutive days the animals were injected with either skin extract or melanoma extract containing the melanocyte chalone (52). This was certainly too short a period of treatment but with optimum dosage, in both the mice and the hamsters, there was an immediate stoppage of tumour growth, a greatly increased cell death rate, ulceration through the overlying skin, and the disappearance of the tumour. All the 75 treated mice and the 200 treated hamsters responded in this way, while in contrast more than 1,000 untreated mice and 3,000 untreated hamsters showed no spontaneous tumour regression. In most of the mice and in all of the hamsters the tumours later recurred; the effect of extending this treatment into a second week still remains to be determined.

Later Mohr et al. (76) concluded that this tumour destruction was due not to the chalone but to the action of contaminating bacteria. This view must be discounted since the mitotic inhibition was observed to begin within minutes of the first injection of a solution freshly prepared from an alcoholprecipitated lyophilised extract; no bacterial spores could have emerged to act in that time. However, it does remain possible that within 5 days the bacterial action could have supported the chalone action.

The second experiments were those of Rytömaa and Kiviniemi (46, 47) using young rats with Shay chloroleukaemia (a myeloid leukaemia) both in its solid and in its dispersed forms. These experiments were better planned: the granulocyte extracts were bacteria-free and the treatment was continued for up to 4 weeks. In the first experiments with rats with solid subcutaneous granulomata the results were the same as those obtained with the melanomata: there was an immediate slackening of tumour growth, a greatly increased cell death rate, ulceration through the overlying skin, and the disappearance of the tumour. In 28 rats out of 42 the tumour did not recur, which, compared with the controls, was statistically highly significant.

The experiments with the dispersed form of the chloroleukaemia were even more dramatic. The survival time was prolonged in all the 40 treated rats and in 9 animals the leukaemia disappeared completely and permanently. By contrast all the control animals died; indeed no spontaneous remissions have been recorded. Considering the lack of any information on the dosage of chalone required, on the best route of administration, on the optimum intervals between injections, and on the necessary duration of treatment, these results are particularly encouraging.

6. Chalone-induced tumour regression

The complete cures that were obtained in these various experiments were unexpected; it had seemed more probable that, at best, chalone treatment would have made the tumour plateau at a smaller mass and that tumour growth would have been resumed as soon as the chalone treatment ended.

The converse situation in which tumour growth is stimulated instead of inhibited illustrates this point. When certain small chronic mammary (77, 78) or epidermal (78–80) neoplasms are stimulated to grow by hormone or irritant treatment, their mitotic responses are merely exaggerations of the responses of the surrounding normal tissues. When treatment ceases they regress to their previous low plateau levels; they do not disappear.

There are at least two possible explanations for the observed elimination of tumours by chalones. First, it is clear that the rate of tumour growth is determined by two conflicting processes: the rate of cell gain due to the distorted dichophase ratio and the rate of cell loss due to normal post-mitotic cell death (e.g., 17–34% of new cells, see Ref. 81), to a possible partial failure of the blood supply (43), and, perhaps most important, to an immune response to the abnormal cell membrane (82). When a tumour appears it is obvious that the mitotic advantage must exceed the inhibition exerted by the other factors, even though their combined action may so damage the cells that the mitotic rate is actually reduced. As Foulds (78) remarked, "in clinical tumours the neoplastic cells are often sick cells that die young and the tumours grow only because the cells proliferate more quickly than they die." Consequently, tumour growth may be very slow.

The eradication of a tumour may therefore follow quickly when the mitotic advantage is reduced by chalone treatment, the actual destruction being due to those other adverse factors, notably the immune response, that were previously too weak to prevail.

The second possible explanation relates to the elimination of the granulocytic leukaemia by the granulocyte chalone (46, 47). Normally each newly formed progranulocyte gives rise by mitosis to a clone of up to perhaps 50 cells, all of which then mature and die. In a granulocyte leukaemia the damage to the progranulocyte is such that mitosis continues to produce a massive and ever-growing clone, which is the leukaemia. If by a raised chalone concentration this leukaemic clone is forced into post-mitosis and death, it may simply die out in the manner of a normal clone.

7. The therapeutic possibilities of chalones

Before these theories can be tested and the therapeutic possibilities of the chalones properly assessed, a considerable effort is needed to produce these substances in large enough quantities and in pure enough form. This is also the necessary preliminary step to a study of chalone chemistry. It is something that can only be done with the resources of the pharmaceutical industry since the yield obtained with normal laboratory extraction methods is too low.

The obvious potential value of chalones is twofold. First, they may be used against any form of hyperplasia caused by chalone lack (*14*) from the benign (*83*) to the malignant (*47*), that is from chronic conditions such as psoriasis to lethal conditions such as acute leukaemia. The advantage of this type of treatment is that each tissue chalone leaves all the other tissues of the body unaffected, while the normal tissue from which the tumour came continues to exist in a hypoplastic condition from which it rapidly recovers when the treatment ceases.

Regarding myeloid leukaemia there is the added advantage over the normal techniques of chemotherapy that although the inhibition of normal granulocyte production opens the way for bacterial infection, the absence of any effect on the lymphocyte system allows for continuing protection against viral infection. Conversely, when the lymphocyte chalone is used against lymphocytic leukaemia there is a continuing normal granulocyte protection against bacterial infection.

It is also possible to envisage the use of chalones together with other anti-tumour agents. Chalone treatment could be combined with a stimulus to the immune response, or a chalone could be used for a period and then suddenly withdrawn so that the tumour cells enter the mitotic cycle synchronously, when they may be destroyed by already established techniques.

The discovery of the lymphocyte chalone has also opened the way to the second possible therapeutic technique. It has already been established that this chalone, by suppressing lymphocyte production, can play a powerful supporting role in tissue and organ transplantation (*84–86*). All other tissues remain unaffected and the animals show no adverse effects of any kind. Further, it has been reported that thymus-dependent (T)-lymphocyte production may be controlled by a separate T-lymphocyte chalone, and this would obviously increase still further the value of this method of inhibiting graft rejection. As with the leukaemias the chances of infection are greatly reduced.

ACKNOWLEDGMENT

It is a pleasure to record my continuing indebtedness to Johanna Deol, who has given so much support during the preparation of this paper.

REFERENCES

1. Bullough, W. S. The control of epidermal thickness. Brit. J. Derm., *87*: 187–199, 347–354, 1972.
2. Bullough, W. S. Mitotic control in adult mammalian tissues. Biol. Rev., *50:* 99–127, 1975.
3. Bullough, W. S. The Evolution of Differentiation, Academic Press, London, 1967.
4. Bullough, W. S. Mitotic and functional homeostasis. Cancer Res., *25*: 1683–1727, 1965.
5. Bullough, W. S. Ageing of mammals. Z. Altersforsch., *27*: 247–253, 1973.
6. Weiss, P. and Kavanau, J. L. A model of growth and growth control in mathematical terms. J. Gen. Physiol., *41*: 1–47, 1957.
7. Iversen, O. H. The regulation of cell numbers in epidermis. A cybernetic point of view. Acta Pathol. Microbiol. Scand., *148* (Suppl.): 91–96, 1961.

8. Mercer, E. H. The cancer cell. Brit. Med. Bull., *18*: 187–192, 1962.

9. Bullough, W. S. and Laurence, E. B. The control of epidermal mitotic activity in the mouse. Proc. Roy. Soc., Ser. B, *151*: 517–536, 1960.

10. Bullough, W. S. The control of mitotic activity in adult mammalian tissues. Biol. Rev., *37*: 307–342, 1962.

11. Rytömaa, T. and Kiviniemi, K. Control of granulocyte production. Cell Tiss. Kinet., *1*: 329–340, 341–350, 1968.

12. Forscher, B. K. and Houck, J. C. Chalones: Concepts and current researches. Natl. Cancer Inst. Monogr., *38*: 1–233, 1973.

13. Bullough, W. S. Epithelial repair. *In;* J. E. Dunphy and W. van Winkle (eds.), Repair and Regeneration, pp. 35–46, McGraw-Hill, New York, 1969.

14. Rohrbach, R. and Laerum, O. D. Variations of mitosis-inhibiting chalone activity in epidermis and dermis after carcinogen treatment. Cell Tiss. Kinet., *7*: 251–257, 1974.

15. Scott, van E. J. and Ekel, T. M. Kinetics of hyperplasia in psoriasis. Arch. Derm., *88*: 373–381, 1963.

16. MacDonald, R. A. Lifespan of liver cells. Arch. Int. Med., *107*: 335–343, 1961.

17. Wessells, N. K. Problems in the analysis of determination, mitosis, and differentiation. *In;* R. Fleischmajer and R. E. Billingham (eds.), Epithelial-Mesenchymal Interactions, pp. 132–151, Williams and Wilkins, Baltimore, 1968.

18. Lawson, K. A. The role of mesenchyme in the morphogenesis and functional differentiation of rat salivary epithelium. J. Embryol. Exp. Morphol., *27*: 497–513, 1972.

19. Alescio, T. and DiMichele, M. Relationship of epithelial growth to mitotic rate in mouse embryonic lung developing *in vitro*. J. Embryol. Exp. Morphol., *19*: 227–237, 1968.

20. Kratochwil, K. Organ specificity in mesenchymal induction demonstrated in the embryonic development of the mammary gland of the mouse. Dev. Biol., *20*: 46–71, 1969.

21. Sigot, M. and Marin, L. Organogenèse de l'estomac de l'embryon de poulet. J. Embryol. Exp. Morphol., *24*: 43–62, 1970.

22. Franks, L. M., Riddle, P. N., Carbonell, A. W., and Gey, G. O. A comparative study of the ultrastructure and lack of growth capacity of adult human prostate epithelium mechanically separated from its stroma. J. Pathol., *100*, 113–119, 1970.

23. Dodson, J. W. The differentiation of epidermis. I. The interrelationship of epidermis and dermis in embryonic chicken skin. J. Embryol. Exp. Morphol., *17*: 83–105, 1967.

24. Billingham, R. E. and Silvers, W. K. Dermoepidermal interactions and epithelial specificity. *In;* R. Fleischmajer and R. E. Billingham (eds.), Epithelial-Mesenchymal Interactions, pp. 252–266, William and Wilkins, Baltimore, 1968.

25. Karasek, M. A. Induction of growth and differentiation in postembryonic epithelial cell cultures. J. Invest. Derm., *52*: 377, 1969.

26. Briggaman, R. A. and Wheeler, C. E. Epidermal-dermal interactions in adult human skin: Role of dermis in epidermal maintenance. J. Invest. Derm., *51*: 454–465, 1968.

27. Briggaman, R. A. and Wheeler, C. E. Epidermal-dermal interactions in adult human skin. II. The nature of the dermal influence. J. Invest. Derm., *56*: 18–26, 1971.

28. Karasek, M. A. and Charlton, M. E. Growth of postembryonic skin epithelial cells on collagen gels. J. Invest. Derm., *56*: 205–210, 1971.

29. Houck, J. C. and Cheng, R. F. Isolation, purification and chemical characterization of the serum mitogen for diploid human fibroblasts. J. Cell. Physiol., *81*: 257–270, 1973.

30. Christophers, E. Kinetic aspects of epidermal healing. *In;* H. I. Maibach and D. T. Rovee (eds.), Epidermal Wound Healing, pp. 53–99, Yearbook Medical Publishers, Chicago, 1972.

31. Bullough, W. S. and Deol, J.U.R. Dermo-epidermal adhesion and its effect on epidermal structure in the mouse. Brit. J. Derm., 1975, in press.

32. Morley, C.G.D. Humoral regulation of liver regeneration and tissue growth. Perspect. Biol. Med., *17*: 411–428, 1974.

33. Bucher, N.L.R. Regeneration of mammalian liver. Int. Rev. Cytol., *15*: 245–300, 1963.

34. Bucher, N.L.R. and Swaffield, M. N. The rate of incorporation of labeled thymidine into the deoxyribonucleic acid of regenerating rat liver in relation to the amount of liver excised. Cancer Res., *24*: 1611–1625, 1964.

35. Bucher, N.L.R., Scott, G. F., and Aub, J. C. Regeneration of the liver in parabiotic rats. Cancer Res., *11*: 457–465, 1951.

36. Leong, G. F., Grisham, J. W., Hole, B. V., and Albright, M. L. Effect of partial hepatectomy on DNA synthesis and mitosis in heterotopic partial autografts of rat liver. Cancer Res., *24*: 1496–1501, 1964.

37. Lajtha, L. G. Review of leukocytes. Natl. Cancer Inst. Monogr., *38*: 111–115, 1973.

38. Rytömaa, T. Chalone of the granulocyte system. Natl. Cancer Inst. Monogr., *38*: 143–146, 1973.

39. Kivilaakso, E. and Rytömaa, T. Erythrocytic chalone, a tissue-specific inhibitor of cell proliferation in the erythron. Cell Tiss. Kinet., *4*, 1–9, 1971.

40. Bullough, W. S. and Deol, J.U.R. Über die Regelung von Gewebeersatz in der Haut. Der Hautarzt, *22*: 174–180, 1971.

41. Sumrall, A. J. and Johnson, W. C. The origin of dermal fibrocytes in wound repair. Dermatologia, *146*: 107–114, 1973.

42. Winter, C. D. Studies, using sponge implants, on the mechanism of osteogenesis. *In;* E. Kulonen and J. Pikkarainen (eds.), Biology of the Fibroblast, pp. 103–125, Academic Press, London, 1973.

43. Bullough, W. S. and Deol, J.U.R. The pattern of tumour growth. Symp. Soc. Exp. Biol., *25*: 255–275, 1971.

44. Bullough, W. S. and Laurence, E. B. Epidermal chalone and mitotic control in the V×2 epidermal tumour. Nature, *220*: 134–135, 1968.

45. Rytömaa, T. and Kiviniemi, K. Control of DNA duplication in rat chloroleukaemia by means of the granulocytic chalone. Eur. J. Cancer, *4*: 595–606, 1968.

46. Rytömaa, T. and Kiviniemi, K. Chloroma regression induced by the granulocytic chalone. Nature, *222*: 995–996, 1969.

47. Rytömaa, T. and Kiviniemi, K. Regression of generalized leukaemia in rat induced by the granulocytic chalone. Eur. J. Cancer, *6*: 401–410, 1970.

48. Elgjo, K. and Hennings, H. Epidermal mitotic rate and DNA synthesis after injection of water extracts made from mouse skin treated with Actinomycin D: Two or

more growth-regulating substances? Virchow Arch. Abtl. B, Zellpathol., *7*: 342–347, 1971.

49. Laurence, E. B. and Elgjo, K. Epidermal chalone and cell proliferation in a transplantable squamous cell carcinoma in hamsters. II. *In vitro* results. Virchow Arch. Abtl. B, Zellpathol., *7*: 8–15, 1971.

50. Bullough, W. S. and Deol, J.U.R. Chalone-induced mitotic inhibition in the Hewitt keratinising epidermal carcinoma of the mouse. Eur. J. Cancer, *7*: 425–431, 1971.

51. Mohr, U., Althoff, J., Kinzel, V., Süss, R., and Volm, M. Melanoma regression induced by chalone: A new tumour inhibiting principle acting *in vivo*. Nature, *220*: 138–139, 1968.

52. Bullough, W. S. and Laurence, E. B. Control of mitosis in mouse and hamster melanomata by means of the melanocyte chalone. Eur. J. Cancer, *4*: 607–615, 1968.

53. Bullough, W. S. and Laurence, E. B. The lymphocyte chalone and its antimitotic action on a mouse lymphoma *in vitro*. Eur. J. Cancer, *6*: 525–531, 1970.

54. Lasalvia, E., Garcia-Giralt, E., and Macieira-Coelho, A. Extraction of an inhibitor of DNA synthesis from human peripheral blood lymphocytes and bovine spleen. Eur. J. Clin. Biol. Res., *15*: 789–792, 1970.

55. Houck, J. C., Irausquin, H., and Leikin, S. Lymphocyte DNA synthesis inhibition. Science, *173*: 1139–1141, 1971.

56. Hinderer, H., Volm, M., and Wayss, K. Spezifische Hemmung der DNS-Synthese von Hela-Zellen durch Endometrium Extrakt. Exp. Cell Res., *59*: 464–468, 1970.

57. Bichel, P. Tumour growth inhibiting effect of JB-I ascitic fluid. Eur. J. Cancer, *6*: 291–296, 1970.

58. Bichel, P. Feedback regulation of growth of ascites tumours in parabiotic rats. Nature, *231*: 449–450, 1971.

59. Bichel, P. Specific growth regulation in three ascitic tumours. Eur. J. Cancer, *8*: 167–173, 1972.

60. Bichel, P. Self-limitation of ascites tumor growth: A possible chalone regulation. Natl. Cancer Inst. Monogr., *38*: 197–203, 1973.

61. Houck, J. C. and Daugherty, W. F. Chalones: A Tissue-specific Approach to Mitotic Control, Medcom Press, New York, 1974.

62. Laird, A. K. Dynamics of tumour growth. Brit. J. Cancer, *18*: 490–502, 1964.

63. Laird, A. K. Dynamics of tumour growth. Brit. J. Cancer, *19*: 278–291, 1965.

64. Laird, A. K. Dynamics of growth in tumors and in normal organisms. Natl. Cancer Inst. Monogr., *30*: 15–28, 1969.

65. Burns, E. R. On the failure of self-inhibition of growth of tumors. Growth, *33*: 25–45, 1969.

66. Steel, G. G. and Lamerton, L. F. The growth rate of human tumours. Brit. J. Cancer, *20*: 74–86, 1966.

67. Steel, G. G. Cell loss from experimental tumours. Cell Tiss. Kinet., *1*: 193–207, 1968.

68. Hewitt, H. B., Chan, D. P.-S., and Blake, E. R. Survival curves for clonogenic cells of a murine keratinizing squamous carcinoma irradiated *in vivo* or under hypoxic conditions. Int. J. Radiat. Biol., *12*: 535–549, 1967.

69. Goodman, G. J. Effects of one tumor upon the growth of another. Proc. Am. Assoc. Cancer Res., *2*: 207, 1957.

70. Trotter, N. L. The effect of partial hepatectomy on subcutaneously transplanted hepatomas in mice. Cancer Res., *21*: 778–782, 1961.

71. Schatten, W. E. An experimental study of post-operative tumor metastases. I. Growth

of pulmonary metastases following total removal of primary leg tumor. Cancer, *11*: 455–459, 1958.

72. Lewis, M. R. and Cole, W. H. Experimental increase of lung metastases after operative trauma. Arch. Surg., *77*: 621–626, 1958.

73. Brown, H. R. The growth of Ehrlich carcinoma and Crocker sarcoma ascites cells in the same host. Anat. Rec., *166*: 283, 1970.

74. Dombernowsky, P., Bichel, P., and Hartman, N. R. Cytokinetic analysis of the JB-1 ascites tumour at different stages of growth. Cell Tiss. Kinet., *6*: 347–357, 1973.

75. Foulds. L. Tumour progression and neoplastic development. *In;* P. Emmelot and O. Mühlbock (eds.), Cellular Control Mechanisms and Cancer, pp. 242–258, Elsevier, Amsterdam, 1964.

76. Mohr, U., Hondius Boldingh, W., and Althoff, J. Identification of contaminating *Clostridium* spores as the oncolytic agent in some chalone preparations. Cancer Res., *32*: 1117–1121, 1972.

77. Bielschowsky, F. Neoplasia and internal environment. Brit. J. Cancer, *9*: 80–116, 1955.

78. Foulds, L. Neoplastic development. vol. I. Academic Press, London, 1969.

79. Rous, P. and Kidd, J. G. A comparison of virus-induced rabbit tumors and tumors of unknown cause elicited by tarring. J. Exp. Med., *69*: 399–424, 1939.

80. Rous, P. and Kidd, J. G. Conditional neoplasms and subthreshold neoplastic states. J. Exp. Med., *73*: 365–389, 1941.

81. Frankfurt, O. S. Mitotic cycle and cell differentiation in squamous cell carcinomas. Int. J. Cancer, *2*: 304–310, 1967.

82. Burnet, F. M. Immunological surveillance in neoplasia. Transplant. Rev., *7*: 3–25, 1971.

83. Frankfurt, O. S. Epidermal chalone. Effect on cell cycle and on development of hyperplasia. Exp. Cell Res., *64*: 140–144, 1971.

84. Kiger, N., Florentin, I., and Mathé, G. A lymphocyte-inhibiting factor (chalone?) extracted from thymus: Immuno-suppressive effects. Natl. Cancer Inst. Monogr., *38*: 135–141, 1973.

85. Chung, A. C. and Hufnagel, C. A. Some *in vivo* effects of chalone (mitotic inhibitor) obtained from lymphoid tissues. Natl. Cancer Inst. Monogr., *38*: 131–134, 1973.

86. Garcia-Giralt, E., Rella, W., Morales, V. H., Diaz-Rubio, E., and Richaud, F. Extraction from bovine spleen of immunosuppressant with no activity on hematopoietic spleen colony formation. Natl. Cancer Inst. Monogr., *38*: 125–129, 1973.

Discussion of Paper of Dr. Bullough

DR. CASTRO: With reference to the inductive phase of tumourigenesis, might oncogenic viruses and chemicals be anti-chalone agents?

DR. BULLOUGH: Probably not. I believe that the most fundamental change involving a tumour cell, by whatever means it has been produced, is an alteration of its cell membrane. Succeeding events are then secondary to this, perhaps centering on the simple outward leakage of chalone at too a high rate.

DR. FROST: If the absence of a chalone is the ultimate cause of neoplastic proliferation, how do tumours become malignant? They should remain as benign lipomas, epitheliomas, *etc.*

DR. BULLOUGH: The distinction is here simple. All tumours showed eventually plateau, but at varying levels. If this cessation of growth due to an accumulated chalone concentration occurs relatively early, the neoplasm is said to be benign, whereas if the plateau cannot be reached before death occurs, the tumour is lethal or malignant.

DR. DRESSER: What is known about the size and chemical structure of chalones. I would suspect that the address portion of the molecules might be quite large in order to encompass sufficient information for the exact tissue specificity you have described. Could it possess a small functional unit, responsible for effecting a change in mitotic rate, attached to a larger carrier portion conferring the tissue specificity? In this way, it would be analogous to diphtheria toxin?

   Do you think these substances act on the cell cycle in a similar manner to that proposed for the action of thymidine, adenosine or cyclic AMP (Thomas, D. B. and Longwood, C. A., Cell, 5: 37, 1975).

DR. BULLOUGH: No chalone has as yet been purified adequately for precise chemical definition, but these substances appear to form two distinct groups, the chalones for erythrocytes, granulocytes, and melanocytes being polypeptides of molecular weight *ca.* 3,000 and those for lymphocytes, fibroblasts, and epidermal cells being *ca.* 30,000–50,000 daltons. The latter proteins may be polymers or contain carriers. Both types may include polysaccharide moieties, and are destroyed by trypsin. The granulocyte chalone, however, is precisely specific for this cell type and yet is only about 2,850 daltons; it lacks an associated carrier. There is some suggestive evidence that chalones act by binding to receptor sites on cell surfaces. If this is true, the succeeding intracellular events might involve cyclic AMP.

DR. HALPERN: It is difficult to conceptualize exactly how these small molecules are genetically coded with such exquisite tissue specificity, and are produced so rapidly under a variety of circumstances.

DR. BULLOUGH: As a cell differentiates during embryogenesis a multitude of tissue-specific molecules are formed. This is merely one such entity. Isolation of these molecules should prove relatively simple as a number of pharmaceutical companies have recently established pilot projects toward this goal.

DR. HALPERN: The urine should serve as a good source of these chalones, as it does for such molecules as the β-2-microglobulin portion of the HL-A antigens. For, they are certainly small enough to be filtered through the glomeruli.

DR. BULLOUGH: I am unsure of their appearance or concentration in the urine, although their presence there has been reported. A group in Helsinki has found that the easiest way to secure a relatively pure chalone preparation is by washing large quantities of leukaemic granulocytes, which lose chalone much more readily than normal granulocytes, in medium and collecting the eluant.

DR. HOBBS: There are several clinical observations which support the chalone concept. The halo nevus consists of a white area about a deeply pigmented tumour. B-lymphocyte tumours selectively suppress normal B cells while T-lymphocyte malignancies suppress normal T cells. However, while recovery from some very progressive forms of multiple myeloma in humans assures complete return of normal B cell function, in 85% of myelomatosis, successfully treated patients being followed for as long as ten years do not exhibit a return of bone marrow cell-derived competency, with normal immunoglobulin synthesis. It is possible that a tumour may produce a modified chalone capable of depressing permanently normal tissues, but I am concerned whether such irreversible tissue loss might not also be observed subsequent to passively administered chalone.

DR. BULLOUGH: Normal tissues, in contrast to tumours, appear to be able to withstand any degree of chalone challenge without irrevocable effects.

HOST DEFENSE AGAINST CANCER AND ITS POTENTIATION, D. MIZUNO ET AL. (EDS.),
UNIV. OF TOKYO PRESS, TOKYO /UNIV. PARK PRESS, BALTIMORE, PP. 337–351, 1975

Immunotherapy of Cancer by Microbial Products

Helen C. Nauts

Cancer Research Institute Inc., New York, N.Y., U.S.A.

Abstract: Historical background. Beneficial effects of bacterial infections, fever and heat, or inflammation. Factors affecting success or failure with Coley toxins (*Streptococcus pyogenes* and *Serratia marcescens*). Significance of delayed hypersensitivity reactions (DHR); therapeutic effect of inducing DHR in tumors; role of streptococci or staphylococci in augmenting these reactions. Role of fever and heat. Potentiation of response of tumor to radiation and protection of normal tissues to radiation induced by bacterial products. *Corynebacterium parvum.* BCG. Yeast extracts. Discussion and conclusions.

For over 200 years physicians have observed dramatic complete or partial regressions of cancer following acute bacterial infections (*1, 24*). One of the first investigators of this phenomenon, Coley, devoted a lifetime to developing a systemic cancer treatment with bacterial vaccines (*2*). After hearing of the "spontaneous regression" of an inoperable recurrent sarcoma following erysipelas, Coley attempted to duplicate this result in a recurrent, metastatic sarcoma of the tonsil by inoculating living streptococcal cultures (*1, 3, 4*). After repeated trials he succeeded, in October 1891, in inducing a severe erysipelas infection which caused complete regression (*1, 4*). During the next year Coley attempted to induce erysipelas in 9 other advanced or terminal patients and thus recognized the difficulties and dangers of using live vaccines (*4*). In December 1892, Coley first combined *Bacillus prodigiosus* (now known as *Serratia marcescens*) with *Streptococcus pyogenes* and produced a more stable and effective filtered preparation.

The first case to receive this product was a male, 19, with inoperable sarcoma of the abdominal wall and pelvis involving the bladder (case 1, Ref. *2*). Complete disappearance occurred in 4 months (traced well 26 years). This first type of "Coley toxins" did not prove potent enough to produce cures in the more resistant types of neoplasms (*5*).

Not until 1940 was an attempt made to evaluate all possible factors which might affect success or failure with this little understood method. Then the studies of Nauts *et al.* (2, 5) led to the founding of the New York Cancer Research Institute Inc. in 1953 (name changed in 1973 to Cancer Research Institute Inc.). This was the first attempt to evaluate the possibilities and limitations of Coley toxins and other agents which could be used to protect and increase host resistance to cancer, and to learn more about the mechanisms of action involved. Beginning in 1953 a series of end result studies were published, which analyzed the relative effectiveness of the 16 different preparations of Coley toxins and the equally important factor of varying techniques of administration (2, 5–17). Detailed histories of 920 microscopically proven cases treated by these various products* indicate that it was not until more potent, stable, unfiltered vaccines were available and properly administered as to site, dosage, frequency and *especially duration* of injections that the more resistant types of neoplasms were successfully treated (2, 5–17). The highest percentage of successes in the toxin treated cases occurred in sarcoma of soft tissues or in malignant lymphomas, especially reticulum cell sarcoma of the bone. The slower growing, more differentiated lesions were not as easily controlled, although remarkable results were obtained in 248 inoperable or metastatic sarcoma of soft tissues, carcinomas of the breast, colon, head and neck, uterus and ovary, lymphosarcoma, Hodgkin's disease, renal and testicular cancer, malignant melanoma, neuroblastoma, and bone tumors. In addition to complete or partial regression of primary or metastatic lesions, reduction or disappearance of lymphedema, ascites, or pleural effusion were observed following toxin therapy; regeneration of bone destroyed by osteolytic bone tumors or bone metastases was also observed (5–17, 46).

Beneficial Effects of Bacterial Infections, Heat, Fever, or Inflammation

During the past 35 years we have analyzed the beneficial effects not only of the Coley vaccines but of many other bacterial products on cancer and allied diseases. These studies included extensive data on the salutary effects of various acute infections (1), heat, fever, or inflammatory episodes on cancer (18–21), and on conditions other than cancer (23); the beneficial effects of one disease upon another, the varying effects of pyogenic, non-pyogenic, or non-pathogenic bacteria, protozoa or viruses or their vaccines. All cases of "spontaneous" regression were analyzed (1, 25). Most of these followed an acute bacterial infection (1), an inflammatory (22) or febrile episode (21), or incomplete removal of the neoplasm. Extensive data on the *deleterious* effects of most viral infections (1), anti-inflammatory agents (26), certain antibiotics (8, 27) and immunosuppressive agents, including most of the cancer chemotherapeutic agents have also been assembled and analyzed (22).

Until recently, many of the questions relating to this study have received little consideration by the medical profession. Why has the incidence of cancer and allied diseases increased much more rapidly since modern aseptic surgery, pasteurization of milk, immunization procedures and antibiotics have largely eliminated

---

* Four hundred fifty-three of these recovered and were followed 5–74 years after onset.

infections and infectious diseases in the developed countries (*1*)? Cancer incidence continues to be much lower in races and countries where infections and infectious diseases continue to be endemic or common (*28–32*). A great deal of experimental data support these clinical observations (*1, 4, 33–36*).

Jacobsen noted the low incidence of malignant disease in patients who had developed a common infectious process, *i.e.*, the actively tuberculous or osteomyelitic, and particularly those with a history of typhoid, paratyphoid, scarlatina, or diphtheria. He concluded that the reticuloendothelial system (RES), when sufficiently active (as when stimulated by one or a number of infectious or inflammatory processes), may thus attain the ability to cope with neoplastic diseases. He believed cancer should be regarded as a disease of the RES, and the hope for prevention and cure lay in microbial vaccines (*36*). Much experimental work has since been reported on the role of the RES in host resistance to neoplasia (*37*). Stern in a recent report stated "Immunocompetence and specific functions of the RES may play decisive roles in the defense of the host against development and progress of malignant tumors" (*39*). Analyses of these data suggest that pathogenic organisms are one of nature's controls of microscopic foci of malignant disease. Incipient cancers, destroyed by bacterial infections before they become clinically apparent, may confer a lasting immunity to the particular type of malignancy involved. In some cases, this host-stimulating effect is not sufficient to prevent onset of clinically apparent cancers. However, in such patients in Africa, *as* Burchenal and others have pointed out, when chemotherapy or radiation is administered, the regression is usually very dramatic and often complete, occurring with far smaller dosage than is required for patients in developed countries whose immune responses have rarely been stimulated (*40*). Anatomically localized infections may play a significant role in decreasing cancer incidence in that particular area. Death rates for pneumonia, influenza, and pulmonary tuberculosis in males have decreased precipitously since 1938, when antibiotics were introduced clinically, but lung cancer has increased from 3.5 per 100,000 to 45.0 per 100,000 population. Increasing and prolonged exposure to cigarette smoke has undoubtedly played a role, but the immunological benefits of respiratory infections have been diminished with infection control (*25, 41*). Moreover, it has been observed that lung cancer patients who develop empyema following lobectomy or pneumonectomy have a considerably higher 5-year survival rate than those without such infections (*25, 41–44*).

In the pre-antibiotic era, surgical patients more often developed wound infections following surgical excision or amputation for malignancy, and appeared to have a higher 5-year survival rate than those reported in later years (*45, 47*).

Factors Affecting Success or Failure with Coley Toxin Therapy

Our Cancer Research Institute has made detailed end result studies of all microscopically proven toxin treated cases of sarcoma of the soft tissues, lymphosarcoma, testicular and colon cancer, malignant melanoma, neuroblastoma, renal cancer, Ewing's sarcoma, osteogenic sarcoma, multiple myeloma and reticulum cell sarcoma of bone (*7–15, 46*). Other studies of giant cell tumor of bone and breast cancer, will appear soon (*6*). Among the significant findings emerging from these studies were the following: (a) variability of preparations of Coley toxins used in the past 82 years; (b) lack of knowledge of optimum technique of administration (site, dosage, frequency, and *especially duration* of therapy); (c) difficulties in obtaining successful results in very far advanced cases or in patients whose immune responses were depleted by old age or prior immunosuppressive therapy; (d) importance of determining the best time to initiate toxin therapy; and (e) better understanding of mechanisms of action involved and how these may be affected by some of the above factors.

The *critical importance of duration of toxin therapy* recently became apparent following analysis of end result studies of several types of tumors, but especially in the 165 cases of osteogenic sarcoma. If injections were given for less than 4 months as an adjuvant to amputation, only 36–43% survived (over twice the expected survival from amputation alone); however, if toxin injections were continued for 4 to 6 months, the 4-year survival rate rose to 100%; and only 2 patients died who received toxins for over 8 months. Calkins was one of the few surgeons who routinely administered Coley toxins for 6 to 12 months in all his operable and inoperable cancer patients and obtained approximately 80% 5-year survivals (*25*).

Delayed Hypersensitivity and Cancer

1. Prognostic significance of intact delayed hypersensitivity reaction (DHR)

The importance of maintaining or stimulating cell-mediated immunity (hypersensitivity) has only recently been recognized as playing an important role in preventing the development of cancer, or in helping to control cancer more effectively (*57*). A patient's ability to respond with a DHR to a standard test is a good prognostic sign. Eilber and Morton noted a significant correlation between cell-mediated immunologic reactivity as measured by a delayed cutaneous hypersensitivity to dinitrochlorobenzene (DNCB) and the course of malignant disease following definitive cancer surgery (*47*).

2. Prognostic significance of infiltrates of lymphoreticular cells

Black and Speer noted an increased survival in breast cancer patients having *sinus histiocytosis of the lymph nodes*. They suggested that cancer tissue may act as an antigen to the host RES (*48, 49*). Berg presented evidence that in human breast cancer the presence of a plasma cell reaction is prognostic of a favorable clinical course: in the group of large anaplastic cured cancers 73% showed a *striking peripheral inflammatory reaction* (*50*). Stewart reported a correlation between the degree of *stromal infiltration of a tumor by lymphocytes* and the presence of a DHR in a patient toward cellular extracts of his own tumor injected intradermally (*51*). A literature review suggested that patients with such lymphocytic infiltration have a better prognosis (*1, 8, 12, 22, 51*).

3. Therapeutic effect of inducing DHR in tumors

Citing Coley's work, Stewart proposed that by administering a non-specific antigenic stimulus one might induce this defense mechanism in patients (52). Stewart caused a recurrent skin lesion to regress following a DHR caused by intradermal injection of the nontoxic extracts of hemolytic streptococci (Varidase); resemblance of this reaction to a small area of erysipelas was very marked (52).

4. Possibility of streptococci and staphylococci augmenting DHR to tumor cell antigens

It would now seem important to adsorb tumor cells removed at biopsy onto killed streptococci, staphylococci, or pseudomonas to produce a more effective immunopotentiating vaccine than is possible with either a bacterial or tumor vaccine alone (53, 54).

5. Stimulation of DHR by chemicals

Klein of Roswell Park Memorial Institute was the first to discover that DHR to a simple chemical, such as DNCB, destroyed tumor foci, particularly those occurring in the skin (55, 56). His dramatic results have now been reported at several conferences. His work has been extensively confirmed by a number of investigators, such as Stjernswärd and Levin, who induced DHR in patients with basal cell carcinoma or lymphomas metastatic to the skin using DNCB. In 13 patients regression of treated tumor nodules compared to untreated nodules was noted; not only primary skin cancer but also carcinomas and lymphomas metastatic to the skin regressed. These findings have relevance to the possible existence of an immunologic surveillance system (57).

Role of Fever and Heat

It was apparent that the most effective infections causing cancer regressions were those accompanied by fever (1). An extensive study of the effects of fever and heat on cancer incidence and control showed that in countries like Japan and Finland, the incidence of cancers of the skin, breast, and testis are significantly lower than in other geographical regions. Bathing habits of the Japanese and Finnish people involve exposure of the whole body to high degrees of heat almost daily (18, 21a). Possibly the excellent end results in Finland with lumpectomy and radiation for breast carcinoma may be attributed to the host-stimulating effects of their sauna bathing (58). Geographic areas where malaria and other fevers are common also tend to have a lower incidence of most types of cancer (1). Of the concurrent infections in cancer patients, it was apparent that the acute febrile, rather than the low grade afebrile type, caused the most dramatic and lasting regressions (1). In extensive studies of the beneficial effects of fever and heat on host resistance, we have analyzed end results according to the type of febrile response in patients receiving bacterial toxin therapy (10, 18, 21, 46). Of patients with inoperable sarcoma of the soft tissues, 60% survived 5 years or more if febrile reactions averaged 102°–103°F, compared with 20% in those having little or no febrile reactions (10). In the operable stage, fever did not seem to be quite so important: 50% survived 5 years or more with little or no reactions, compared to 71% in those having average reactions of 102°–103°F.

Microbial Products and Radiation or Chemotherapy

Critical attention has been increasingly directed to the adverse effects of excessive radiation, including damage to normal tissue and function, diminished immunologic and hematologic integrity, and even subsequent production of other neoplasms, especially lymphomas (25, 59). Experimental studies indicate that either prior bacterial infection (1) or injections of microbial products, such as Coley toxins, protect the body against the deleterious effects of irradiation, while a potentiated response of the tumor to radiation occurs, thus making a smaller radiation dose possible (60–65). Coley toxins, and other bacterial endotoxins also potentiate the response to chemotherapy (25).

1.   Corynebacterium parvum

In the past decade an increasing number of physicians in France, England, and the United States have been using injections of heat-killed C. parvum as an immunopotentiator (67, 68). At a recent CIBA Foundation Conference on Immunopotentiation, Medawar stated "The promising results obtained with C. parvum in human cancer stress the interest of this group of immunopotentiators in general and of C. parvum in particular" (69).

Israel has treated over 400 patients with C. parvum in the last 7 years. Such therapy protects the patient against the immunosuppressive effects of chemotherapy (70, 71). Israel has used many different sites of injection, and in 1974 began using the intravenous route with very encouraging results. He concluded that the possibilities of C. parvum therapy and immunopotentiation in general are far from being fully explored. The optimal dose, frequency and duration of therapy are not yet known, nor which types of tumors may be most sensitive to such therapy. He concluded that it is now time for clinicians to answer these questions and to develop better methods of monitoring immunotherapy.

2.   BCG

There has been increasing interest in Europe, Canada, and the United States in the use of BCG as an immunopotentiator in the treatment of cancer or leukemia, as a result of the pioneering efforts of Old and Benacerraf in New York, and Halpern, Mathé and their colleagues in France (75, 76). Widespread clinical studies are now in progress and a beginning has been made in understanding the problems and potentialities of BCG.

3.   Yeast extracts and polysaccharides

As early as 1896 De Backer reported the beneficial effects of yeast extracts in cancer (77). Maisin noted that yeast-fed mice showed only 1.2% incidence as compared to 23.2% in the controls (78). Lewisohn noted that the addition of either pantothenic acid or riboflavin to an active yeast extract appeared to improve its effectiveness in preventing the development of carcinoma (79). Bradner noted the importance of dosage of zymosan in stimulation of host defense against cancer; low doses stimulated resistance, and very high doses (1,000 mg/kg) could block the low-dose effect completely. Timing was also important (80). Forssberg noted that zymosan accelerates hematopoietic recovery after radiation (81). Diller tested the oncolytic activity of zymosan and hydroglucan against a number of well-established mouse tumors, achieving 90–95% total regression of Sarcoma 180, and 83% of Krebs-2 Carcinoma with *no lethality*, using hydroglucan intravenously, and believed the host-mediated reaction involved stimulation of phagocytic elements of the liver and spleen (82). Martin used zymosan combined with surgery and chemotherapy, producing 70–80% cure rates, which could be nullified by an immunosuppressive agent (cortisone), and concluded that a combined immunologic and chemotherapeutic approach to the treatment of neoplastic disease seems indicated (83, 84). Nagy recently reported on 10 years' experience using a yeast extract (mannozym) for cancer of the breast, genitalia, alimentary tract, and lung; those receiving mannozym showed a 52.3% 5-year survival compared to 28.6% for the controls receiving "classical therapy" (85).

Lentinan, a polysaccharide derived from mushrooms, has proved to be an immunopotentiator according to Maeda *et al.* (86).

An excellent study has been made in Japan by Okamoto *et al.*, in Kanazawa, using a Beta hemolytic streptococcus preparation known as PCB45 (87). Hattori and Kurokawa at the Cancer Institute Hospital are using another streptococcal preparation (88).

It is hoped that these two groups of investigators will not limit their studies to advanced cancer patients whose immune responses have been suppressed by age, extent of disease, or prior chemotherapy or radiation. All such clinical studies should avoid the use of antipyretics or anti-inflammatory drugs since fever and inflammatory reactions are beneficial.

The recent work of Homma and his colleagues in the University of Tokyo, using a *Pseudomonas aeruginosa* purified protein moiety is encouraging. This preparation exerts excellent tumor inhibitory effects while protecting the host against *P. aeruginosa* infections which can be a serious problem in immunodeficient cancer and leukemia patients. It is hoped that these Japanese preparations will now be available for clinical trials in other countries (89, 90).

DISCUSSION AND CONCLUSIONS

(a) There is urgent need for more widespread cooperative studies of the immunological role of microbial products. (b) Coley's mixed toxins, *C. parvum*, staphylococcal, pseudomonas, and streptococcal or *Escherichia coli* vaccines or yeast extracts have little or no side effects compared with chemotherapeutic agents (2, 5–16, 46, 75–90). (c) *Technique of administration* of microbial products is of the utmost importance, especially regarding duration of therapy, but also timing, site, dosage, and frequency. (d) The possible beneficial effect of *streptococcal enzymes* (*hyaluronidase, streptodornase,* and *streptokinase*) should probably receive study at this time (*91–94*). (e) *Large scale clinical trials* should now be carried out in many countries using carefully planned protocols for many microbial products alone or used sequentially as immunopotentiators, not only in recurrent or inoperable cases, but as an adjuvant before and after surgery, radiation, or chemotherapy. (f) Prevention: At least two investigators have recently observed a significantly increased survival in leukemia patients who had concurrent infections or who had received a *Pseudomonas* vaccine to avoid or control *Pseudomonas* infection (*25*). A recent report suggests a diminished leukemia incidence in children who received BCG to prevent tuberculosis in Canada (*95*). A few physicians who have routinely administered mixed bacterial or respiratory vaccines in treating infections, sinusitis, allergies, or arthritis have observed a lower incidence of cancer in such patients (*25, 96*). These findings suggest that in due time *preventive* injections of microbial products may be warranted to maintain immunological responses at a proper level of efficiency, despite the effects of aging, stress or carcinogens in our environment. Possibly one reason why more dramatic results seem to have occurred with Coley toxins in the earlier years is that many more patients in that period had had prior exposure to infections and were better able to respond immunologically to the Coley toxin injections. Modern man has been overprotected and his immunological responses may be far less sensitive, except in certain areas where infections and infectious diseases are still endemic. (g) *The bacterial characteristics* of the streptococci now available may have been changed by the long term, widespread use of antibiotics since 1940. *The first priority* now is to obtain the best possible preparations of many bacterial vaccines and to use them in the most effective way, based on present knowledge of techniques and modes of action.

REFERENCES

1. Nauts, H. C. The apparently beneficial effects of bacterial infections on host resistance to cancer: End results in 435 cases. Monograph No. 8, p. 822, New York Cancer Research Institute, New York, 1969.
2. Nauts, H. C., Fowler, G. A., and Bogatko, F. H. A review of the influence of bacterial infection and of bacterial products (Coley's toxins) on malignant tumors in man. Acta Med. Scand., *145* (Suppl. 276): p. 103, 1953.
3. Coley, W. B. Contribution to the knowledge of sarcoma. Ann. Surg., *14*: 199–220, 1891.
4. Coley, W. B. Treatment of malignant tumors by repeated inoculations of erysipelas, with a report of 10 cases. Med. Rec., *43*: 60–61, 1893.
5. Nauts, H. C., Swift, W. E., and Coley, B. L. The treatment of malignant tumors by bacterial toxins as developed by the late William B. Coley, M. D., reviewed in the light of modern research. Cancer Res., *6*: 205–216, 1946.
6. Nauts, H. C. Bibliography of reports concerning the clinical or experimental use of Coley toxins (*Streptococcus pyogenes* and *Serratia marcescens*), p. 22, 383 references 1891–1975.
7. Fowler, G. A. Enhancement of natural resistance to malignant melanoma with special reference to the beneficial effects of concurrent infections and bacterial toxin therapy. Monograph No. 9, p. 85, New York Cancer Research Institute, New York, 1969.

8. Fowler, G. A. Beneficial effects of acute bacterial infections or bacterial toxin therapy on cancer of the colon and rectum. Monograph No. 10, p. 57, New York Cancer Research Institute, New York, 1969.

9. Fowler, G. A. and Nauts, H. C. The apparently beneficial effects of concurrent infections, inflammation or fever and of bacterial toxin therapy on neuroblastoma. Monograph No. 11, p. 82, New York Cancer Research Institute, New York, 1970.

10. Nauts, H. C., Pelner, L., and Fowler, G. A. Sarcoma of the soft tissues, other than lymphosarcoma, treated by toxin therapy. End results in 186 determinate cases with microscopic confirmation of diagnosis: 49 operable, 137 inoperable. Monograph No. 3, p. 80, New York Cancer Research Institute, New York, 1959.

11. Nauts, H. C. and Fowler, G. A. End results in lymphosarcoma treated by toxin therapy alone or combined with surgery and/or radiation or with concurrent bacterial infection. Monograph No. 6, p. 119, New York Cancer Research Institute, New York, 1969.

12. Nauts, H. C. Enhancement of natural resistance to renal cancer: Beneficial effects of concurrent infections and immunotherapy (bacterial vaccines). Monograph No. 12, p. 96, New York Cancer Research Institute, New York, 1973.

13. Nauts, H. C. Multiple myeloma: Beneficial effects of concurrent infections or immunotherapy (bacterial vaccines). Monograph No. 13, p. 69, Cancer Research Institute,* New York, 1975.

14. Nauts, H. C. Ewing's sarcoma; end results following immunotherapy (bacterial toxins) combined with surgery and/or radiation. Monograph No. 14, p. 108, Cancer Research Institute, New York, 1974.

15. Nauts, H. C. Osteogenic sarcoma: End results following immunotherapy (bacterial vaccines) 165 cases, or concurrent infections, inflammation or fever, 41 cases. Monograph No. 15, p. 120, Cancer Research Institute, New York, 1975.

16. Nauts, H. C. Giant cell tumor of bone: End results following immunotherapy (Coley toxins) alone or combined with surgery and/or radiation (66 cases) or with concurrent infection (4 cases). Monograph No. 4, 2nd ed., Cancer Research Institute, New York, 1975.

17. New York Cancer Research Institute. Progress Report, 1972–73.

18. Nauts, H. C. The beneficial effects of heat on malignant tumors in plants, animals and man. Brief abstracts of 170 references. Unpublished.

19. Strauss, A. A. Immunologic resistance to carcinoma produced by electro-coagulation, based on 57 years' experience and clinical results. Charles C. Thomas, Springfield, Illinois, 1969. (Also in Surg. Gyn. Obst., *121*: 989–996, 1965).

20. Stehlin, J. S., Jr. Hyperthermic perfusion with chemotherapy for cancers of the extremities. Surg. Gyn. Obst., *129*: 305–308, 1969.

21. Nauts, H. C. The beneficial effects of fever on cancer and other diseases. Unpublished.

21a. Nauts, H.C.: Pyrogen therapy of cancer: a historical overview and current activities. Read at an International Symposium on Cancer Therapy by Hyperthermia and Radiation, April 1975. Unpublished.

22. Nauts, H. C. Host resistance to cancer. Review of the early and recent literature. Monograph No. 5, p. 403, 2nd ed., New York Cancer Research Institute, New York, 1970.

23. Nauts, H. C. The beneficial effects of concurrent bacterial infection or bacterial products on conditions other than cancer. Unpublished.

---

* Name changed from New York Cancer Research Institute in August, 1973.

24. Everson, T. C. and Cole, W. H. Spontaneous Regression of Cancer. W. B. Saunders Co., Philadelphia/London, 1966.

25. Cancer Research Institute Records (founded in 1953 as New York Cancer Research Institute). Personal communications from patients or their families, physicians or hospitals.

26. Kelly, M. Corticosteroids and carcinogenesis, a clinical survey. Acta Rheum. Scand., 5: 286–290, 1959; 7: 315–320, 1961.

27. Zwaveling, A. Implantation metastases. Chemotherapeutic prophylaxis and tumor growth in an infected milieu. Cancer, 15: 790–796, 1962.

28. Smith, R. C., Salsbury, C. G., and Gilliam, A. G. Recorded and expected mortality among the Navajo; with special reference to cancer. J. Natl. Cancer Inst., 17: 77–89, 1956.

29. Smith, R. L. Recorded and expected mortality among the Indians of the United States with special reference to cancer. J. Natl. Cancer Inst., 18: 385–396, 1957.

30. Warwick, O. H. and Phillips, A. J. Cancer among Canadian Indians. Brit. J. Cancer, 8: 223–230, 1954.

31. Davies, J.N.P., Knowelden, J., and Wilson, B. A. Incidence rates of cancer in Kyadondo County, Uganda, 1954–1960. J. Natl. Cancer Inst., 35: 789–821, 1965.

32. Teutschlander. Tuberculose und Krebs. Zentralbl. Bakteriol., 122: 57–62, 1931.

33. Shwartzman, G. Effect of spontaneous and induced infections upon the development of mouse sarcoma 180 (preliminary report). Proc. Soc. Exp. Biol. Med., 32: 1603–1605, 1935; Arch. Pathol., 21: 284–297, 1936.

34. Havas, H. F., Donnelly, A. J., and Porreca, A. V. The cytotoxic effect of hemolytic streptococci on ascites tumor cells. Cancer Res., 23: 700–706, 1963.

35. Christensen, E. A. Infection and malignant tumors. I. Growth of Brown-Pearce carcinoma in rabbits treated with living or killed hemolytic streptococci. Acta Pathol. Microbiol. Scand., 46: 285–295, 1959.

36. Jacobsen, C. Der chronische Reis des reticuloendothelialen Systems—eine Krebshemmung. Arch. Dermatol. Syphilol., 169: 562–576, 1934.

37. Halpern, B. N., Biozzi, G. and Stiffel, C. Role du Système Réticulo-endothélial dans l'immunité antibactérienne et antitumorale, 221–236, Centre National de la Recherche Scientifique, Paris, 1963.

38. Old L. J., Benacerraf, B., Clarke, D. A., Carswell, E. Q., and Stockert, E. The role of the reticuloendothelial system in the host reaction to neoplasia. Cancer Res., 21: 1281–1300, 1961.

39. Stern, K. Experimental models for evaluation of host defenses in cancer. Israel J. Med. Sci., 7: 42–51, 1971.

40. Burchenal, J. H. Geographic chemotherapy—Burkitt's tumor as a stalking horse for leukemia: Presidential address. Cancer Res., 26: 2393–2405, 1966.

41. Davidson, M. Cancer of the Lung and Other Intrathoracic Tumors, pp. 40–42, William Wood & Co., New York, 1930.

42. Sensenig, D. M., Rossi, N. P., and Ehrenhaft, J. L. Results of surgical treatment of bronchogenic carcinoma. Surg. Gyn. Obst., 116: 229–284, 1963.

43. Takita, H. Effect of postoperative empyema on survival of patients with bronchogenic carcinoma. J. Thorac. Cardiovasc. Surg., 59: 642–644, 1970.

44. Virkula, L. and Kostiainen, S. Post pneumonectomy empyema in pulmonary carcinoma patients. Scand. J. Thorac. Cardiovasc. Surg., 4: 262–270, 1970.

45. Da Costa, J. C. Modern Surgery, 10th ed., p. 293, W. B. Saunders Co., Philadelphia, 1931.

46. Miller, T. N. and Nicholson, J. T. End results in reticulum cell sarcoma of bone treated by toxin threapy alone or combined with surgery and/or radiation (47 cases) or with concurrent infection (5 cases). Cancer, *27*: 524–548, 1971.

47. Eilber, F. R. and Morton, D. L. Impaired immunologic reactivity and recurrence following cancer surgery. Cancer, *25*: 362–367, 1970.

48. Black, M. M. and Speer, F. D. Sinus histiocytosis of lymph nodes in cancer. Surg. Gyn. Obst., *106*: 163–175, 1958.

49. Black, M. M., Freeman, C., Mork, T., Harvei, S., and Cutler, S. J. Prognostic significance of microscopic structure of gastric carcinomas and their regional lymph nodes. Cancer, *27*: 703–711, 1971.

50. Berg, J. W. Inflammation and prognosis in breast cancer. A search for host resistance. Cancer, *12*: 714–720, 1959.

51. Stewart, T.H.N. The presence of delayed hypersensitivity reactions in patients toward cellular extracts of their malignant tumors. 2. A correlation between the histologic picture of lymphocyte infiltration of the tumor stroma, the presence of such a reaction and a discussion of the significance of this phenomenon. Cancer, *23*: 1380–1387, 1969.

52. Stewart, T.H.M. and Tolnai, G. The regression of an inflammatory skin lesion by the induction of a delayed hypersensitivity reaction. A case report. Cancer, *24*: 201–205, 1969.

53. Burky, E. J. The production in the rabbit of hypersensitive reactions to lens, rabbit muscle and low ragweed extracts by the action of staphylococcus toxin J. Allergy, *4*: 466–476, 1933–1934.

54. Glynn, L. E. and Holborrow, E. J. The production of complete antigens from polysaccharide haptens by streptococci and other organisms. J. Pathol. Bacteriol., *64*: 775–783, 1952.

55. Klein, E. Hypersensitivity reactions at tumor sites. Cancer Res., *29*: 2351–2362, 1969.

56. Klein, E. Progress in immunotherapeutic approaches to the management of neonlasms. *In;* Perspectives in Cancer Research and Treatment, pp. 51–58, Alan R. Liss, New York, 1973.

57. Stjernswärd, J. and Levin, A. Delayed hypersensitivity-induced regression of human neoplasms. Cancer, *28*: 628–640, 1971.

58. Mustakallio, S. Conservative treatment of breast cancer. Clin. Radiol., *23*: 110–116, 1972.

59. Woodward, A. H., Ivins, J. C., and Soule, E. H. Lymphangiosarcoma arising in chronic lymphedatous extremities. Cancer, *30*: 562–572, 1972.

60. Ainsworth, E. J. and Forbes, P. D. The effect of *Pseudomonas pyrogen* on survival of irradiated mice. Radiat. Res., *14*: 767–774, 1961.

61. Hollcraft, J. W. and Smith, W. W. Endotoxin treatment and X-irradiation in mice bearing transplanted tumors. J. Natl. Cancer Inst., *21*: 311–330, 1958.

62. Smith, W. W., Alderman, I. M., and Gillespie, R. E. Increased survival in irradiated animals treated with bacterial endotoxins. Am. J. Physiol., *191*: 124–130, 1957.

63. Smith, W. W., Alderman, I. M., and Gillespie, R. E. Hematopoietic recovery induced by bacterial endotoxin in irradiated mice. Am. J. Physiol., *192*: 549–556, 1958.

64. Zweifach, B. W., Kivy-Rosenberg, E., and Nagler, A. L. Resistance to whole-body X-irradiation in rats made tolerant to bacterial endotoxins. Am. J. Physiol., *197*: 1364–1370, 1959.

65. Chandler, J. J., Stark, D. B., Allen, C. V., and Fletcher, W. S. Observations on the treatment of cancer by bacterial toxins. Am. Surg., *31*: 443–449, 1965.

66. Halpern, B. B., Prévot, A. R., Biozzi, G., Stiffel, C., Mouton, D., Morard, J. D., Boutillier, Y., and Decreuesefond, C. Stimulation de l'activité phagocytaire du système reticuloendothéliale provoquée par *Corynebacterium parvum*. J. Reticuloendothel., *1*: 77–96, 1964.

67. Halpern, B. N., Biozzi, G., Stiffel, C., and Mouton, D. Inhibition of tumor growth by administration of killed *Corynebacterium parvum*. Nature, *212*: 853–854, 1966.

68. Halpern, B. N., Fray, A., Crepin, Y., Platica, O., Lorinet, A. M., Rabourdin, A., Sparros, L., and Isac, R. *Corynebacterium parvum*, a potent immunostimulant in experimental infections and in malignancies. *In;* G.E.W. Wolstenholme and J. Knight (eds.), Immunopotentiation (Ciba Foundation Symposium), vol. 18, Elsevier/Excerpta Medica/North Holland, Amsterdam/London/New York, 1973.

69. Israel, L. and Halpern, B. N. Le *Corynebacterium parvum* dans les cancers avancés. Première évaluation de l'activité thérapeutique de cette immuno-stimuline. N. Presse Méd., *1*, 19–23, 1972.

70. Israel, L. On 414 cases of human tumors treated with *Corynebacteria*. Read at symposium on *Corynebacterium parvum*, Paris, May 9–10, 1974, in press.

71. Israel, L. Preliminary results of non-specific immunotherapy for lung cancer. Cancer Chemother. Rep., *4*: 283–286, 1973.

72. Israel, L., Depierre, A., and Chahinian, P. Combination chemotherapy for 418 cases of advanced cancer. Cancer, *27*: 1089–1093, 1971.

73. Israel, L., Depierre, A., and Edelstein, R. Local and systemic effects of intranodular B.C.G. in 25 cases of recurrent melanoma. Proc. Am. Soc. Clin. Oncol., March 27–28, 1974.

74. Old, L. J., Clark, D. A., and Benacerraf, B. Effect of Bacillus Calmette-Guérin injection in transplanted tumors in the mouse. Nature, *184*: 291–292, 1959.

75. Halpern, B. N., Biozzi, G., Stiffel, C., and Moulton, D. Effet de la stimulation du système reticulo-endothélial par l'inoculation de bacille de Calmette-Guérin sur le développement de l'épitheliome atypique T-8 de Guérin chez le rat. Compt. Rend. Soc. Biol., *153*: 919–923, 1959.

76. Mathé, G., Schwarzenberg, L., Amiel, J. L., Schneider, M., Caltan, A., and Schlumberger, J. R. The role of immunology in the treatment of leukemias and hematosarcomas. Cancer Res., *27*: 2542–2553, 1967.

77. De Backer. De la cancérose et de son traitement au moyens de ferments purs. J. de Med. de Paris, *2*: 276–279, 1897.

78. Maisin, J., Pourbaix, V., and Caeymaex, P. Influence de l'alimentation à base de levure bouillé sur le cancer experimental. Compt. Rend. Soc. Biol., *127*: 1477–1478, 1938.

79. Lewisohn, R., Leuchtenberger, C., Leuchtenberger, R., Laszlo, D., and Block, K. Action of yeast extract on transplanted and spontaneous malignant tumors in mice. Cancer Res., *1*: 799–806, 1941.

80. Bradner, W. T. and Clarke, D. A. Stimulation of host defense against cancer. II. Temporal and reversal studies of zymosan effect. Cancer Res., *19*: 673–678, 1959.

81. Forssberg, A., Lingen, C., Ernster, L., and Lindberg, O. Modification of the X-irradiation syndrome by lycopene. Exp. Cell. Res., *16*: 7–14, 1959.

82. Diller, I. C., Mankowski, Z. T., and Fisher, M. E. The effect of yeast polysaccharides on mouse tumors. Cancer Res., *23*: 201–208, 1963.

83. Martin, D. S., Hayworth, P., Fugmann, R. A., English, R., and McNeil, H. W. Combination therapy with cyclophosphamide and zymosan on a spontaneous mammary cancer in mice. Cancer Res., *24*: 652–654, 1964.

84. Martin, D. S., Fugmann, R. A., and Hayworth, P, Surgery, cancer chemotherapy, host defenses and tumor size. J. Natl. Cancer Inst., *29*: 817–834, 1962.

85. Nagy, I., Jeno, A., and Koszoru, M. Complementary immunotherapy in tumorous diseases. A ten years' survey of mannozym therapy. Arch. Italiano di Patologia e Clinica dei Tumori, *14*: 29–35, 1971.

86. Maeda, Y. Y., Hamuro, J., Yamada, Y. O., Ishimura, K., and Chihara, G. The nature of immunopotentiation by anti-tumor polysaccharide, lentinan, and the significance of serotonin, histamine and catecholamines in its action. *In;* G.E.W. Wolstenholme and J. Knight (eds.), Immunopotentiation (Ciba Foundation Symposium), vol. 18, Elsevier/Excerpta Medica/North Holland, Amsterdam/London/New York, 1973.

87. Okamoto, H., Koshimura, S., Shoin, S., and Shimizu, R. B-Hemolytic Streptococcus as a Cancer Controller. A Commentary on PC-B-45. Chugai Pharmaceutical Company, Ltd., Tokyo, Japan, 1973.

88. Kurokawa, T., Hattori, T., and Furue, H. Clinical experiences with Streptococcal anticancer preparation, O.K.-432 (NSC-B116209). Cancer Chem. Rep., *56*: 211–220, 1972.

89. Homma, J. T., Abe, C., Okada, K., Tanamoto, K., and Hirao, Y. The biological properties of the protein moiety of the endotoxin of *Pseudomonas aeruginosa*. Proc. 4th Int. Symp. on Animal, Plant and Microbial Toxins, Tokyo, Sept. 8–13, 1974, in press.

90. Homma, J. Y., Kawaharajo, K., Okada, K., and Shimizu, T. *Pseudomonas aeruginosa* infection and its serodiagnosis. Proc. on Bacterial Resistance, Organized by the Commission of Chemoresistance, Tokyo, Oct. 24–26, 1974, in press.

91. Duran Reynals, F. Studies on a certain spreading factor existing in bacteria and its significance for bacterial invasiveness. J. Exp. Med., *58*: 161–181, 1933.

92. Duran Reynals, F. Further studies on the influence of testicle extract upon the effects of toxins, bacteria and viruses, and on the Shwartzman and Arthus phenomena. J. Exp. Res., *58*: 451–463, 1933.

93. Johnson, A. J. Cytological studies in association with local injections of streptokinase —streptodornase in patients. J. Clin. Invest., *29*: 1376–1386, 1950.

94. Miller, J. M. Proteolytic enzymes in inflammation. Rationale for use. Postgrad. Med., *19*: 16–22, 1956.

95. Davignon, L., Lemond, P., St. Pierre, J., and Frappin A. BCG vaccination and leukemia mortality. Lancet, *II*: 638, 1970; *I*: 80–81, 1971.

96. Baird, K. A. The Human Body and Bacteria. A Study of Their Actions and Reactions, pp. 182, Bruce Publ. Co., U.S.A., 1968.

Discussion of Paper of Dr. Nauts

DR. SIMMONS: If one were to organize a cooperative clinical study to investigate the effect of a microbial product on cancer, which such substance would you advise selecting, and which type of neoplasm would be most efficacious to examine?

DR. NAUTS: While the data is presently insufficient to choose a single microbial substance for analysis, I believe the commercially available mixed staphylococcus-streptococcus and the pseudomonas vaccines would be suitable candidates. Our review of spontaneous infections in cancer patients has revealed that while streptococcal diseases accompany the most dramatic regressions, this state is often only temporary. Significant staphylococcal infections appear to accompany the greatest number of *permanent* regressions. Most viral infections probably suppress a host's defense against a tumor, despite a recent report in Cancer from a group in Japan indicating that mumps vaccine may be an effective anti-cancer therapy.

DR. ALEXANDER: In the cases you've reported, was there objective evidence for the disappearance of proven distant metastases along with the primary lesion? Many of these anecdotes appeared when accurate means for the following of such secondaries may not have been available.

Also, is hemorrhagic necrosis involved in the regression of tumors after certain systemic infections?

DR. NAUTS: A number of the dramatic permanent recoveries occurred in the presence of obvious massive secondaries. The significance of hemorrhagic necrosis in these individuals depends on the degree of tumor vascularity. Injection of a bacterial toxin directly into a tumor leads to the greatest necrosis. As the antigenicity of a neoplasm can sometimes be augmented if the appropriate microorganism or its toxin reach the target cells early in the course of therapy, a series of injections should thus be made in or near the tumor.

DR. JERNE: Has administration of allogeneic lymphocytes been tried in human cancer therapy?

DR. NAUTS: Our group hasn't attempted this, and I am unaware of such reports in the literature.

Dr. Nishioka: In East Africa, malarial infections are often accompanied by lowered immune responses and a precipitous drop in levels of C3. Yet, you described tumor suppression concomitant with malaria. How do you reconcile these observations?

Dr. Nauts: We have actually found only two cases of tumor regression directly following acute concurrent cases of malaria.

Dr. Simmons: In fact, Burkitt's lymphoma occurs almost exclusively in those areas of Africa with high incidences of malaria.

Dr. Mizuno: Is the intradermal administration of the vaccines you mentioned effective as cancer therapies?

Dr. Nauts: Yes. This route is much more efficient than subcutaneous injection. Intravenous administration is also effective. One of the important parameters appears to be the induction of fever by these agents.

HOST DEFENSE AGAINST CANCER AND ITS POTENTIATION, D. MIZUNO ET AL. (EDS.),
UNIV. OF TOKYO PRESS, TOKYO / UNIV. PARK PRESS, BALTIMORE, PP. 353-364, 1975

Humoral Resistant Factors from the Resistant Mouse against Allogeneic and Syngeneic Tumor Cells

Den'ichi MIZUNO, Masatoshi YAMAZAKI, Shoji OHKUMA, and
Hirotaka SHINODA

Faculty of Pharmaceutical Sciences, University of Tokyo, Tokyo, Japan

Abstract: The antitumor effect of bacterial lipopolysaccharide (LPS) has been studied. The stimulation of macrophage as well as lymphocyte was observed by detecting the increase with time of ^{32}P-labeled RNA and DNA of mouse spleen. By intradermal injection of LPS in the presence of tumor cells, new resistant humoral factors were isolated. They are $\alpha \sim \beta$-globulins.

Attenuated cells of syngeneic tumor MM46 were given to C3H/He forming a high titer of IgG both in ascitic fluid and serum. This titration can be done in the presence of either resistant or normal macrophage without complement. The conventional technique using complement could not have detected the presence of this IgG.

We have been studying on the mechanism of therapeutic effect of bacterial lipopolysaccharide (LPS), especially from *Proteus vulgaris* OX 19. The emphasis has been put on humoral factors and macrophage both of which seem to be less highly evaluated than lymphocytes. The present report will cover two topics (*1–5*) on this problem in a brief sketch and the recent new findings in which we could find a humoral resistant activity, possibly ascribed to IgG, in the host challenged with a syngeneic tumor cell apart from the problem of LPS. This activity was shown more clearly when macrophage was employed.

LPS as a Stimulator of Reticular Cells (*1–3*)

The LPS obtained from *P. vulgaris* by the method of Westphal could show a marked therapeutic effect on the solid type of Ehrlich carcinoma as well as Sarcoma 180 (S 180) (Table 1). At that time the most effective route of injection was intradermally (Table 1). Therefore, since 1968 we have been studying the effect always by intradermal route. The phagocytic activity as observed by carbon clearance was markedly stimulated (Fig. 1). The primary effect we found was the

TABLE 1-1. Antitumor Effect of LPS against Ehrlich Carcinoma

Sample	Dose (μg) and route of LPS	Wt. difference[a]	Survivors	Tumor wt. (mg)	Percent (treated/ control $\times$100)
Control			9/ 9	763	100
Mitomycin	50, 7 times, i.p.	−8.0	7/10	225	29.5
Mitomycin	100, 3 times, i.d. (days 2, 4, 6)	−7.0	10/10	168	22.0
LPS	100, 3 times, i.d. (days 2, 4, 6)	0.3	9/9	143	18.7
LPS	10, 3 times, i.d.	−4.4	9/9	159	20.8
LPS	1, 3 times, i.d.	−2.3	10/10	303	39.7

Antitumor effect of LPS of *P. vulgaris* injected intradermally (i.d.) on solid-type of Ehrlich carcinoma cells. i.p.: intraperitoneally. [a] Animal weight difference: average weight change of treated host minus average weight change of control host.

TABLE 1-2. Antitumor Effect of LPS against S 180

Sample	Dose (μg) and route of LPS 3 times	Wt. difference[a]	Survivors	Tumor wt. (mg)	Percent (treated/ control $\times$100)
Control			10/10	1,510	100
LPS	100, i.p. (days 2, 4, 6)	−4.8	9/10	864	57.2
LPS	10, i.p.	−0.9	10/10	868	57.5
LPS	1, i.p.	−2.4	10/10	903	59.8
LPS	100, i.d. (days 2, 4, 6)	−2.6	10/10	383	25.3
LPS	10, i.d.	−1.1	10/10	831	54.9
LPS	1, 3 times, i.d.	−2.3	9/9	712	47.3

Antitumor effect of LPS of *P. vulgaris* injected i.d. on the solid-type of S 180 carcinoma cells. [a] Same as in Table 1-1.

stimulation of reticuloendothelial system (Fig. 2). An additional mechanism was found to show a direct cytotoxic effect of LPS on the tumor cells (Fig. 3).

We studied the dynamic change of cells in mouse spleen when injected with LPS. That is to say the effect was examined *in vivo* in normal mouse spleen. The change of DNA and RNA in spleen was followed (Figs. 4 and 5). The marker isotope was ^{32}P. A remarkable change with time was observed in RNA and then in DNA. Based on these findings together with the change as observed histochemically we concluded that when LPS is given, the reticular cells are stimulated first and successively the mitotic cells appear abundantly in the spleen of mice.

Humoral Factors Found in Tumor-resistant Mouse (4, 5)

The conventional approach in cancer immunotherapy is to seek for the cytotoxicity of lymphocytes or macrophages. Contrary to this tendency our primary attention has been focused to seek for some humoral factors which are resistant against tumor either specifically or non-specifically. We seeked for resistant factors

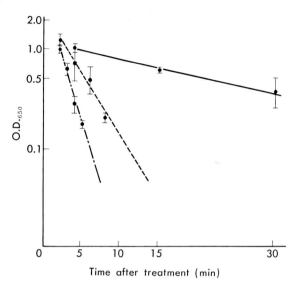

FIG. 1.   Rates of removal of intravascular colloidal carbon in mice treated with the LPS of *P. vulgaris*. ——— control; — · — intradermal (i.d.) treatment, 100 μg/mouse; - - - - intraperitoneal (i.p.) treatment, 100 μg/mouse. Half times of removal: control, 16.5 min; i.d. treatment, 70 sec; i.p. treatment, 2.8 min.

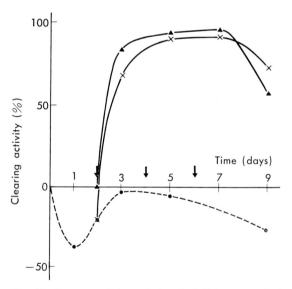

FIG. 2.   Response of the reticuloendothelial system of mice of injection of LPS of *P. vulgaris* and Ehrlich ascites carcinoma cells. Ehrlich carcinoma cells (3×10^6 cells/mouse) were injected subcutaneously (s.c.), and 100 μg of LPS were administered i.d. 3 times, 2, 4, and 6 days after cell inoculation.   Carbon clearance was measured 1, 2, 3, 5, 7, and 9 days after cell inoculation.   ▲ LPS only; × cells and LPS; ● Ehrlich carcinoma cells (s.c.); ↓ injection of LPS (i.d.).

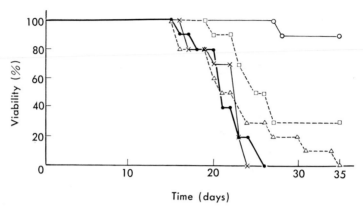

Fig. 3. Antitumor effect of LPS of *P. vulgaris* on the ascites form of Ehrlich carcinoma cells, as revealed by the survival curve after direct contact with the cells. Drugs were prepared as solutions of 100 μg/ml, mixed with the cell suspension, and incubated for 1 hr at 37°C and then inoculated into mice by the i.p. route. ○ Mitomycin; □ Bleomycin; △ LPS; × 8-azaguanine; ● control.

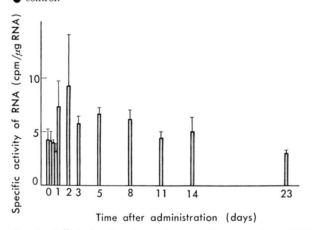

Fig. 4. Effect of endotoxin on the rate of incorporation of ^{32}Pi into RNA at intervals after administration of endotoxin. Each bar represents the average of the values of 6 mice with the standard deviation.

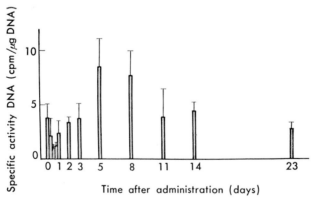

Fig. 5. Effect of endotoxin on the rate of incorporation of ^{32}Pi into DNA at intervals after administration of endotoxin. Each bar represents the average of the values of 6 mice with the standard deviation.

TABLE 2. Behaviors of Humoral Resistant Factor (4, 5)

1. Neutralizing activity without specificity
2. Inability of complement-dependent cytotoxic activity
3. Not adsorbed to tumor cells
4. Not absorbed by anti-IgG or -IgM sera
5. Non-dialyzable
6. $\alpha \sim \beta$-globulin fraction
7. Heat labile (65°C 30 min)
8. Sensitive to sodium periodate (0.01 M)
9. Resistant to mercaptoethanol (0.1 M)

produced in the serum of resistant mouse against Ehrlich carcinoma by intradermal injection of LPS. Factors were obtained as revealed by the neutralization test. The serum of resistant mouse was mixed with the tumor cells and given to the normal mouse intraperitoneally to observe the survival. The resistance was observed in the fraction of $\alpha \sim \beta$-globulin. The absorption of these resistant factors with rabbit anti-mouse-γ-globulin serum cannot abolish the activity. These factors have no cytotoxicity against tumor cells in the presence of complement. The activity was not specific (Table 2).

We do not know at present whether this activity is ascribed to alloantigen on the Ehrlich carcinoma cells or not. However, we would like to say that in the resistant mouse serum we can obtain some humoral resistant factors apart from antibodies.

The increase of factors like these have been reported by other authors, when mice are treated with lentinan (6) and when mice become resistant against ascitic tumor cells which have been discarded (7).

Presence of Cytotoxic Factor in the Ascitic Fluid and the Serum of Resistant Mouse

Apart from the resistant mouse against tumor cells induced by LPS, we have been examining the cytotoxic factors in the resistant mouse induced by the con-

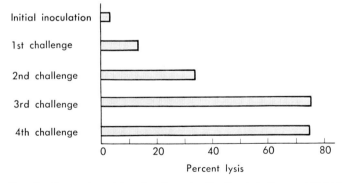

FIG. 6. Cytotoxic activity of peritoneal cells after 4 challenges. MM 46 cells were attenuated by Mitomycin-C (40 μg/ml, incubated at 37°C for 20 min) and given to the mouse C3H. Challenges were performed by fresh tumor cells at 3-week intervals. Cytotoxic activity of peritoneal cell was determined by the ^{51}Cr release from labeled tumor cells.

TABLE 3. Specificity of Target Cell Destruction

Target cell	% lysis	MM antigen
MM 46	70	+
47	6	±
48	10	−
102	22	−
MH134	3	−
FM3A 78	63	+

Target cells were labeled with ^{51}Cr, mixed with the peritoneal cells obtained from resistant mouse and incubated for 8 hr. The ratio of tumor to peritoneal cells is 1/100.

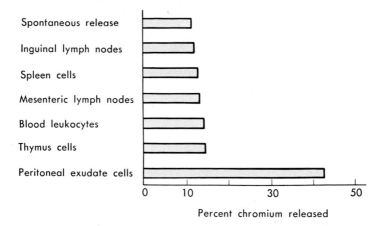

FIG. 7. Cytotoxic activity of various resistant lymphoid cells. MM 46 cells were labeled with ^{51}Cr, mixed with various lymphoid cells from resistant mouse and incubated for 8 hr at 37°C.

ventional techniques. In this case C3H/He mouse and MM 46, syngeneic tumor cells, are employed.

The cells were attenuated by Mitomycin-C and transplanted to mouse intraperitoneally followed by 4 successive challenges with 3-week intervals. The peritoneal cells were tested to induce the isotope release from ^{51}Cr-labeled tumor cells after the incubation of 8 hr (Fig. 6). The cytotoxic activity runs parallel with the content of the MM antigen which was elucidated by Nishioka's group (Table 3). Also, we found that the responsible cells were confined to the peritoneal cells as compared with other lymphoid cells derived from the same resistant mice (Fig. 7).

We noticed at that time that the incubated medium was essential for this cytotoxicity (Table 4). Peritoneal cells from resistant mice were incubated for 90 min. This was called preincubation. After the preincubation the cells were divided into two, one is glass adherent, the other is nonadherent. The preincubated medium was tested for the cytotoxicity in the presence or absence of either or both cells. The adherent cells and the preincubated medium were found to be two essential factors for the cytotoxicity.

As shown in Table 5 the adherent cells were treated with rabbit anti-θ serum

TABLE 4. Cytotoxic Activity of Adherent and Nonadherent Peritoneal Cells with or without the Preincubated Medium

Cells	Medium	% lysis	
		Exp. I	Exp. II
Undisturbed	Preincubated	82	64
Nonadherent	Preincubated	11	12
	Fresh	1	2
Adherent	Preincubated	77	51
	Fresh	8	0
Reconstituted	Preincubated	86	—
	Fresh	5	—
None	Preincubated	—	2

Peritoneal cells from resistant mouse were washed and incubated in the medium (PRMI 1640 with 10% fetal calf serum) for 90 min. The supernatant of this preincubation was called preincubated medium which was tested for the cytotoxic activity in the presence of glass-adherent and -nonadherent cells.

TABLE 5. Inhibition of Adherent Cell Activity by Antibody

Adherent	Treatment	% released
+	Anti-θ+C	30
+	Anti-γ-globulin+C	29
+	—	37
−	—	12

Adherent cells were treated with antibody and complement (C) at 37°C for 60 min. After washing, ascitic fluid from resistant mice was added and the cytotoxic activity was observed.

or with anti-mouse-γ-globulin serum (Table 5). The activity of those treated cells remained at the level of nontreated control. We would like to say that the glass adherent cells, we should say macrophage, are responsible for the reaction. The possible contamination of lymphocytes, if any, either bone marrow-derived cells (B cells) or thymus-derived cells (T cells) do not play a main role in the cytotoxic reaction. The carbon uptake by adherent and nonadherent cells were compared to give a result that 94% of the adherent cells were phagocytes.

The preincubated medium and the cells derived from resistant mouse were compared with those from normal mouse. Even the normal macrophage is active, if preincubated medium derived from sensitized cells is present, although the activity is about 50% compared to the complete system (Table 6).

The macrophage which is preferably sensitized and the ascitic fluid derived from resistant mouse can provoke the cytotoxicity. The minimal ratio for tumor cells *versus* macrophage was 1/25.

The ascitic fluid from resistant mouse was tested. It was found to contain cytotoxic factor in a great amount, if it is tested in the presence of macrophage. We wanted to identify this humoral cytotoxic factor. The ascitic fluid as diluted in Fig. 8 showed significant activity by about 1/64 (Fig. 8). The conventional complement-dependent cytotoxicity without macrophage was 1/2. The absorption of

TABLE 6. Cytotoxic Activity of Normal and Resistant Peritoneal Cells

Macrophage	Lymphocyte	Preincubated medium	% lysis
R	R	R	61
N	R		0
N		R	32
	N	R	4
R	N		0
R		N	2
	R	N	0

R : resistant peritoneal cells. N : normal peritoneal cells. Macrophages from the resistant mouse were compared with those from the normal for the cytotoxic activity in the presence of preincubated medium.

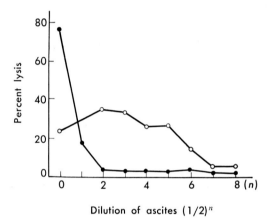

FIG. 8. Cytotoxic activity of ascitic fluid from the resistant mice. ● complement-dependent; ○ macrophage-dependent.

TABLE 7. Inhibition of Cytotoxic Activity of Ascitic Fluid by Anti-γ-globulin Serum

Treatment	% lysis
None	75.1
Absorption	1.2

The ascitic fluid from resistant mouse was incubated with rabbit anti-mouse-γ-globulin serum overnight at 4°C. After absorption, the supernatants were assayed for cytotoxic activity.

this ascitic fluid with rabbit anti-mouse-γ-globulin serum abolished the activity (Table 7).

The resistant ascitic fluid was fractionated by ammonium sulfate and the 70% precipitates were further fractionated by column chromatography with Sephadex G-200. The activity appeared in the second peak which is known as 7S γ-globulin (Fig. 9).

This γ-globulin fraction was further fractionated by the DEAE-cellulose chromatography. The flow through fraction contains the major activity. This shows also that the major activity in γ-globulin fraction is IgG (Fig. 10).

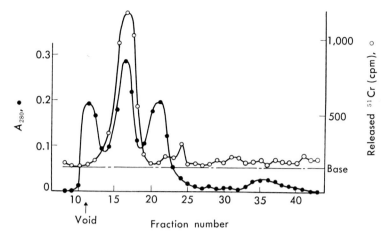

FIG. 9. Sephadex G-200 column profile of the 70% precipitates of ammonium sulfate.

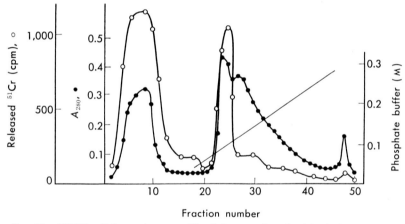

FIG. 10. DEAE-cellulose column profile of the second peak of Sephadex G-200.

The γ-globulin fraction from the normal and the present preparations were compared in sodium dodecylsulfate (SDS) gel electrophoresis (Fig. 11). The same patterns were obtained to show that new identities in this farction did not appear.

In Fig. 12 the existence of macrophage-dependent cytotoxic antibody is also shown in the serum of the resistant mouse, unexpectedly in a big amount (Fig. 12).

Thus we can say that the cytotoxic factor may be IgG, but its activity can be positively detected when the macrophage is present.

DISCUSSION

We have been seeking for new humoral factors which are responsible for the resistance against tumor cells in the resistant mouse. By the potentiation with LPS we could find resistant factors in the serum apart from γ-globulin. These are non-specific and fall in the fraction of α∼β-globulin. Another resistant factor was

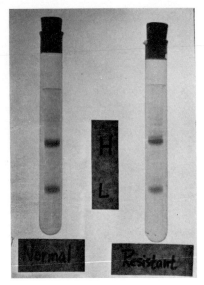

FIG. 11. SDS gel patterns of flow through fractions of DEAE-cellulose column chromatography.

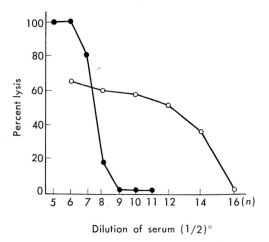

FIG. 12. Cytotoxic activity of resistant mice sera. ● complement-dependent; ○ macrophage-dependent.

found in the serum and also in ascitic fluid from the resistant mouse against its syngeneic tumor cells. This factor was now proposed to be IgG.

Now I should like to point out the significances of this finding. First, the assay of this humoral activity is important. The macrophage was used to increase the cytotoxicity against tumor cells sensitized with the syngeneic antibody either from serum or from ascitic fluid of resistant mouse. Our purpose in the beginning was to seek for the resistant factor. But the clarification of the experiment revealed the need of macrophage and, in turn, it converted to give a new assay method to identify the IgG present in the humoral fluid. The amplification of this cytotoxic system is about 50 times.

Second, I should like to point out the presence of specific antibody in a big amount in the humoral fluid of resistant mouse at least in the present case. By the conventional immunological method this activity would have been observed in a lesser extent. We cannot tell further at present, but it is probable that the resistant animals against syngeneic tumor cells have specific antibody in the humoral fluid and that this activity can be assayed by this macrophage-dependent cell lysis which has been now proposed.

During the session of this symposium existence of the antibody has been very frequently discussed. I should like to say that this antibody is really present at least in this case, although the identity of this antibody is not clear as to whether the conventional antibody is equal to this or not.

REFERENCES

1. Mizuno, D., Yoshioka, O., Akamatsu, M., and Kataoka, T. Antitumor effect of intracutaneous injection of bacterial lipopolysaccharide. Cancer Res., *28*: 1531–1537, 1968.
2. Takano, T. and Mizuno, D. Dynamic state of the spleen cells of mice after administration of the endotoxin of *Proteus vulgaris*. I. Cellular proliferation after administration of the endotoxin. Japan. J. Exp. Med., *38*: 171–183, 1968.
3. Takano, T., Yoshioka, O., Mizuno, D., Watanabe, K., Ohtani, T., and Kageyama, K. Dynamic state of the spleen cells of mice after administration of the endotoxin of *Proteus vulgaris*. II. Cellular differentiation into RE-cells 48 hours after administration of endotoxin. Japan. J. Exp. Med., *38*: 241–249, 1968.
4. Kato, N., Ito, S., Yamazaki, M., and Mizuno, D. Effect of *Proteus vulgaris* lipopolysaccharide on resistance of mice inoculated with tumor cells sensitized to Ehrlich carcinoma transplantation. Gann, *64*: 111–120, 1973.
5. Yamazaki, M., Ohkuma, S., and Mizuno, D. Humoral anti-Ehrlich carcinoma factor found in mice with tumor resistance acquired by intradermal lipopolysaccharide administration. Gann, *65*: 337–344, 1974.
6. Maeda, Y. Y., Chihara, G., and Ishimura, K. Unique increase of serum proteins and action of antitumour polysaccharides. Nature, *252*: 250–252, 1974.
7. Egawa, K., Tanino, T., and Saito, M. Biphasic immunoreaction against tumor antigen. Japan. J. Exp. Med., *45*: 53–54, 1975.

Discussion of Paper of Drs. Mizuno et al.

DR. JERNE: Does your cytocidal factor adsorb onto normal macrophages?

DR. MIZUNO: No, as when macrophages are incubated with this factor and washed no lysis is obtained.

DR. SIMMONS: It thus appears not to be a cytophilic antibody.

DR. H. OKADA: Do you believe one can readily generalize from the phenomena you observed using the MM46 mouse mammary carcinoma to other tumor systems, for most serum transfers from tumor-bearing animals lead to a tumor-enhancing effect, rather than the inhibition which you here report?

DR. MIZUNO: As yet we have not tried to extend our findings to other tumor systems.

DR. HOBBS: Fakhri and I, using a spontaneous peritoneal tumor not thought to be virus induced, gathered results very similar to yours. Antibody from these animals is cytotoxic, but only in high concentrations, and is supported by non-adherent cells, most effectively by macrophages. The antibody could be adsorbed out by the host's tumor cells but not by normal cells. So I do feel that one might be permitted to generalize from your system.

DR. ALEXANDER: Currie and Evans noted that IgG_1 and IgG_2 obtained from the serum of patients, as well as mice and rats, with a variety of neoplasms will lyse tumor cells in the presence of macrophages at one-hundredth the concentration of complement needed to accomplish comparable cytotoxicity.

DR. NISHIOKA: You might be able to determine which of the two surface receptors macrophages possess for C3b and IgG is functioning in your system by attempting to block the receptor for C3b by macrophage trypsinization, and by blocking that for IgG with aggregated IgG.

DR. MIZUNO: Thank you. I will follow your suggestions.

HOST DEFENSE AGAINST CANCER AND ITS POTENTIATION, D. MIZUNO ET AL. (EDS.), UNIV. OF TOKYO PRESS, TOKYO / UNIV. PARK PRESS, BALTIMORE, PP. 365–377, 1975

Fundamental Approaches to Cancer Immunotherapy Using a Protein-bound Polysaccharide, PS-K, with Special Reference to Its Clinical Application

Shigeru TSUKAGOSHI

Cancer Chemotherapy Center, Japanese Foundation for Cancer Research, Tokyo, Japan

Abstract: We have isolated a polysaccharide, termed PS-K, from *Coriolus versicolor* (FR.) QUÉL. of Polyporaceae (*Basidiomycetes*), differing from other antitumor polysaccharides in that it contains tightly bound protein (about 15%) and exhibited antitumor activity against animal tumors after oral administration. The structure of polysaccharide portion of PS-K has been studied by Hirase *et al.* as having main chain structure of α- or β-$(1\rightarrow4)$ glucan with branching. PS-K was most effective against sarcoma-180 by intraperitoneal administration, but oral administration was also effective. Intraperitoneal or oral pretreatment of mice or rats with PS-K before inoculation of sarcoma-180 or ascites hepatoma AH-13 cells was effective, showing the host-mediated activity of this preparation like other polysaccharides. Intraperitoneal growth of AH-13 cells was considerably suppressed in the group in which both PS-K pretreatment and subcutaneous inoculation of AH-13 cells admixed with PS-K, which were carried out before intraperitoneal inoculation of the tumor cells, were combined. Against a syngeneic mouse tumor, leukemia P388, the life prolongation of the tumor-bearing mice treated with PS-K was best in the group in which the interval between pre- and posttreatment was 6 weeks, indicating a 50% increase of average life span. This result also shows that PS-K has a host-mediated activity on a syngeneic mouse tumor. From current results, PS-K seemed to stimulate either non-specific or specific immune responses. In animal experiments PS-K could prevent in some extent leukopenia, loss of body weight and immuno-suppression caused by cyclophosphamide. In the clinical studies on PS-K, it has been given orally to various cancer patients with or without surgery, radiation, or chemotherapy, and the therapeutic results are under investigation.

There are numerous papers concerning the antitumor effect of polysaccharides isolated from various natural sources. For example, hemicellulose fractions (*1–4*) from various plants and polysaccharide from bamboo (*5*), fungi (*6–9*), bagasse (*10*), lichen (*11*), and yeast (*12–14*), and bacterial lipopolysaccharides (*15*) have been examined for their antitumor properties mostly against mouse sarcoma-180. Recently we have isolated a similar polysaccharide from *Basidiomycetes*, which differed from other antitumor polysaccharides in that it contained a tightly bound protein and exhibited antitumor action against mouse sarcoma-180 and rat ascites hepatomas after its oral administration. The physical and chemical properties and the antitumor activity of this polysaccharide have been studied, and it has almost no appreciable toxicity (*16, 17*). In Japan, some fungi belonging to *Basidiomycetes* have been used for the treatment of malignant neoplasms as folk remedies and this polysaccharide was also isolated from one such fungus.

Chihara and others (*8, 18*) isolated lentinan from *Lentinus edodes* (BERK) SING. and reported that the antitumor effect of lentinan against mouse sarcoma-180 might be due to the stimulation of cell-mediated immune responses (*19–21*).

Preparation and Characteristics of Protein-bound Polysaccharide, PS-K

Protein-bound polysaccharide, PS-K, was obtained as follows: Mycelia of *Coriolus versicolor* (FR.) QUÉL. of Polyporaceae family (*Basidiomycetes*) were first extracted with hot water and then the precipitate was separated from the clear supernatant by saturation of ammonium sulfate, and used for experiments after desalting. Structure of the polysaccharide portion has been studied by Hirase *et al.* (*22*), as having a main chain structure of an α- or β-$(1\rightarrow4)$ glucan with branching at the 3- or 6-position of the carbon atoms of glucose at the rate of one branch chain per 5 glucose units and containing about 15% protein. Conventional deproteinization procedures such as the treatment of PS-K with trichloroacetic acid, trifluorotrichloroethane, pronase, Sephadex column (G-75, G-100), DEAE-cellulose column, and $CHCl_3$-amyl alcohol were all unsuccessful, proving that protein binding was considerably tight. PS-K occurs as an odorless, tasteless, water-soluble and brownish powder, having a molecular weight greater than 10,000. For experimental use, it was dissolved in sterilized physiological saline before use but water solution was used for oral administration. As have been reported by Tsukagoshi and others (*16*), PS-K revealed almost no appreciable toxicity by various routes of administration, and showed some cytostatic activity *in vitro* against rat ascites hepatoma, AH-13, cells.

Animal and Tumors

Animals used for the leukemia P388 were female CDF_1, (C57BL/6 female $\times$ DBA/2 male)F_1 mice, 8–10 weeks old and weighing 22–27g. The mice and leukemia P388 were supplied by Drug Research and Development (DR & D), Division of Cancer Treatment National Cancer Institute, N.I.H., U.S.A. Leukemia P388 cells were maintained in DBA/2 male mice and 5- or 6-day-old ascites cells were used for experiments. Rat ascites hepatomas (AH-13, AH-7974, AH-66F) in the ascites forms were those maintained in our laboratory, and Donryu rats, weighing 100–130 g used were from Nihon Rat Co., Ltd., Saitama, Japan.

The rat tumor cells obtained from 5-day-old ascites were suspended in physiological saline and 1.0 ml (10⁶ cells) was inoculated intraperitoneally or subcutaneously. Mouse sarcoma-180 was maintained in our laboratory in the ascites form and 0.1 ml (10⁶ cells) of 7-day-old ascites tumors was transplanted subcutaneously into the right axillary region of ICR-JCL mice, weighing about 20 g (CLEA Japan Inc., Tokyo, Japan). For sarcoma-180 experiments, PS-K was injected intraperitoneally or orally from 3 days after tumor inoculation. After 32 days, all the mice were killed, tumors were extirpated, and their weights were compared with those of control tumors to calculate the inhibition ratio.

Antitumor Effect on Sarcoma-180

From 24 hr after subcutaneous inoculation of sarcoma-180 cells to ICR-JCL mice (10 mice/group), PS-K was administered every other day.

As shown in Table 1, PS-K was effective by intraperitoneal administration. Of interest was that PS-K was also quite effective by oral administration, indicating that PS-K possesses quite a different characteristic from other antitumor polysaccharide preparations which are ineffective by oral use.

TABLE 1. Effect of PS-K on Mice Bearing Sarcoma-180

Route of administration	Dose (mg/kg)	No. of administration	Average tumor weight (g)	Inhibition (%)
Intraperitoneal	Control	—	2.56 ± 1.20[a]	—
(8 mice/group)	10	11	0.16 ± 0.56	93.7
	100	11	0.06 ± 0.17	97.6
	600	11	0.03 ± 0.17	99.3
Oral	Control	—	2.36 ± 1.42	—
(10 mice/group)	500	20	1.01 ± 1.18	57.1
	1,000	20	0.57 ± 0.99	75.9
Intramuscular	Control	—	2.37 ± 1.27	—
(10 mice/group)	100	11	0.50 ± 0.40	78.0
Intravenous	Control	—	3.52 ± 1.97	—
(8 mice/group)	58	11	1.80 ± 1.33	48.3

ICR-JCL mice were inoculated subcutaneously with sarcoma-180 (10⁶ cells/mouse). Administration of PS-K started 7 days after inoculation of sarcoma-180. Body and tumor weights were measured on the 32nd day after inoculation. [a] Values are means ± standard deviation (SD).

Effect on Rat Ascites Hepatomas by Treatment before Tumor Inoculation

PS-K (250 mg/kg) was injected intraperitoneally to normal rats once a day for 10 days at a dose of 250 mg/kg and tumor cells were transplanted 8 days after the last injection. In case of AH-13, PS-K was given intravenously, subcutaneously, or orally as well as intraperitoneally.

Results of this experiment are shown in Table 2, in which PS-K was found effective by oral administration against AH-13, and somewhat effective against AH-7974 and AH-66F which are strongly and moderately resistant to the conventional antitumor alkylating agents. From these results it was shown that PS-K possesses a host-mediated antitumor activity.

TABLE 2.   Effect of Pretreatment of Rats Bearing Ascites Hepatomas with PS-K

	Treatment (mg/kg × times)	Route	60-Day survivors	Average life span in days: T/C
AH-13	250 × 10	i.p.	7/10	8.5/ 8.0
	,,	p.o.	2/10	12.0/ 8.0
	,,	s.c.	0/10	8.0/ 8.0
	,,	i.v.	0/10	8.0/ 8.0
AH-7974	250 × 10	i.p.	2/10	20.0/23.0
AH-66F	250 × 10	i.p.	4/10	8.5/ 9.0

PS-K (250 mg/kg) was given intraperitoneally (i.p.), subcutaneously (s.c.) intravenously (i.v.), or orally (p.o.) for 10 days to Donryu rats (10 rats/group) and rats were inoculated i.p. with ascites hepatoma, AH-13, AH-7974, or AH-66F (10^6 cells/rat), 8 days after the last injection.   Figures in parentheses indicate average life span (days) of the dead rats in the treated group (T) to that in the control (C).

Effect of Pretreatment of Rats with PS-K on the Growth of Intraperitoneally Inoculated AH-13 Cells

Before intraperitoneal inoculation of AH-13 cells (10^6 cells/rat) 250 mg/kg of PS-K was injected intraperitoneally once daily for 5 days (10 rats/group), and 8 days after the last injection, AH-13 cells (10^6 cells/ml) were mixed with PS-K (25 mg/ml/10^6 cells), and 1 ml of tumor suspension with or without PS-K was inoculated subcutaneously in the dorsum. Seven days after subcutaneous inoculation, AH-13 ascites cells (10^6 cells/rat) were inoculated intraperitoneally. Peritoneal ascites cells were washed out 5 times with a small amount (about 1 ml) of physiological saline and cell counts were made after Giemsa staining using a hemocytometer 5 days after inoculation. Total peritoneal ascites cells of each animal were calculated by multiplying cell counts/ml and total volume of the suspension. These results are shown in Table 3.

As shown in this table, intraperitoneal growth of AH-13 ascites cells was considerably suppressed in the group in which both PS-K pretreatment and subcutaneous inoculation of AH-13 cells mixed with PS-K were combined. In the case of experiments shown in Table 3, both subcutaneously and intraperitoneally inoculated AH-13 cells grew gradually making it difficult to judge the antitumor effect of PS-K from the prolongation of life span of the treated animals.

This result, together with the host-mediated action of PS-K as shown in Table 2, indicates that PS-K seems to stimulate non-specific and/or specific host immu-

TABLE 3.   Effect of PS-K Pretreatment and Subcutaneous Inoculation of AH-13 Cells Admixed with PS-K on the Growth of Ascites Tumor Cells

Group	Pretreatment	Subcutaneous inoculation	Intraperitoneal inoculation	Average total cell count	T/C[a] (%)
1	—	AH-13	AH-13	201 ± 258	100
2	—	AH-13+PS-K	AH-13	214 ± 181	107
3	PS-K	AH-13	AH-13	39 ± 67	19
4	PS-K	AH-13+PS-K	AH-13	6 ± 10	3

[a] T/C = (average total cell count in group 2, 3, or 4/average total cell count in group 1) × 100.

nity. In this case, tumor cell inoculated subcutaneously grew gradually, together with the growth of peritoneal ascites cells.

In order to reconfirm this effect of PS-K with a syngeneic tumor system, the mouse leukemia P388 was used in a similar experiment and the effect of PS-K was examined by the prolongation of survival time of the treated mice.

Effect of Pre- and Posttreatment with PS-K on Mice Inoculated with P388

As in the preceding experiment, the following protocol was used with mouse leukemia P388 implanted in groups of ten CDF_1 mice.

	2 weeks	2 weeks	2 weeks		
(A)	(B)	(B)		(C)	(E)
	(D_1)	(D_1)			
	(D_2)	(D_2)			

(A)   Mice (10 mice/group) were pretreated intraperitoneally with 500 mg/kg of PS-K daily for 5 days.

(B)   One-tenth milliliter of P388 cells (10^8 cells/ml) irradiated with 10,000 rads of X ray was inoculated subcutaneously in the dorsum. X-ray irradiation was delivered at 10 MV with source tumor distance (STD) 100 cm, field of 16×10 cm², and 300 rads/min, for each exposure with Toshiba Linac, LMR-13.

(D_1) X-ray irradiated P388 cells as in (B) were mixed with PS-K 25 mg/ml/10^8 cells and 0.1 ml of the cell suspension were inoculated subcutaneously.

(D_2) Same as (D_1), but 12.5 mg/ml of PS-K was mixed.

(C)   Intraperitoneal inoculation of P388 (10^6 cells/mouse).

(E)   Mice were injected intraperitoneally 500 mg/kg of PS-K daily for 5 days starting 1 day after intraperitoneal inoculation of P388 cells.

These results are shown in Table 4, and it will be seen that the life prolongation was the best in the group in which the interval between pretreatment and posttreatment was 6 weeks, showing a 50% prolongation in average life span. Subcutaneous inoculation of the attenuated P388 cells did not show any special benefit for the prolongation of life span. This result also indicates that PS-K definitely possesses a considerable host-mediated activity, since posttreatment alone with PS-K exhibited only 25% increase of average life span.

In the experiments given in Table 4, various radiation doses ranging from 2,500 to 10,000 rads were applied to P388 cell suspension before inoculation, and it was found that 10,000 rads was just sufficient to prevent *in vivo* tumor growth after subcutaneous inoculation to CDF_1 mice. All other doses caused the death of all or some of mice inoculated subcutaneously with the irradiated cells showing metastases to various organs in a separate experiment. However, the best result was obtained in the group which did not receive subcutaneous inoculation of tumor cells. It is rather difficult to give any explanation on the difference in antitumor effect of PS-K's between the two experiments shown respectively in Tables 3 and 4, but one possible explanation is that the difference of immunological responses might be coming from that between allogeneic AH-13 and syngeneic P388 cells.

TABLE 4.   Effect of PS-K Pre- and/or Posttreatment on the Life Span of Mice Inoculated with P388

Treatment	MST[a] (day)	T/C[b] (%)
C	10.0	100
CE	12.5	125
AC	10.5	105
ACE	15.0	150
BC	10.5	105
BCE	12.5	125
ABC	10.0	100
ABCE	13.5	135
D_1C	9.0	90
D_1CE	12.5	125
AD_1C	11.0	110
AD_1CE	14.0	140
D_2C	9.0	90
D_2CE	14.0	140
AD_2C	10.0	100
AD_2CE	13.0	130

[a] MST : median survival time.   [b] T/C=(MST in treated mice/MST of control mice)×100.

Immunological Studies on PS-K

Bacille Calmett-Guérin (BCG), *Corynebacterium* preparations, polyinosinic-poly-cytidylic acid, and polyadenylic-polyuridylic acid have been found by one or several experiments to be able to stimulate immune responses (*23*), and Mathé mentioned that some of these agents are capable of exerting immunostimulation in reactions that require the cooperation of thymus-dependent (T) and bone marrow-derived (B) lymphocytes.

Present experimental results showed that PS-K also possesses host-mediated antitumor activity like other polysaccharide preparations. However, one of the distinguishing characteristics of PS-K from other polysaccharide preparations is that its antitumor activity can be obtained by oral use. The antitumor activity of lentinan, is reported as elicited by T-cell stimulation (*17*). The action mechanism of PS-K has not been fully elucidated yet. However, Nakano and others (*24*) studied delayed skin reaction using hapten-type antigen, picryl chloride, in mice either in tumor-bearing mice or by the administration of conventional antitumor agents, and found that the decrease of skin reaction in mice bearing sarcoma-180 or Ehrlich ascites tumor or in mice given antitumor agents, 838D or L-asparaginase, was prevented by oral administration of PS-K.

The effect of antilymphocyte serum (ALS) on the antitumor activity of PS-K was reduced by intraperitoneal inoculation of ALS prepared by the method of Gray *et al.* (*25*). The result is shown in Table 5.

On the contrary, PS-K did not accelerate various immune responses such as phagocytic activity (*26*) and delayed hypersensitivity (*27*) as indicated in Tables 6 and 7.

TABLE 5. Effect of Antilymphocyte Serum on the Antitumor Activity of PS-K

Exp.	Samples	Dose	Average tumor weight (g)	D/T	Inhibition ratio (%)	Complete regression
1[a]	PS-K	50 mg/kg × 10 i.p.	0.25	1/8	94.7	5/7
	PS-K ALS	50 mg/kg × 10 0.1 ml × 10 i.p.	3.03	1/8	35.3	0/7
	ALS	0.1 ml × 10	3.67	1/8	21.6	0/7
	PS-K NRS	50 mg/kg × 10 0.1 ml × 10	1.15	1/8	75.4	1/7
	Control		4.68	0/8		
2[b]	PS-K	50 mg/kg × 10	0.25	1/8	94.7	5/7
	PS-K ALS	50 mg/kg × 10 0.1 ml × 10	1.44	1/8	69.2	0/7
	ALS	0.1 ml × 10	3.14	3/8	32.9	0/7
	PS-K NRS	50 mg/kg × 10 0.1 ml × 10	0.76	0/8	83.8	4/8
	Control		4.68	0/8		0/8

D/T: number of dead mice/number of total mice (ICR-JCL). NRS: normal rabbit serum. [a] PS-K and antilymphocyte serum were injected i.p. 24 hr after transplantation of sarcoma-180. [b] PS-K was injected 24 hr after tumor transplantation, and antilymphocyte serum injected 12 days after tumor transplantation.

TABLE 6. Effects of PS-K on the Carbon Clearance

	Dose (mg/kg × days)	Average phagocytic index (K)[a]
PS-K	5 × 10	0.0222 ± 0.0038
PS-K	50 × 10	0.0282 ± 0.0070
Control		0.0217 ± 0.0010

PS-K was injected i.p. to 3 groups of ICR/JCL mice. The carbon clearance activity was examined 24 hr after the last day of PS-K injection. [a] $K = (\log C_1 - \log C_2)/(T_2 - T_1)$. C_1 is Indian ink concentration in blood at the time of T_1 and C_2 is that at the time of T_2.

TABLE 7. Effects of PS-K on Cutaneous Delayed Type Hypersensitivity in Guinea Pig

Sample	Dose (mg/kg × days)	Skin reaction to antigen in mm² at 24 hr after challenge	
		Egg albumin	Saline
PS-K	1,000 × 6 p.o.	207.0 ± 37.8[a]	0
Control	1.0 ml × 6	212.7 ± 85.6	0

A solution of 3 g of the egg albumin dissolved in 0.25 ml of physiological saline was emulsified with an equal volume of Freund's adjuvant without mycobacteria and 0.5 ml of this emulsion was distributed to the 4 foot pads of the guinea pigs. In one group, 1,000 mg/kg of PS-K was given p.o. for 6 days from the day after sensitization. In another control group, only the saline solution was injected. [a] Values are means ± SE.

Ohno, Yamada, and their associates reported that antibody formation against sheep red blood cells (SRBC) measured by hemolytic plaque formation method increased significantly by PS-K administration when 2.1 ml of 0.5% SRBC suspension was injected (*28*). From the present studies, it can be seen that PS-K stimulates either non-specific or specific immune responses but immunological behaviors are probably the same as in lentinan.

Prevention of Side Effects of Antitumor Agents by PS-K

1) When PS-K was administered orally in a daily dose of 1,000 mg/kg together with or without intraperitoneal daily injection of cyclophosphamide (Endoxan, 25 mg/kg), decreases of peripheral leukocyte counts of ICR-JCL mice (10 mice/ group), and body weight due to cyclophosphamide were fairly prevented by PS-K administration. The results were shown in Figs. 1 and 2.

In another similar experiment, oral administration of PS-K prevented the decrease of humoral antibody production caused by intraperitoneal injection of cyclophosphamide (*29*).

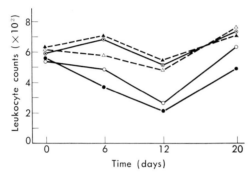

FIG. 1.   Change of average leukocyte counts of mice treated with Endoxan and/or PS-K. Animals: ICR-JCL mice. ⊙ PS-K 1,000 mg/kg p.o.; ○ PS-K+Endoxan 25 mg/kg i.p.; ● Endoxan; △ control; ▲ normal.

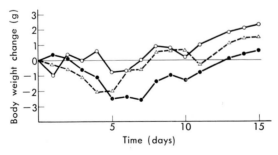

FIG. 2.   Effect of PS-K on the body weight of mice given Endoxan. Animals: ICR-JCL mice. ○ PS-K+Endoxan 25 mg/kg i.p.; ● Endoxan 25 mg/kg i.p.; △ control.

2) When PS-K was given orally in daily doses of 500–1,000 mg/kg to Donryu rats inoculated intraperitoneally with DBLA-6 rat leukemia, which is a sensitive tumor strain against vincristine, time of toxic death caused by intravenous injection of vincristine 0.5 mg/kg for 3 times were prolonged as shown in Fig. 3.

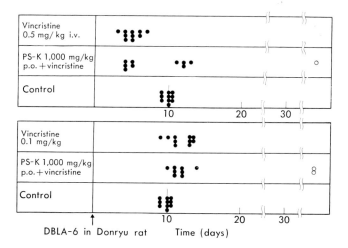

Fig. 3. Effect of PS-K on the life span of rats inoculated with DBLA-6 cells and treated i.v. with vincristine. DBLA-6 rat leukemia (10^6 cells/rat) was inoculated intraperitoneally to Donryu rats (10 rats/group) and from the day after inoculation vincristine (0.1 or 0.5 mg/kg) was injected every other day for 3–10 times i.v. with or without p.o. daily administration of PS-K (1,000 mg/kg). Rats which received i.v. vincristine alone (0.5 mg/kg/day for 3 times) died before day 10 due to the toxicity of vincristine. ● death of individual rat; ○ long survivor.

Clinical Trials of PS-K

PS-K has been given orally to various cancer patients with or without other treatments and the therapeutic responses are under investigation. Following are two examples of such cases reported by Drs. Itoh and Kondo.

1) A 63-year-old woman with esophagus cancer received radical operation in March, 1971 and was found to have vertebral metastasis in October, 1971. During these 7 months, cyclophosphamide was administered orally, resulting in the appearance of severe alopecia. Since October, 1971, PS-K 3 g/day have been given orally up to present, totaling in more than 1,800 g. Severe rachialgia and paresthesia of the lower extremities disappeared gradually, and the patient is now enjoying her normal life (by Dr. I. Ito, National Cancer Center Hospital, Tokyo).

2) A woman with breast cancer received radical mastectomy in August, 1961, and the bilateral ovaries and adrenals were extirpated. In May, 1972, lymph node metastasis in the right neck was found and daily oral administration of PS-K alone was started. Thirty days later, two remaining tumor nodules disappeared (by Dr. T. Kondo, Nagoya University).

Clinical effect of PS-K has been examined in various hospitals by immunological parameters. Kondo and his associates of Nagoya University reported that there was a good correlationship between the rate of blastogenesis of peripheral lymphocytes and the clinical responses after PS-K administration (31).

The reason why PS-K could prevent the side effects of antitumor drugs is not clear yet, but this phenomenon might be somewhat related to the immunopotentiating activity of PS-K or other biological activities of polysaccharides as have been shown by lentinan (*30*).

ACKNOWLEDGMENTS

This study was supported in part by a Grant-in-Aid for Scientific Research from both the Ministry of Education and Ministry of Health and Welfare, Japan.

This paper is dedicated to Prof. Yoshiaki Miura of Chiba University in celebration of his 60th birthday.

We are grateful to the staff of Research Laboratory of Kureha Chemical Industries, Ltd., Tokyo, for supplying us PS-K preparation.

REFERENCES

1. Nakahara, W., Fukuoka, F., Maeda, Y., and Aoki, K. The host-mediated antitumor effect of some plant polysaccharides. Gann, *55*: 283–288, 1964.
2. Tanaka, T., Fukuoka, F., and Nakahara, W. Mechanism of antitumor action of some plant polysaccharides. Gann, *56*: 529–536, 1965.
3. Nakahara, W., Tokuzen, R., Fukuoka, F., and Wistler, R. L. Inhibition of mouse sarcoma-180 by a wheat hemicellulose B preparation. Nature, *216*: 347–375, 1967.
4. Tanaka, T. Mechanism of antitumor action of polysaccharide fraction prepared from bagasse. II. Immunological reactivity of their sera. Gann, *58*: 451–457, 1967.
5. Suzuki, S., Saito, T., Uchiyama, M., and Akiya, S. Studies on the antitumor activity of polysaccharides. I. Isolation of hemicelluloses from Yakushima-bamboo and their growth inhibitory activities against sarcoma-180 solid tumor. Chem. Pharm. Bull. (Tokyo), *16*: 2032–2039, 1968.
6. Shibata, S., Nishikawa, Y., Cheng, F. M., Fukuoka, F., and Nakanishi, M. Antitumor studies of some extracts of *Basidiomycetes*. Gann, *59*: 159–161, 1968.
7. Ikekawa, T., Nakanishi, M., Uehara, N., Chihara, G., and Fukuoka, F. Antitumor action of some *Basidiomycetes*, especially *Phellinus linteus*. Gann, *59*: 155–157, 1968.
8. Chihara, G., Maeda, Y., Hamuro, J., Sasaki, T., and Fukuoka, F. Inhibition of mouse sarcoma-180 by polysaccharides from *Lentinus edodes* (BERK.) SING. Nature, *222*: 687–688, 1969.
9. Ikekawa, T., Uehara, N., Maeda, Y., Nakanishi, M., and Fukuoka, F. Antitumor activity of aqueous extracts of edible mushrooms. Cancer Res., *29*: 734–735, 1969.
10. Oka, S., Okamura, N., Kato, S., Sato, K., Tamari, K., Matsuda, K., and Shida, M. Antitumor activity of some plant polysaccharides. I. Fractionation and antitumor activity of bagasse polysaccharide. Gann, *59*: 35–42, 1968.
11. Shibata, S., Nishikawa, Y., Tanaka, M., Fukuoka, F., and Nakanishi, M. Antitumour activities of lichen polysaccharides. Z. Krebsforsch., *71*: 102–104, 1968.
12. Bradner, W. J., Clarke, D. A., and Stock, C. C. Stimulation of host defense against experimental cancer. I. Zymosan and sarcoma-180 in mice. Cancer Res., *18*: 347–351, 1958.
13. Bradner, W. J. and Clarke, D. A. Stimulation of host defense against experimental cancer. II. Temporal and reversal studies of zymosan effect. Cancer Res., *19*: 673–678, 1959.
14. Oka, S., Kumano, N., Sato, K., Tamari, K., Matsuda, K., Hirai, H., Oguma, T.,

Ogawa, K., Kiyooka, S., and Miyao, K. Antitumor activity of some plant polysaccharides. II. Chemical constituents and antitumor activity of yeast polysaccharide. Gann, *60*: 287–293, 1969.

15. Mizuno, D., Yoshioka, O., Akamatsu, M., and Kataoka, T. Antitumor effect of intracutaneous injection of bacterial lipopolysaccharide. Cancer Res., *28*: 1531–1537, 1968.

16. Tsukagoshi, S., Sakurai, Y., Otsuka, S., Ueno, S., Yoshikumi, C., and Fujii, T. Antitumor activity of protein-bound polysaccharide, PS-K, isolated from *Basidiomycetes*. Proc. 8th Int. Congr. Chemother., 1974.

17. Tsukagoshi, S. and Ohashi, F. Protein-bound polysaccharide preparation, PS-K, effective against mouse sarcoma-180 and rat ascites hepatoma AH-13 by oral use. Gann, *65*: 557–558, 1974.

18. Chihara, G., Hamuro, J., Maeda, Y. Y., Arai, Y., and Fukuoka, F. Fraction and purification of the polysaccharides with marked antitumor activity, especially lentinan, from *Lentinan edodes* (BERK.) SING. (an edible mushroom). Cancer Res., *30*: 2776–2781, 1970.

19. Maeda, Y. Y. and Chihara, G. The effect of neonatal thymectomy on the antitumor activity of lentinan, carboxymethylpachymaran and zymosan, and their effects on various immune responses. Int. J. Cancer, *11*: 153–161, 1973.

20. Maeda, Y. Y. and Chihara, G. Lentinan, a new immunoaccelerator of cell-mediated responses. Nature, *229*: 634, 1971.

21. Maeda, Y. Y., Hamuro, J., and Chihara, G. The mechanisms of antitumor polysaccharides. I. The effect of antilymphocyte serum on the antitumor activity of lentinan. Int. J. Cancer, *8*: 41–46, 1971.

22. Hirase, S., Otsuka, S., Uneno, S., Yoshikumi, C., Ohara, M., Hirose, F., Fujii, T., Omura, Y., Wada, T., Matsunaga, K., Aoki, T., and Furusho, T. Study on chemical nature of the antitumor polysaccharide fractions isolated from *Basidiomycetes* (9). Abstr. Papers, Pharm. Soc. Japan, *IV*: 5, 1974 (in Japanese).

23. Mathé, G. Attempt at using systemic immunity adjuvants in experimental and human cancer therapy. *In;* G.E.W. Wolstenholme and J. Knight (eds.), Immunopotentiation (Ciba Foundation Symposium), vol. 18, pp. 305–330, Elsevier/Excerpta Medica/North-Holland, Amsterdam/London/New York, 1973.

24. Nakano, Y., Taguchi, T., Shiba, S., and Arakawa, Y. Influence of protein polysaccharide (PS-K) isolated from *Basidiomycetes* on delayed hypersensitivity in sarcoma-180 bearing mice. Proc. Japan Cancer Assoc. 32nd Annu. Meet., 282, 1973.

25. Gray, J. G., Monaco, A. P., Wood, M. L., and Russell, P. S. J. Immunol., *96*: 217, 1966.

26. Biozzi, G., Benacerraf, B., and Halpern, B. N. Quantitative study of the granulopectic activity of the reticulo-endothelial system. II: A study of the kinetics of the granulopectic activity of the RES in relation to the dose of carbon injected. Relationship between the weight of the organs and their activity. Brit. J. Exp. Pathol., *34*: 441–457, 1953.

27. Uhr, J. W., Salvin, S. B., and Pappenheirer, A. M., Jr. Delayed hypersensitivity. II. Induction of hypersensitivity in guinea pigs by means of antigen-antibody complexes. J. Exp. Med., *105*: 11–24, 1957.

28. Ohno, R., Imai, K., Yokomaku, S., Nagata, K., Sugiura, S., Yamada, K., and Hirabayashi, N. The effect of PS-K on mice lymphoid tissue. Proc. Japan Cancer Assoc., *33*: 149, 1974.

29. Tsukagoshi, S. Host-mediated antitumor activity of polysaccharides, with special reference to the effect of PS-K, Cancer Chemother., *1*: 97–103, 1974.
30. Maeda, Y. Y., Hamuro, J., Yamada, Y., Ishimura, K., and Chihara, G. The nature of immunopotentiation by the antitumor polysaccharide lentinan and the significance of biogenic amines in its action. *In;* G.E.W. Wolstenholme and J. Knight (eds.), Immunopotentiation (Ciba Foundation Symposium), vol. 18, pp. 259–286, Elsevier/Excerpta Medica/North Holland, Amsterdam/London/New York, 1973.
31. Kondo, T., Kamei,H., Momoi, T., and Sugimoto, K. Activation of non-specific immunological resistance against malignant tumor. Cancer Chemother., *5*: 81–89, 1974.

Discussion of Paper of Dr. Tsukagoshi

DR. KENNEDY: In the clinical case report you presented of a 63-year-old woman being treated with PS-K following radical surgery for an esophageal carcinoma, there appeared to be increased osteolytic areas in the vertebrae in the face of continued subjective improvement.

DR. I. ITOH (National Cancer Center Hospital, Tokyo):   Yes. Areas of her vertebral column have gradually been destroyed over the past 4 years, but the patient remains comfortable.

DR. NOMOTO: PS-K shares certain properties with lentinan, in that it completely restores the suppressed helper cell function of mice bearing sarcoma-180, while it has minimal effect on such function in normal animals.

DR. H. OKADA: In the investigation of the possible clinical efficacy of combined immunopotentiation and chemotherapeutic regimenes, it is important to determine the appropriate timing of the administration of these two therapies. For, an immunopotentiator often leads to lymphocyte proliferation, a stage at which these cells would be especially susceptible to the toxic effects of chemotherapeutic drugs.

DR. TSUKAGOSHI: I completely agree with your analysis.

HOST DEFENSE AGAINST CANCER AND ITS POTENTIATION, D. MIZUNO ET AL. (EDS.),
UNIV. OF TOKYO PRESS, TOKYO / UNIV. PARK PRESS, BALTIMORE, PP. 379–388, 1975

Antitumor Antibiotics Carrying Immunopotentiating Capacity

Tadashi YAMAMOTO

Institute of Medical Science, University of Tokyo, Tokyo, Japan

Abstract: Rather an ectobiological approach designed for screening antitumor
antibiotics by means of possible normalization of the increased sugar transport in
cell membranes of Rous sarcoma virus-infected and -transformed chick embryo
cells resulted in probably by chance to have picked up an antitumor antibiotic
which carried some immunopotentiating capacity. Secalonic acid D obtained from
culture filtrates of *Penicillium oxalicum* was an active principle. Tetrahydropyranylization of alcoholic OH groups reduced the toxicity in mice 6–10 times, giving both
antitumor and immunopotentiating capacities. Since the pyranyl secalonic acid was
provided with the inflammation-inducing capacity, possible immunotherapeutic
experiments similar to BCG treatment were undertaken. Ascites sarcoma 180 at
the level of 10^6 tumor cells was mixed with 50 μg of pyranyl secalonic acid and
injected intradermally into $(DDD \times BALB/c)F_1$ mice. Three to 4 weeks later when
the local tumor regressed, 10^6 tumor cells of sarcoma 180 were challenge-injected.
All the mice thus-treated acquired the resistance to the challenge. In case of syngeneic tumor system such as ascites mastocytoma P815 in CDF_1 mice such a protecting effect could not be observed, but in the case of Rous sarcoma virus Schmidt-
Ruppin strain D-induced C57BL/6 mouse ascites sarcoma in BDF_1 mice, almost
all the mice pretreated survived the challenge-injection. A possible new way of
hunting such immunotherapeutic antitumor antibiotics was discussed.

It has been often claimed that most of the effective cancer chemotherapeutics
including antitumor antibiotics have indelible side effects of immunosuppression.
At the opening remarks of this symposium Dr. Mizuno also referred to this point
expressing as the modern cancer chemotherapy somehow facing a deadrock. We
had considered it rather natural consequence of the intended screening for anti-
mitotica such as radiomimetica which could affect not only the vigorously dividing
tumor cells but also the normal cell division partly included in the host defence
against cancer. Another approach, focussed on the possible normalization of the

characteristic increase in sugar transport of sarcoma virus-transformed cell membranes (1), made us pick up an antitumor antibiotic from *Penicillium oxalicum* which was later confirmed as secalonic acid D. It was probably by chance that this secalonic acid D had some immunopotentiating capacity as well as inflammation-inducing activity. Upon this we have attempted an immunochemotherapeutic use of this low molecular substance, particularly of its chemically modified derivative, pyranyl secalonic acid, with which the present paper will mainly be concerned.

Secalonic Acid D and Pyranyl Secalonic Acid

Hatanaka and Hanafusa (2) clearly demonstrated that the increased sugar transport in cell membranes was sequentially associated with the process of cell transformation of chick embryo cells after infection with Schmidt-Ruppin strain of Rous sarcoma virus subgroup D (SR-RSV-D). Kawai and Hanafusa (3) confirmed the parallel relationship between sugar transport and transformed morphology by the use of their temperature-sensitive mutant, TS-68, isolated from Schmidt-Ruppin strain of Rous sarcoma virus subgroup A (SR-RSV-A). With an aim of possible normalization of this increased ^{14}C-glucose transport in chick embryo cells transformed by SR-RSV-A (4) we made screening of 2,000 samples of microbial culture filtrates and a light yellow crystalline product of *P. oxalicum* was obtained as an active principle. It was later confirmed as secalonic acid D, at first reported by Steyn as a mycotoxin in Africa (5). As shown in Fig. 1 on its chemical structure, this substance belongs to a group of ergot pigments, ergochromes, which are produced in the sclerotia of the fungus *Claviceps purpurea* when grown on rye (6). Secalonic acid D, which we have isolated from *P. oxalicum*, showed an anti-bacterial activity against *Bacillus subtilis* at the level of 1 μg/ml in concentration. To test the mode of action of this crystalline secalonic acid D, an SR-RSV-D-induced virus-non-producing mouse sarcoma cell line, SR-C3H 2127 (7, 8), previously ascertained its increased sugar transport of cell membranes probably as a direct expression of the existing whole genome of Rous sarcoma virus in the cell (9), was treated with 10 μg/ml of the substance for 2 hr at 37°C and the sequential analysis of the incorporation of ^{14}C-glucose into cells and ^{14}C-leucine, ^{14}C-uridine, and ^{14}C-thymidine

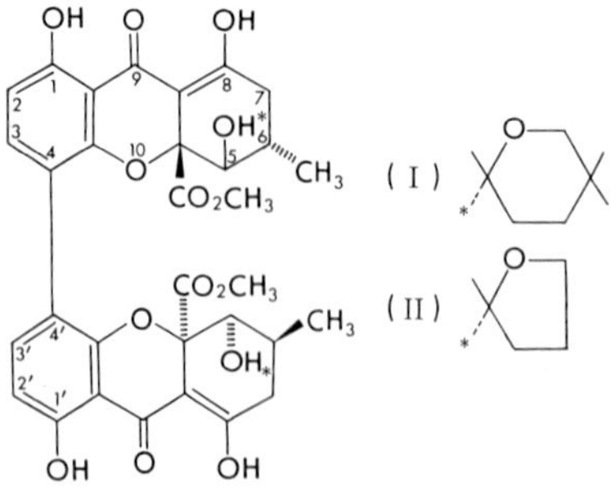

FIG. 1. Chemical structure of secalonic acid D and its tetrahydropyranyl (I) and tetrahydrofuranyl (II) derivatives.

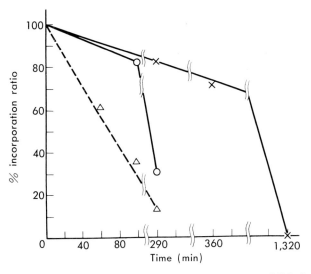

FIG. 2.   Effects of secalonic acid D on incorporation of ¹⁴C-glucose into SR-C3H-2127 cells and of ¹⁴C-uridine and ¹⁴C-leucine into TCA-insolubles. Each 10 μg/ml of secalonic acid D was added at 0 time. The petri dishes were incubated at 37°C for several minutes and washed at indicated points. Pulse labellings of ¹⁴C-glucose were for 10 min and those of ¹⁴C-uridine and ¹⁴C-leucine for 60 min.   × ¹⁴C-glucose; △ ¹⁴C-uridine; ○ ¹⁴C-leucine.

into trichloroacetic acid (TCA)-insolubles was undertaken. In order of time the incorporation of ¹⁴C-uridine was first affected and then of ¹⁴C-leucine followed by that of ¹⁴C-glucose as shown in Fig. 2. Incorporation of ¹⁴C-thymidine was not at all affected during the first 2 hours' observation period. The reason why the increased sugar transport in this cell line was not markedly affected is not clear. Nevertheless the secalonic acid D inhibited or retarded the tumor growth of several strains of mouse transplantable tumors in *in vivo* tests. Due to the different toxicity in different mouse strains, however, we had to undertake the chemical modification

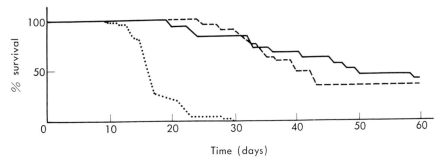

FIG. 3.   Treatment of Ehrlich ascites carcinoma with pyranyl secalonic acid as compared with mitomycin C. —— pyranyl secalonic acid dissolved in olive oil, 8 mg/kg/day intraperitoneally (i.p.) on day 1 and 3. - - - mitomycin C, 1 mg/kg/day i.p. on day 1, 2, 3, 4, and 5. ··· control, 2×10⁶ cells of Ehrlich ascites carcinoma inoculated i.p. on day 0.

of this secalonic acid D. Tetrahydropyranylization of the alcoholic OH-groups reduced the toxicity in mice 6 to 10 times; LD_{50} of this pyranyl secalonic acid was 300 to 500 mg/kg, though the solubility in water decreased. Antitumor activity was well reserved in *in vivo* test with Ehrlich ascites tumor. Intraperitoneal injections of 8 mg/kg of pyranyl secalonic acid dissolved in olive oil on day 1 and 3 gave very similar survival curve to those of 1 mg/kg of mitomycin C on day 1, 2, 3, 4, and 5 as shown in Fig. 3.

Immunochemotherapeutic Use of Pyranyl Secalonic Acid

One of the characteristics of pyranyl secalonic acid was its same immuno-potentiating capacity. When 10^8 sheep red blood cells (SRBC) were injected intra-peritoneally into mice together with 160 μg of pyranyl secalonic acid in olive oil, the number of plaque-forming cells (PFC) in mouse spleen increased 2 to 5 times more than that of control group mice injected with 10^8 SRBC, as shown in Fig. 4. It appeared necessary, however, that the pyranyl secalonic acid was injected into the same site of peritoneal cavity simultaneously with antigenic substances; when pyranyl secalonic acid was injected intraperitoneally and SRBC intravenously, such adjuvant activity of pyranyl secalonic acid could not be observed.

Another characteristic of pyranyl secalonic acid was its inflammation-inducing capacity. When the substance was suspended in 0.1% carboxymethylcellulose containing phosphate buffer saline and injected intradermally into an auricle of mice, the inflammation process could be observed quantitatively by measuring the thickness of the auricle with a Peacock type dial thickness gauge. Moreover, when

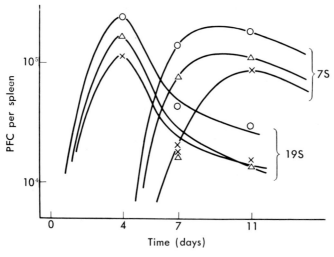

Fig. 4. Immunostimulation of pyranyl secalonic acid. 10^8 SRBC were injected i.p. into mice together with 160 μg pyranyl secalonic acid (SA) at day 0 and spleen PFC were counted. ○ 10^8 SRBC with 160 μg pyranyl SA in 0.2 ml olive oil; △ 10^8 SRBC with 0.2 ml olive oil; × 10^8 SRBC.

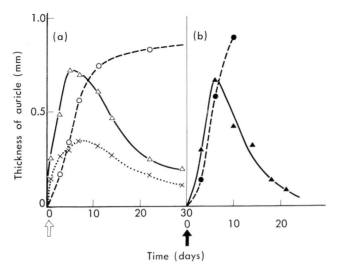

Fig. 5. Changes in thickness of mouse auricles after local injections of tumor cells with or without pyranyl secalonic acid (a) and after rechallenge injections of tumor cells at another auricles into the mice pretreated with tumor cells and pyranyl secalonic acid (b). (a) Left auricle : ○ tumor cells alone ; △ tumor cells with pyranyl SA ; × pyranyl SA alone. (b) Right auricle : ● control ; ▲ pretreated mice. ⇧ sarcoma 180 10⁶ cells with or without pyranyl SA 50 μg ; ⬆ sarcoma 180 10⁶ cells.

50 μg of pyranyl secalonic acid were mixed with 10^6 cells of Crocker sarcoma 180 and injected into the left auricle, we could find out the subsequent suppression of tumor growth, as shown in Fig. 5. And of more interest when the thus-treated mice were challenge-injected with 10^6 cells of the sarcoma 180 intradermally into the right auricle about 3 to 4 weeks after the first treatment, the tumor in the right auricle did not grow well and regressed completely, suggesting that the mice were systemically immunized by the previous treatment.

With the use of several kinds of mouse ascites tumors, the possible immuno-chemotherapeutic use of pyranyl secalonic acid was explored. The procedures employed were those in the suppression studies with living BCG by Zbar et al. (10): the primary intradermal injection of the mixture of pyranyl secalonic acid and tumor cells into the right leg and the secondary intradermal challenge injection of the tumor cells into the left leg at the interval of 3–4 weeks. Results obtained are summarized in Table 1. In case of non-specific tumors such as sarcoma 180 ascites and/or Ehrlich ascites carcinoma in $DDD \times BALB/c$ F_1 mice the most favorable results were obtained. Almost all of the treated mice survived the challenge injection of the same tumor. Cross resistance, however, was not well inducible between the two ascites tumors. In case of specific tumors, no such protecting effects were inducible in case of ascites plasmocytoma P815 in CDF_1 mice, but some protecting effects were observed in case of SR-RSV-induced CDF_1 mouse ascites glioma in CDF_1 mice. The tumor cells were previously confirmed to carry the virus-induced tumor specific transplantation antigen (TSTA) (11). Rather promising effects were obtained in case of SR-RSV-induced C57BL/6

TABLE 1. Intradermal (i.d.) Inoculations of Several Kinds of Tumor Cells Mixed with Pyranyl Secalonic Acid and Their Protecting Effects to Subsequent Tumor Cell Challenge

Mixture inoculated i.d.		No. of tumor-free mice / No. of mice inoculated	Challenge	No. of tumor-free mice/ No. of mice inoculated
Tumor cells	Pyranyl SA			
(I) (DDD×BALB/c)F$_1$ mice				
Sarcoma 180 10^6 cells	50 μg	26/26	Sarcoma 180 10^6 cells	21/21
Sarcoma 180 10^6 cells	—	0/21	—	—
—	—	—	Sarcoma 180 10^6 cells	0/18
Sarcoma 180 10^6 cells	50 μg	7/7	Ehrlich ca. 10^6 cells	2/7
Ehrlich ca. 10^6 cells	50 μg	24/24	Ehrlich ca. 10^6 cells	16/18
Ehrlich ca. 10^6 cells	—	2/18	—	—
—	—	—	Ehrlich ca. 10^6 cells	1/18
Ehrlich ca. 10^6 cells	50 μg	5/5	Sarcoma 180 10^6 cells	2/5
(II) CDF$_1$ mice				
Mastocytoma P815 2×10^6 cells	100 μg	0/5	—	—
Mastocytoma P815 2×10^6 cells	50 μg	0/5	—	—
Mastocytoma P815 2×10^6 cells	—	0/5	—	—
Mastocytoma P815 2×10^5 cells	100 μg	4/5	Mastocytoma P815 2×10^4 cells	0/4
Mastocytoma P815 2×10^5 cells	50 μg	4/5	Mastocytoma P815 2×10^4 cells	0/4
Mastocytoma P815 2×10^5 cells	—	0/3	—	—
Mastocytoma P815 2×10^4 cells	50 μg	16/16	Mastocytoma P815 2×10^4 cells	0/7
Mastocytoma P815 2×10^4 cells	—	0/7	—	—
—	—	—	Mastocytoma P815 2×10^4 cells	0/9
(III) BDF$_1$ mice				
SR-C57BL/6 2008B ascites sarcoma 10^6 cells	50 μg	38/40	SR-C57BL/6 2008B 5×10^4 cells	13/17
			SR-C57BL/6 2008B 2×10^5 cells	2/15
SR-C57BL/6 2008B 10^6 cells	—	0/14	—	—
—	—	—	SR-C57BL/6 2008B 5×10^4 cells	1/11
			SR-C57BL/6 2008B 2×10^5 cells	0/10

mouse ascites sarcoma, SR-C57BL/6 ascites sarcoma 2008B strain (12), in BDF_1 mice. Almost all of the pretreated mice resisted to the challenge injection of the specific tumor cells.

DISCUSSION

Our work probably indicates the possible existence of low molecular antitumor antibiotics which also carry some immunopotentiating capacities. Diketocoriolin B, an oxidated derivative of coriolin B, a sesquiterpene compound, at first isolated from *Coriolus consors* by Umezawa and his associates (13), is one of the very few antitumor antibiotics carrying an immunopotentiating capacity (14). It is of interest that diketocoriolin B has a potent inhibitory action of Na-K-ATPase activity of tumor cell membranes resulting in the cessation of tumor cell growth (15). We have examined the inflammation-inducing activity of diketocoriolin B as compared with pyranyl secalonic acid but no remarkable activity was observable in the auricle test. Nevertheless it was recently informed us that when the mixture of 20 μg of diketocoriolin B and 10^7 L1210 leukemia cells was injected intradermally into CDF_1 mice, some mice survived the subsequent intradermal challenge injection of 10^3 leukemia cells. There may exist so many different points of attack in immunopotentiation, either specific or non-specific, particularly in relation to the modern concept of A-, B-, and T-cell interaction, that we could expect more active antitumor antibiotics carrying immunopotentiating capacities. The procedures we have employed may be used in screening such new antibiotics.

REFERENCES

1. Hatanaka, M. Transport of sugars in tumor cell membranes. Biochim. Biophys. Acta, *355*: 77–104, 1974.
2. Hatanaka, M. and Hanafusa, H. Analysis of a functional change in membrane in the process of cell transformation by Rous sarcoma virus: Alteration in the characteristics of sugar transport. Virology, *41*: 647–652, 1970.
3. Kawai, S. and Hanafusa, H. The effects of reciprocal changes in temperature on the transformed state of cells infected with a Rous sarcoma virus mutant. Virology, *46*: 470–479, 1971.
4. Kawai, S. and Yamamoto, T. Isolation of different kinds of non-virus producing chick cells transformed by Schmidt-Ruppin strain (subgroup A) of Rous sarcoma virus. Japan. J. Exp. Med., *40*: 243–256, 1970.
5. Steyn, P. S. The isolation, structure and absolute configuration of secalonic acid D: The toxic metabolite of *Penicillium oxalicum*. Tetrahedron, *26*: 51–57, 1970.
6. Franck, B. Structure and biosynthesis of the ergot pigments. Angew. Chem. Int. Edit., *8*: 251–260, 1970.
7. Yamaguchi, N., Takeuchi, M., and Yamamoto, T. Rous sarcoma virus production in mixed cultures of mammalian Rous sarcoma cells and chick embryo cells. Int. J. Cancer, *4*: 678–689, 1969.
8. Yamamoto, T. and Takeuchi, M. Studies on Rous sarcoma virus in mice. I. Establishment of an ascites sarcoma induced by Schmidt-Ruppin strain of Rous sarcoma virus in C3H/He mouse. Japan. J. Exp. Med., *37*: 35–50, 1967.

9. Hino, S. and Yamamoto, T. Expression of the sarcoma genome in a Rous mouse tumor cell line, SR-C3H-2127. Gann, *62*: 539–544, 1971.

10. Zbar, B., Bernstein, I., Tanaka, T., and Rapp, H. J. Tumor immunity produced by the intradermal inoculation of living tumor cells and living *Mycobacterium bovis* (strain BCG). Science, *170*: 1217–1218, 1970.

11. Kumanishi, T. and Yamamoto, T. Brain tumors induced by Rous sarcoma virus Schmidt-Ruppin strain. II. Brain tumor specific transplantation antigen in subcutaneously passaged mouse brain tumors. Japan. J. Exp. Med., *40*: 79–86, 1970.

12. Takeuchi, M., Hino, S., and Yamamoto, T. Studies on Rous sarcoma virus in mice. III. Three strains of SR-RSV-induced mouse ascites sarcomas. Japan. J. Exp. Med., *39*: 239–251, 1969.

13. Takeuchi, T., Takahashi, S., Inuma, H., and Umezawa, H. Diketocoriolin B, an active derivative of coriolin B produced by *Coriolus consors*. J. Antibiot., *24*: 631–635, 1971.

14. Ishizuka, M., Inuma, H., Takeuchi, T., and Umezawa, H. Effect of diketocoriolin B on antibody formation. J. Antibiot., *25*: 320–321 1972.

15. Kunimoto, T. and Umezawa, H. Mechanism of action of diketocoriolin B. Biochim. Biophys. Acta, *298*: 513–525, 1973.

Discussion of Paper of Dr. Yamamoto

DR. MIZUNO: In screening for potential cancer chemotherapeutic agents, it is important to be able to differentiate the mitotic poison from the immunopotentiator. We have developed an assay method to accomplish this, involving the comparison of the anti-tumor effect of a substance with its ability to evoke a delayed hypersensitivity reaction in the mouse foot pad. In this regard, such agents appear to fall into two categories; mitotic poisons which have high anti-tumor capacities with little ability to induce a delayed hypersensitivity reaction (DHR), such as mitomycin C; and the immunopotentiators, which are able to induce both tumor regression and a DHR.

DR. YAMAMOTO: Could we directly test substances in this scheme by an intradermal injection of a mixture of tumor cells and the agent, followed by intradermal or subcutaneous injection of the same tumor cells 2–3 weeks later?

DR. MIZUNO: I agree it's possible.

DR. ALEXANDER: Have you determined the mechanism of action of secalonic acid on nucleic acid metabolism? Also, is its action on sugar transport direct or a consequence of the inhibition of RNA synthesis and intracellular damage it produces?

DR. YAMAMOTO: The crude *P. oxalicum* product first isolated did have an inhibitory effect on glucose transport by RSV-transformed chick embryo cells. However, crystallization at this material to yield secalonic acid D abolished this effect. From the data shown in Fig. 2, I have inevitably to consider the sequence of the inhibition obtained with this secalonic acid D in RSV-induced mammalian tumor cells which do not produce viruses might be mRNA synthesis, then protein synthesis, and finally glucose transport.

   We have not examined further the mode of action of secalonic acid on the inhibition of RNA synthesis.

DR. M. HOZUMI: Have you examined the effect of secalonic acid on tumor cells *in vitro*? I would be especially interested to know it could restore contact inhibition to such cells.

DR. YAMAMOTO: *In vitro*, we have only recognized the effects of secalonic acid on RNA and protein synthesis and glucose transport. *In vivo*, its most important function seems to be the establishment of inflammatory loci where the accumulation of lymphocytes and macrophages in large numbers facilitates contact with tumor cells.

DR. HALPERN: Have you determined whether the decreased glucose transport you observed is due to a suppression of glucosyl transferase activity or a blocking of the glucose cell surface receptor? This differentiation can be made by employing an artificial receptor molecule such as ovomucoid.

DR. YAMAMOTO: No, but Dr. Eckhart of the Salk Institute reported that increased sugar transport in cell membranes was also associated with polyoma virus-induced cell transformation, and here a phosphorylization process was apparently not involved as 3-O-methylglucose could be transported into the cells.

HOST DEFENSE AGAINST CANCER AND ITS POTENTIATION, D. MIZUNO ET AL. (EDS.),
UNIV. OF TOKYO PRESS, TOKYO / UNIV. PARK PRESS, BALTIMORE, PP. 389-396, 1975

Approaches to the Immunotherapy of Experimental Tumors[*1]

George S. TARNOWSKI

Memorial Sloan-Kettering Cancer Center, New York, N.Y., U.S.A.

Abstract: Effects of biological products and synthetic chemicals on the induction
of complete regression of tumors or prevention of their growth has been examined
in sarcoma-180 (S-180) and Meth A mouse sarcomas, allogeneic and syngeneic
tumor-host systems, respectively. These tests are a part of a much broader program
designed to investigate various approaches to immunotherapy of tumors and to
combination therapy involving the use of materials capable of stimulation of host
defense against tumors.

Regression of Meth A and S-180 has been observed after administration of
Corynebacterium parvum vaccines, mixed bacterial vaccines and bacterial lipopolysaccharides; effects of BCG were less pronounced and varied from test to test. BCG
prolonged survival time of mice bearing the ascites form of Meth A.

Plant polysaccharides lentinan and zymosan have caused regression of S-180
in either CD-1 or C3H/He mice but did not induce rejection of Meth A. Regression of S-180 was observed even when therapy with polysaccharides had started
when tumors were 6–18 days old. Combined treatment of S-180 with zymosan and
a number of biologically active amines and their antagonists did not result in a
clear-cut potentiation or blocking of the tumor regression-inducing capacity of
polysaccharides.

Among the small molecular synthetic chemicals tilorone dihydrochloride and
related compounds induced regression of S-180 after oral or intraperitoneal administration; no effects were observed against Meth A.

For several years study of the stimulation of host defense mechanisms against
experimental tumors has been a part of a larger program seeking effective immunomodulators.[*2] Two transplanted tumor-host systems—the allogeneic system of

---

[*1] This work is supported in part by NCI Grant CA-08748.

[*2] The broader aspects of this program are presented by C. C. Stock in the discussion of this paper.

sarcoma-180 (S-180)* growing in the ICR/Ha-derived CD-1 female mice and the syngeneic system of Meth A fibrosarcoma—served as the main test systems in which all the materials were examined for their ability to act as immunomodulating agents capable of stimulation of the host defense against tumors. Meth A, which was induced in a BALB/c mouse (2), is carried as an ascites tumor in these mice and used for tests in the (BALB/cJ × C57BL/6J)F$_1$ female mice, subsequently designated as the CB6 mice.

The test materials examined have included: intact bacterial cells in the form of attenuated or killed vaccines, bacterial lipopolysaccharides, plant polysaccharides, tilorone and related dibenzfurans, fluorenes and xanthenes, some thiazoles and other miscellaneous chemicals, and biological products. Many of these have been tested to provide base line information for the systems as we have employed them. Variables, such as dose-response relationships, dose schedules, and routes of administration have been examined for a number of the agents. For the effective immunostimulants the nature of the action will be determined if not already known, and they will be used in combination therapy with chemotherapeutic agents.

Several categories of biological products and synthetic chemicals have been examined by previous investigators for their ability to retard growth of tumors or to cause their regression by indirect action involving stimulation of host defenses against tumors. Early studies on zymosan reported effectiveness in causing regression of S-180 in mice (3) and were followed by Diller (4) and Sakai (5). Other investigators have shown the value of BCG (6, 7). Numerous studies with Coley's toxin or mixed bacterial vaccines had their origin in the early observations of Coley (reviewed by Nauts (8)) as will be reported in this Symposium (9). More recently, suspensions of killed *Corynebacterium parvum* were found to be potent stimulants of the host defense against a variety of animal tumors (10, 11).

The following examples of the results obtained with these and other groups of chemicals and biological products in our studies in S-180 and Meth A illustrate this approach to immunotherapy of tumors.

Intact Bacterial Cells

BCG vaccines from three different sources were administered in single intravenous (i.v.) doses 7 days prior to the intradermal (i.d.) inoculation of 7.5×10^5 viable cells of Meth A. Response of treated tumors, expressed as the frequency of complete tumor regression observed on day 28 of tumor growth was small and did not show dose dependence (Table 1). Large variability of response between tests has been observed: 2×10^7 BCG cells (Chicago) have caused 4 of 11 regressions in one test, 1 of 10 in another, and none in the other 3 tests.

When Chedid *et al.* (12) administered BCG or other mycobacterial preparations intraperitoneally (i.p.) 14 days before inoculation of Ehrlich ascites i.p., a

---

* The line of S-180 used in this study has been kindly supplied by Dr. G. Chihara of the National Cancer Center Research Institute, Tokyo. It was selected because of the reported absence of spontaneous regression in the ICR-derived JCL line of mice (1).

TABLE 1.   Effect of BCG Vaccines on Meth A Fibrosarcoma[a]

BCG dose[b] (cells/ mouse)	Source of BCG vaccine					
	Chicago		Pasteur		Phipps	
	No. of tests	R[c]	No. of tests	R	No. of tests	R
0	9	0/74	2	0/22	2	0/22
1×10^6	4	0/28	1	0/10	1	4/10
1×10^7	2	1/22	2	2/22	2	1/22
2×10^7	9	5/74	2	0/22	2	1/17

[a] Tumor load: 7.5×10^5 cells, i.d. on day 0.   [b] Single i.v. dose on day -7.   [c] Tumor regression frequency observed on day 28.

TABLE 2.   Effect of BCG Vaccines on the Ascites Form of Meth A[a]

BCG source	BCG dose[b] (cells/mouse)	Male mice		Female mice	
		MST[c] (days)	Tumor-free mice on day 56	MST (days)	Tumor-free mice on day 56
	0	16	0/8	21	0/8
Chicago	1×10^4	15	0/8	>56	5/8
	1×10^5	28	1/8	>56	7/8
	1×10^6	28	2/8	>56	8/8
	1×10^7	25	1/8	46	3/8
Connaught	1×10^4	17	1/8	27	4/8
	1×10^5	17	1/8	>56	7/8
	1×10^6	32	3/8	>56	5/8
	1×10^7	31	2/8	45	3/8

[a] Tumor load: in males 2×10^5 cells, i.p.; in females 1×10^5 cells, i.p.   [b] Single i.p. dose on day -14.   [c] MST: median survival time.

substantial prolongation of the survival time of hosts has been achieved. In the ascitic form of Meth A a similar pretreatment with as little as 1×10^4 BCG cells from two different sources induced a marked increase of the survival time of treated hosts bearing tumors derived from inocula of 1×10^6 cells; at the low dose levels of BCG the effect was more pronounced in the females than in the male hosts (Table 2).

Suspensions of killed *C. parvum* (Burroughs Wellcome Co.) produced regression of Meth A following an i.d. administration of vaccine at the time of tumor inoculation or one day thereafter; other time schedules proved to be ineffective. On the other hand, regression of S-180 could be induced by administration of *C. parvum* from 3 days prior to 3 days following tumor inoculation (Table 3). Intraperitoneal, but not the intravenous, administration of *C. parvum* also caused regression of some Meth A solid tumor. Preliminary tests of the effect of combination therapy of Meth A with bleomycin and single i.d. doses of *C. parvum* administered at the beginning of therapy with bleomycin or 7 days later are sufficiently encouraging (Table 4) to justify further concentration on this line of investigation, and its exten-

TABLE 3. Effect of the Timing of Therapy[a] of Mouse Sarcomas with *C. Parvum* on Regression Frequency[b]

Therapy on day	Meth A		S-180	
	Control	Treated	Control	Treated
−7	0/12	0/12	0/6	0/6
−3	0/12	1/12	0/6	2/6
−1	0/12	0/12	0/6	3/6
0	0/12	5/12	1/6	5/6
1	0/12	2/12	0/6	3/6
3	0/12	0/12	0/6	3/6
7	0/12	0/12	0/6	1/6

[a] Tumor load: 7.5×10^5 cells, i.d. on day 0. *C. parvum*: single i.d. dose of 210 μg/mouse. [b] R on day 42.

TABLE 4. Combination Therapy of Meth A[a] with Bleomycin and *C. parvum*

Therapy	Day 14		Day 28		
	Mice with tumors (N)	Aver. weight change[b] (g)	Survivors	Tumor regression (R)	R/N (%)
Saline, pyrogen-free	12	+2.3	11	0	0
Bleomycin[c]	12	−0.4	12	1	8
C. parvum,[d] day −7	12	+3.3	11	0	0
C. parvum, day 0	12	+2.8	11	0	0
C. parvum, day 7	12	+3.7	12	0	0
Bleomycin+*C. parvum*, day −7	12	−1.1	12	1	8
Bleomycin+*C. parvum*, day 0	12	−0.6	11	7	58
Bleomycin+*C. parvum*, day 7	12	−0.4	12	4	33

[a] Tumor load: 7.5×10^5 cells i.d., on day 0. [b] Day 14 − day 0. [c] Bleomycin: 5 mg/kg/day, i.p., qd (qustidie: every day), $10 \times$, from day 1. [d] *C. parvum*: 10 mg/kg/day, i.d., $1 \times$ as indicated.

TABLE 5. Regression of Meth A and S-180 Treated with MBV[a]

Tumor	Dilution of MBV	Day 7	Day 8			Final day of observation[c]		
		No. of tumor-bearing mice (N)	No. of dead mice	No. of tumor hemor-rhages	Aver. weight change[b] (g)	No. of		
						Survi-vors	Mice without tumor (R)	R/N (%)
Meth A	Saline	22	0	0	+0.5	21	0	0
	1 : 1,000	22	0	8	−1.4	22	5	23
	1 : 100	22	0	14	−1.9	22	6	27
	1 : 10	22	3	9	−1.2	15	6	27
S-180	Saline	6	0	0	0.0	6	0	0
	1 : 10,000	6	0	1	−1.7	6	0	0
	1 : 1,000	6	0	1	−1.8	6	0	0
	1 : 100	6	0	3	−3.1	6	3	50
	1 : 10	6	1	2	−2.6	5	2	33

[a] One i.v. dose on day 7, 0.5 ml volume. [b] Day 8 − day 7. [c] Day 28 for Meth A, day 42 for S-180.

sion to other combinations of chemotherapeutic agents and immunomodulators and to different tumor-host systems.

Mixed bacterial vaccine (MBV) (Coley's toxin (*8*)) is a mixture of a culture of *Streptococcus pyogenes* in its growth medium and of a suspension of *Serratia marcescens* cells in saline. When administered i.v. to mice bearing 7-day-old Meth A or S-180, MBV produced hemorrhagic necroses in a considerable proportion of treated tumors and caused one-third to one-half of tumors to regress completely. Regressions of Meth A occur in the course of 1–2 weeks after therapy and no further regressions are observed after 1 month. Treated S-180 tumors regress at a later time and over a longer period of time so that observation period is extended to 6 weeks when S-180 is tested in CD-1 mice (Table 5).

Lipopolysaccharides

Lipopolysaccharides, commercially prepared by the method of Westphal (*13*) from such gram-negative bacterial species as *Escherichia coli*, *Salmonella typhimurium*, *S. marcescens*, and *Shigella flexneri* have been tested in both Meth A and S-180 for their ability to produce regression in treated tumors (*14*). It is well known that these materials produce hemorrhagic necroses in tumors and shock in treated hosts which limits their usefulness for the treatment of human tumors. Dose-response relationship of both toxic and antitumor effects of tumor-bearing mice treated with lipopolysaccharide from *E. coli* 0127 : B8 on the 7th day of the growth of Meth A is shown in Table 6. Effective doses extended over an 8- to 16-fold range and instances have been observed of tumors regressing in animals in which no macroscopic signs of hemorrhagic necrosis in tumors have been observed. Such rare combinations of regression without preceding tumor necrosis have been observed in 3% of mice with Meth A and in 7% of those with S-180 which were treated with the four varieties of lipopolysaccharides.

All the above-described categories of tested materials have produced, under

TABLE 6.   Regression of Meth A Treated with Lipopolysaccharide from *E. coli* 0127 : B8[a]

Dose (µg/ mouse)	Day 7	Day 8			Day 28		
	No. of tumor-bearing mice (N)	No. of dead mice	No. of tumor hemor-rhages	Aver. weight change[b] (g)	No. of Survivors	No. of Without tumor (R)	R/N (%)
0	34	0	0	0.0	29	0	0
6.25	16	1	8	−0.8	15	0	0
25	16	0	11	−1.5	16	0	0
50	18	0	13	−2.4	15	4	22
100	18	0	14	−2.2	16	6	33
200	18	0	15	−2.2	18	8	44
400	18	0	11	−2.6	17	11	61
800	26	13	11	—	8	4	50

[a] Therapy: a single i.v. dose on day 7.   [b] Day 8–day 7.

appropriate conditions, regression of both Meth A and S-180. Only S-180 responded to therapy with substances to be reported in subsequent paragraphs.

Plant Polysaccharides

Effects of plant polysaccharides have been examined in S-180 using the assay procedure described by Chihara et al. (1). Therapy was started one day after inoculation of 8×10^6 S-180 cells subcutaneously (s.c.) into the right groin of CD-1 mice (an ICR/Ha-derived line) and consisted of 10 daily doses injected i.p. Comparison of the dose-response relationship of lentinan and zymosan administered to mice bearing S-180 (Table 7) shows that lentinan caused regression of S-180 in

TABLE 7.   Dose Dependence of Regression Frequency of S-180 Growing in Two Different Mouse Strains and Treated with Lentinan or Zymosan[a]

Dose (mg/kg/day)	Regression frequency[b] after treatment with			
	Lentinan	Zymosan	Lentinan	Zymosan
	S-180 in CD-1 mice		S-180 in C3H/HeJ mice	
0	0/12	0/12	0/6	0/6
0.032	0/12		0/6	
0.1	6/12		0/6	0/6
0.32	9/12	0/20	0/6	0/6
1	9/12	10/20	3/6	2/6
3.2	11/12	16/20	5/6	5/6
10	11/12	13/20	5/6	5/6
32	5/6	12/28	5/6	3/6
100	1/6	8/20		4/6
320		4/9[c]		

[a] Tumor load: 8×10^6 cells, s.c. on day 0.   Therapy: 10 i.p. doses, qd, from day 1.   [b] Regression frequency = No. CD-1 mice without tumor on day 42 (on day 70 in C3H/He mice)/No. mice with tumor on day 7.   [c] 11/20 mice died before day 7 (toxicity deaths).

TABLE 8.   Combination Therapy of S-180 with Zymosan and Various Amines[a]

Amines			Saline	Zymosan[b]	Zymosan and amines	
Name	Dose[c]	R[d]	R	R	Dose	R
Carbachol	0.3	8	8	25	0.5+0.3	0
Chlorpheniramine	50	8	0	50	0.5+50	42
Histamine	100	0	8	25	0.5+100	25
5-Hydroxy-L-tryptophan	150	0	8	17	0.5+150	8
Isoproterenol	40	0	0	50	0.5+40	27
Norepinephrine	5	0	8	33	0.5+5	33
Propranolol	80	0	8	25	0.5+80	8
Regitine	80	0	0	50	0.5+80	42
Serotonin	250	25	8	25	0.5+250	58

[a] Therapy: 10 i.p. doses of each chemical, qd, from day 1; both chemicals injected at the same time but as separate solutions.   [b] Dose of zymosan: 0.5 mg/kg/day.   [c] Doses in mg/kg/day.   [d] Regression frequency (%); groups of 12 mice.

CD-1 mice in the lowest doses which were 10 times smaller than the lowest effective dose of zymosan; the latter polysaccharide was toxic in very high doses. Both lentinan and zymosan have produced numerous regressions of S-180 growing in C3H/HeJ mice from the Jackson Laboratory, Bar Harbor, Maine. Regressions of S-180 in CH/HeJ mice were slow and required an observation period of 70 days for confirmation. In a preliminary test both lentinan and zymosan have induced regression of S-180 even when therapy started as late as 14–18 days after implantation. Zymosan was less effective than lentinan against the more advanced tumors.

Following observation by Maeda *et al.* (*15*) of antitumor activity of 5-hydroxytryptophan and serotonin against S-180 and of the partial blocking of action of lentinan by antihistamines, a number of amines and their antagonists have been examined for their activity against S-180 when administered alone or in combination with zymosan (Table 8). Doses of chemicals were those used by Maeda *et al.* No clear-cut evidence of either increased or decreased activity of zymosan could be obtained. We were also unable to confirm the capacity of chlorpheniramine to block the tumor regression-inducing capacity of lentinan.

Small Molecular Synthetic Chemicals

Tilorone dihydrochloride, 2,7-bis[2-(diethylamino)ethoxy]fluoren-9-one, has previously been shown to have antitumor activity against Walker carcinosarcoma-256 and some other tumors (*16*). In the case of S-180 four oral doses of 250 mg/kg/day administered on days 1, 4, 7, and 11 have caused regression of 4 of 6 tumors in a preliminary test. A similar regression rate was produced by i.p. treatment with 50 mg/kg/day of this chemical (10 doses from day 1).

Levamisole, L-(−)2,3,5,6-tetrahydro-6-phenylimidazo(2,1-b)thiazole hydrochloride, a veterinary anthelmintic, which was used by Renoux and Renoux (*17*) for induction of a decrease of primary tumors and lung metastases of the Lewis lung tumor of the mice, induced inconsistently only a few regressions of S-180 upon either oral or i.p. administration. Another thiazole, thiabendazole, 2(4-thiazolyl)benzimidazole, on the contrary, though inactive when administered i.p. to mice with S-180, produced regression of this tumor when given orally in a low dose of 0.8 mg/kg/day.

None of these small molecular synthetic chemicals have induced regression of Meth A but it is not excluded that they may be useful in combination with chemotherapeutic agents. Studies along these lines are planned.

REFERENCES

1. Chihara, G., Hamuro, J., Maeda, Y. Y., Arai, Y., and Fukuoka, F. Fractionation and purification of the polysaccharides with marked antitumor activity, especially lentinan, from *Lentinus edodes* (BERK.) SING. (an edible mushroom). Cancer Res., *30*: 2776–2781, 1970.
2. Old, L. J., Boyse, E. A., Clarke, D. A., and Carswell, E. A. Antigenic properties of chemically induced tumors. Ann. N. Y. Acad. Sci., *101*: 80–106, 1962.

3. Bradner, W. T., Clarke, D. A., and Stock, C. C. Stimulation of host defense against experimental cancer. I. Zymosan and sarcoma 180 in mice. Cancer Res., *18*: 347–351, 1958.

4. Diller, I. C., Mankowski, Z. T., and Fisher, M. E. The effect of yeast polysaccharides on mouse tumors. Cancer Res., *23*: 201–208, 1963.

5. Sakai, S., Takada, S., Kamasuka, T., Momoki, Y., and Sugayama, J. Antitumor action of some glucans, especially on its correlation to their chemical structure. Gann, *59*: 507–512, 1968.

6. Old, L. J., Clarke, D. A., and Benacerraf, B. Effect of Bacillus Calmette-Guerin (B.C.G.) infection on transplanted tumors in the mouse. Nature, *184*: 291–292, 1959.

7. Halpern, B. N., Biozzi, G., Stiffel, C., and Mouton, D. Effet de la stimulation du système reticulo-endothélial par l'inoculation du bacille de Calmette-Guérin sur le developpement d'épithelioma atypique T-8 du Guérin chez le rat. Compt. Rend. Soc. Biol., *153*: 919–923, 1959.

8. Nauts, H. C., Swift, W. E., and Coley, B. L. The treatment of malignant tumors by bacterial toxins as developed by the late William B. Coley, M. D. reviewed in the light of modern research. Cancer Res., *6*: 205–216, 1946.

9. Nauts, H. C. Immunotherapy of cancer by microbial products. *In;* D. Mizuno *et al.* (eds.), Host Defense against Cancer and Its Potentiation, pp. 335–349, Univ. of Tokyo Press, Tokyo, 1975.

10. Halpern, B., Fray, A., Crepin, A., Platica, O., Lorinet, A. M., Rabourdin, A., Sparros, L., and Isac, R. *Corynebacterium parvum,* a potent immunostimulant in experimental infections and in malignancies. *In;* G.E.W. Wolstenholme and J. Knight (eds.), Immunopotentiation (Ciba Foundation Symposium), vol. 18, pp. 217–236, Elsevier/Excerpta Medica/North Holland, Amsterdam/London/New York, 1973.

11. Woodruff, M.F.A., McBride, W. H., and Dunbar, N. Tumour growth, phagocytic activity and antibody response in *Corynebacterium parvum*-treated mice. Clin. Exp. Immunol., *17*: 509–518, 1974.

12. Chedid, L., Lamensans, A., Parant, F., Parant, M., Adam, A., Petit, J. F., and Lederer, E. Protective effect of delipidated mycobacterial cells and purified cell walls against Ehrlich carcinoma and a syngeneic lymphoid leukemia in mice. Cancer Res., *33*: 2187–2195, 1973.

13. Westphal, O., Lüderitz, O., and Bister, F. Über die Extraktion von Bakterien mit Phenol/Wasser, Z. Naturforsch., *7b*: 148–155, 1952.

14. Tarnowski, G. S., Mountain, I. M., Old, L. J., and Stock, C. C. Regression of transplanted mouse sarcomas treated with bacterial endotoxins. Unpublished.

15. Maeda, Y. Y., Hamuro, J., Yamada, Y. O., Ishimura, K., and Chihara, G. The nature of immunopotentiation by the antitumour polysaccharide lentinan; the significance of biogenic amines in its action. *In;* G.E.W. Wolstenholme and J. Knight (eds.), Immunopotentiation (Ciba Foundation Symposium), vol. 18, pp. 259–286, Elsevier/Excerpta Medica/North Holland, Amsterdam/London/New York, 1973.

16. Munson, A. E., Munson, J. A., Regelson, W., and Wampler, G. L. Effect of tilorone hydrochloride and congeners on reticuloendothelial system, tumors, and the immune response. Cancer Res., *32*: 1397–1403, 1972.

17. Renoux, G. and Renoux, M. Levamisole inhibits and cures a solid malignant tumour and its pulmonary metastases in mice. Nature, *240*: 217–218, 1972.

HOST DEFENSE AGAINST CANCER AND ITS POTENTIATION, D. MIZUNO ET AL. (EDS.),
UNIV. OF TOKYO PRESS, TOKYO / UNIV. PARK PRESS, BALTIMORE, PP. 397-404, 1975

Discussions of Presentation by Dr. George Tarnowski

C. Chester STOCK

Sloan-Kettering Institute for Cancer Research, New York, N.Y., U.S.A.

Mr. Chairman, I am most grateful for the added time that I have been given to extend the remarks of Dr. Tarnowski by discussing the broader aspects of the program under the direction of Dr. L. Old and myself. In this program both chemotherapeutic and immunotherapeutic agents are sought and various phenomena encountered in the course of our studies are investigated. Dr. Tarnowski has described methods and given detailed results in a study of immunopotentiating agents in two tumor systems. These antitumor tests are part of a number of immunotherapy projects that have been grafted onto an experimental cancer chemotherapy program, long in existence and one to which Dr. K. Sugiura has made so many contributions. Some of our current investigations represent extensions of our earlier studies on zymosan (*1*) and on BCG (*2*). Dr. Tarnowski's presentation shows clearly that the two tumor systems we are using reveal greatly different degrees of responsiveness to immunopotentiation. Nearly all of the materials quite effective on sarcoma-180 in ICR/Ha derived CD-1 mice have failed to cause regressions of the fibrosarcoma Meth A in BALB/cJ × C57BL/6J mice. His report has emphasized what has appalled me, as an old cancer chemotherapist, namely, the large numbers of parameters that are so critical in detecting the immunopotentiation capacity of immunomodulators. The vagaries of dosage, routes, timing, and response curves are so much more in need of examination than in experimental cancer chemotherapy studies. It raises even more prominently questions of the carry over of experimental results to clinical practice.

Our program seeking immunopotentiating agents has included determinations of influence on carbon clearance in CD-1 mice as conducted by Biozzi *et al.* (*3*) and of skin graft rejection of male skin on isogeneic C57BL/6 females according to the technique of Billingham and Medawar (*4*). Treatment has been given on day −7, +1, or +7 with respect to grafting. The median survival time of untreated grafts has been 40.5 days. The results thus far obtained by Dr. M. Teller in both systems suggest to us their use to extend information about active substances rather than using the systems for initial detection of such materials.

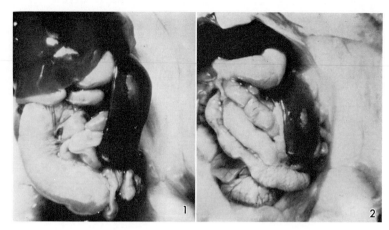

Fig. 1. Regression of leukemic tissue in an AKR mouse treated with normal serum. (1) Control: untreated AKR mouse with advanced leukemia; note massive enlargement of liver, spleen, and mesenteric lymph nodes. (2) Matched leukemic AKR mouse treated with normal horse serum 48 hr previously. Liver, spleen, and mesenteric nodes are markedly reduced in size by comparison with control.

Our program has also included a number of attempts to induce regression of established Meth A fibrosarcomas by active immunization. Numerous modifications of antigen, use of different treatment schedules, and addition of any of a number of immunopotentiators have failed to yield consistently as good results as those reported in his system by Dr. Simmons in this Symposium.

One of the phenomena investigated by Kassel and Old has been a further examination of the dramatic effect reported by Graff et al. (5) on the effect of interferon on primary spontaneous leukemias in mice. Questions on the nature of the factor in the earlier interferon preparations capable of cell destruction in 1 1/2 hr and resolution of leukemic nodes and spleen within 24 hr were raised by the accomplishment of these beneficial results also from an infusion of normal serum from a number of species (Fig. 1) (6). The rather rapid and marked resolution of lymphosarcomas in cats was also observed (6). A number of facts pointed to the active principle as being the C5 component of complement (7). It has also been observed by Kassel and associates by immunofluorescence that leukemic but not normal AKR lymphocytes possess C5-binding surface receptors (8).

Another phenomenology example is the intensive investigation by Green and Old and associates on a factor designated "tumor hemorrhagic necrosis inducing agent" (THN) (6, 9). It was observed that mice sensitized with BCG and shocked with endotoxin had present in their serum a factor causing hemorrhagic necrosis of Meth A fibrosarcoma (Fig. 2) (6). The factor appearing in the α_2-globulin fraction (Fig. 3) has been purified as outlined in Table 1. It exhibits the characteristics detailed in Table 2 and chemical analysis shown in Table 3. Additional information will be presented at the 1975 AACR meeting (10, 11). My earlier questions on the reports of Mizuno and of Chihara were seeking to determine whether the THN might be similar or the same as the active principles they described. Their responses

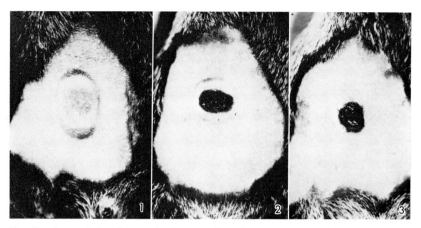

Fig. 2. Serum-induced necrosis of a transplanted mouse sarcoma. (1) An untreated mouse. (2) A mouse treated with endotoxin. (3) A mouse that received serum from nontumorous mice; the serum-donor mice had been infected with BCG and subsequently treated with endotoxin.

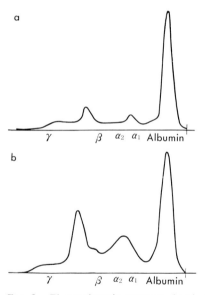

Fig. 3. Electrophoretic patterns showing increase in α_2, containing THN, in the BCG-endotoxin serum. Cellulose acetate electrophoresis: a, normal mouse serum; b, BCG-endotoxin serum.

and the information I have reported for Dr. Green appear to indicate a lack of identity.

One of the better agents we have studied is *Corynebacterium parvum*. Dr. Tarnowski mentioned effects upon tumors from injection of *C. parvum* at sites distant from the tumor. As Dr. Halpern will be speaking more extensively on *C. parvum*, I will illustrate Dr. Tarnowski's point with one figure (Fig. 4) taken from data of Kassel. He has found that injections of *C. parvum* into one of a pair of Meth A tumors per mouse usually, but not always, cause regression also in the non-injected tumor.

TABLE 1. Isolation of THN from Serum of BCG-endotoxin Ttreated Mice

No.	Sample	Protein (mg)	Treatment	Fraction	Protein (%)	THN activity[a]
1	Serum	5,850		Whole	—	0.033
2	Serum	5,850	$(NH_4)_2SO_4$	35–70%	56	0.061
3	35–70%	3,276	G-100 Sephadex	Peak 1	35	0.105
4	Peak 1	1,147	G-200 Sephadex	Peak 2	53	0.154
5	Peak 2	604	Acryl. electro.	Center segment 3.5 cm	33	0.250
6	Center segment	200	Extraction ; acryl. electro.	Band 1	14	0.526
7	Band 1	21	Centrifugation 16.5 hr ; 150,950 g	Pellet	84	0.540

[a] One unit THN activity : lowest concentration of protein producing hemorrhagic necrosis in 100% of Meth A tumors.

TABLE 2. Other Properties of THN

1)	Molecular weight (Sephadex G-200)	115,000–175,000
2)	$s_{20,w}$ (52,000 rpm, 66 min)	6.0–8.0
3)	Heating at 56°C, 1 hr	No loss in activity
4)	Heating at 70°C, 1 hr	Complete loss in activity
5)	Freeze-thaw ($5\times$)	No loss in activity
6)	Limulus sensitivity	$ca.$ 1.0 μg endotoxin
7)	Enzyme determinations	
	a) Acid phosphatase	
	b) Alkaline phosphatase	
	c) β-Glucuronidase	
	d) β-Glucosidase	Not present in measurable amounts
	e) α-Galactosidase	
	f) NAD glycohydrolase	
	g) Non-specific esterase	
	h) Lysozyme	

TABLE 3. Characteristics of the Factor (THN) Isolated from the Sera of BCG-endotoxin Treated Mice (G-200-II, B_1)

Component	Total (μg)	Percent of dry weight
Protein	3,000	90.3
Carbohydrate		
Glucose	15	0.5
Galactose	0	0
Galactosamine	90	2.7
Sialic acid	98	3.0
Fatty acids		
Lauric (C_{12})	0	0
Myristic (C_{14})	3.2	0.10
Palmitic (C_{16})	15.6	0.52
Oleic (C_{18})	3.4	0.11
Stearic (C_{18})	4.6	0.15

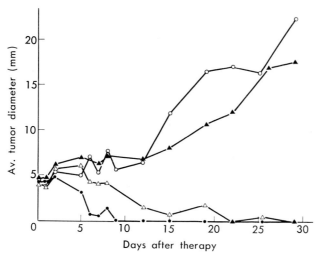

Fig. 4. Responsiveness of contralateral tumors injected and non-injected with *C. parvum*. ○ untreated double-tumor controls; ● injected contralateral tumors; △ non-injected contralateral tumors—responsive; ▲ non-injected contralateral tumors—resistant.

The occasional failures in response raise interesting questions on the basis for the lack of response.

As a final point I wish to stress the further consideration that must be given to the type of cancer chemotherapy that is employed in the light of possible different

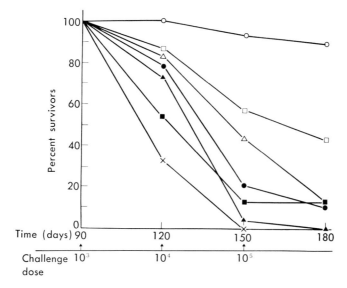

Fig. 5. Survival of mice cured of LPC-1 plasma cell tumor by various chemotherapeutic regimens and then subjected to successive challenges at 30-day intervals. ○ DAU+5-FUseq.; ● DAU+5-FUcon.; □ 5-FU; ■ AM+5-FUseq.; △ CY; ▲ CY+5-FUseq.; × AM. DAU: 1,3-diallylurea. FU: 5-fluorouracil. AM: aniline mustard. CY: cytoxan. seq: sequential treatment with drugs. con: concurrent injection of drugs.

effects upon the tumor and on the host defenses. When there are a number of effective agents against a cancer, it should be recognized that some may provide better protection against subsequent challenge. This is illustrated in Fig. 5 in which marked differences in resistance to a series of challenges are observed in groups of mice cured of the plasma cell tumors, LPC-1, by different chemotherapy regimens (12). It can be seen that mice cured by 5-fluorouracil and 1,3-diallylurea given sequentially were markedly resistant whereas those cured with aniline mustard were little resistant to subsequent challenge.

In conclusion, I wish to say how appropriate it has been to have as a speaker Mrs. Nauts, daughter of Dr. W. B. Coley. He was among the very early investigators of the stimulation of host defenses in humans with cancer (13).

REFERENCES

1. Bradner, W. T., Clarke, D. A., and Stock, C. C. Stimulation of host defense against experimental cancer. Cancer Res., 18: 347–351, 1958.
2. Old, L. J., Clarke, D. A., and Benacerraf, B. Effect of bacillus Calmette-Guerin infection on transplanted tumors in the mouse. Nature, 184: 291–292, 1959.
3. Biozzi, G., Benacerraf, B., and Halpern, B. N. Quantitative study of the granulopectic activity of the reticuloendothelial system. Brit. J. Exp. Pathol., 34: 441–457, 1953.
4. Billingham, R. F. and Medawar, P. B. The technique of free skin grafting in mammals. J. Exp. Biol., 28: 385–402, 1951.
5. Graff, S., Kassel, R., and Kastner, D. Interferon. Trans. N. Y. Acad. Sci., Ser. II., 32: 545–556, 1970.
6. Old, L. J. and Boyse, E. A. Current enigmas in cancer research. Harvey Lecture, Ser. 67, 273–315, 1973.
7. Kassel, R. L., Hardy, W. D., Old, L. J., Hess, P. W., MacEwen, G., Day, N.K.B., Merigan, T. C., and Muller-Eberhard, H. J. Serum mediated leukemia cell destruction in mouse and cat. Proc. Am. Assoc. Cancer Res., 15: 120, 1974.
8. Kassel, R. L., Stackpole, J. M., and Christopher, W. Unpublished.
9. Green, S., Carswell, E., Old, L. J., Fiore, N., Mamaril, F., Dobrjansky, A., and Schwartz, M. K. Mechanism of endotoxin-induced tumor hemorrhagic necrosis. Proc. Am. Assoc. Cancer Res., 15: 139, 1974.
10. Fiore, N., Green, S., Williamson, B., Carswell, E., and Old, L. J. Tumor necrosis factor: Further studies. Proc. Am. Assoc. Cancer Res., 1975, in press.
11. Hoffmann, M. K., Green, S., Fiore, N., Carswell, E., and Old. L. J. BCG-endotoxin treated mice on immune parameters in vitro. Proc. Am. Assoc. Cancer Res., 1975, in press.
12. Teller, M. N., Bowie, M., Mountain, I. M., and Stock, C. C. Combination chemotherapy of advanced murine myeloma and subsequent resistance to tumor cell challenge. J. Natl. Cancer Inst., 52: 667–671, 1974.
13. Coley, W. B. Treatment of inoperable malignant tumors with toxins of erysipelas and the Bacillus prodigious. Am. J. Med. Sci., 108: 50–66, 1894.

Discussion of Papers of Drs. Tarnowski and Stock

DR. T. TANAKA: Does BCG treatment alone alter the serum protein pattern in your animals?

DR. STOCK: No, and our BCG lots are free of endotoxin.

DR. H. OKADA: We administered 50 mg/kg tilorone-HCl i.p. to C3H/He mice one day after the s.c. inoculation of 1×10^6 syngeneic FM3A tumor cells and noted that up to day 10 to 12, tumors grew progressively in both control and treated groups, whereas subsequently those animals given tilorone exhibited sudden regressions from mean tumor diameters of 10 mm. Can you suggest why tilorone has such a relatively long latent period?

DR. TARNOWSKI: I'm unsure of the reason for this latency, but thiabendazole and other related chemicals reveal suppression of tumor growth in a similar manner. As oral administration of tilorone is often necessary, an effect related to the biliary system, or perhaps stimulation of macrophages in the peritoneal cavity, must be considered.

DR. TSUKAGOSHI: Some of your results are directly opposed to those of Dr. Chihara, who observed that lentinan was ineffective against sarcoma-180 in C3H/He mice. Can you explain this discrepancy?

DR. TARNOWSKI: The immunogenicity of the Sloan-Kettering Institute line of sarcoma-180 is evidently different from that of Dr. Chihara, as ours regresses in 50% of C3H/He mice while no such regressions appear using Dr. Chihara's line of sarcoma-180. We have also found lentinan to be effective against Dr. Chihara's line of sarcoma-180 in BALB/c mice, a strain in which this tumor does not spontaneously regress. Substrain differences among various breeding colonies must be considered.

DR. T. TOKUNAGA: I would like to emphasize the fact that the genetic background of the host mice used in such studies is often of critical importance in examining potential immunopotentiating agents. We observed prophylactic and therapeutic responses with BCG using an autochthonous methylcholanthrene-induced tumor in Swiss mouse/MS, but no such response with a similar tumor grown in C3H/He mice. Also, Swiss mouse/MS is a high responder in a delayed hypersensitivity reaction to BCG, while C3H/He exhibits a poor delayed hypersensitivity reaction to this bacillus.

DR. FACHET: A report in the Proc. Soc. Exp. Biol. Med. noted that tilorone treatment results in a substantial depletion of cells from the lymphatic system of the thymus, leading to a selective impairment of thymus-dependent immunologic processes. How do you rationalize this fact with the antitumor activity of this substance?

DR. TARNOWSKI: Little is known about the mechanism of antitumor action of tilorone. Regelson, Munson, and others have conducted several studies on the effect of this agent on immunologic parameters, but these effects may be irrelevant to the antitumor properties we observe. The doses of tilorone we have employed, 250 mg/kg, are much higher than those used by others, resulting in significant loss of body weight and even death among treated animals.

DR. NISHIOKA: You discussed complement deficiency as a possible limiting factor in the potency of an immunotherapeutic. Certain complement components, notably C5a and C7, 8, 9, are chemotaxic. Did you look for leukocyte infiltration of your tumors and the surrounding tissues?

DR. STOCK: No. It is interesting to note, however, that while normal AKR lymphocytes do not bind C5, as determined by immunofluorescence techniques, AKR spontaneous leukemia cells do bind this factor. Chemotaxic effects have not been investigated for the THN.

HOST DEFENSE AGAINST CANCER AND ITS POTENTIATION, D. MIZUNO ET AL. (EDS.),
UNIV. OF TOKYO PRESS, TOKYO / UNIV. PARK PRESS, BALTIMORE, PP. 405-419, 1975

Inhibition of Tumour Invasion by *Corynebacterium parvum* and Its Mechanisms

Bernard HALPERN

Department of Experimental Medicine, Collège de France, Institute of Immunobiology of the Ministry of Health, Paris, France

Abstract: YC8 lymphoma (isogenic tumour) is particularly virulent in Balb/c mouse strain since a dose of 100 cells, given intraperitoneally, determines 100 per 100 of lethality in about 30–40 days.

Treatment with *Corynebacterium parvum* affords 100 per 100 of protection against this dose and even against inocula which contain 10, 100 and 1,000 100 per 100 lethal dose. About 50 per 100 of mortality have been observed with a dose 10^4 times of the minimal 100 per 100 lethal dose.

The results are also highly significant when *C. parvum* is given intravenously but not when *C. parvum* is administered subcutaneously. Time factors are important.

C. parvum-treated animals display a significant prolongation of survival time and, in a certain range of tumour cell/*C. parvum* dosages, definitive survival can be obtained. The most dramatic action was observed on metastatic dissemination with both YC8 and Lewis tumours.

When injected intratumourally *C. parvum* produces, in all cases, a slowing down of the tumour growth followed by total regression of the tumour. The animals so treated display a hightened resistance to the reimplantation of the same tumour. The mechanisms of action and the nature of the immunocompetent cells involved were investigated *in vivo* and *in vitro*.

The effects of *C. parvum* on YC8 tumour were comparable in control and in "B mice" (thymectomized-irradiated and bone marrow-restored), suggesting that thymus-dependent (T) lymphocytes are, but little, involved in the increased host resistance induced by *C. parvum*.

From the *in vitro* studies evidence has been gained that *C. parvum* is stimulating the growth of the macrophages population, as macrophage antitumour cytostatic activity and macrophage antitumour cells cytotoxicity.

The first immunological property of *Corynebacterium parvum*, which we discovered when we started to explore about 10 years ago the possible use of this bacterium as an immunostimulant, was the activation of the reticulo-endothelial system (RES) (*1*). This could be evidenced in two manners: (1) The cellular hyperplasia of the reticulo-endothelial structures as evidenced by the increase in the weight of the spleen and of the liver; for the spleen, it was about 8- to 10-folds and for the liver, 2-folds; (2) the concomitant stimulation of the phagocytic activity of the reticulo-endothelial cells, as measured by the now classical techniques, once developed in my laboratory, *i.e.*, the blood clearance rate of colloidal suspensions.

As to the kinetics of these phenomena, three points deserve to be stressed: (1) a lag period, which lasts 2–3 days, preceeds activation of the reticulo-endothelial cells. (2) The activation of the RES is reflected by a progressive and parallel increase of the three parameters: the phagocytic index, the weight of the liver, and the weight of the spleen, culminating on about the 8–10th day after intravenous or intraperitoneal injection. (3) The progressive and long-lasting decay of this activity, which subsides about 20–25 days following the injection of *C. parvum*.

The increase in the weight and in the phagocytic activity of the reticulo-endothelial organs reflects a highly proliferative process of the phagocytic macrophages. This proliferative effect, which is regularly obtained *in vivo*, could never been reproduced when the *in vivo* activated macrophages were cultured *in vitro*. This suggests either that a factor responsible for the macrophage proliferation is lacking *in vitro* cultures, or as it was more recently shown (*2*) that the hyperplasia of the organs is due to the influx of cells originating from other sites. Actually total body inactivation preceeding injection of *C. parvum* suppresses the activation of the RES.

Some Immunological Features

Like other so-called adjuvants, *C. parvum* is stimulating delayed hypersensitivity and antibody synthesis. We recently found that these effects could be obtained not only, as in the classical Freund's method, by incorporating the antigen in emulsifying agents and by injecting the mixture in the same site, but also when *C. parvum* and antigens were injected separately in different sites and at different times.

I shall consider successively the effect of *C. parvum* on delayed type of hypersensitivity and on antibody synthesis.

1. Delayed type of reactivity

Delayed type of hypersensitivity to a variety of particulate and soluble antigens could be induced in the guinea pig when the antigens were administered incorporated in Freund's *complete* adjuvant (FCA). However, when Freund's *incomplete* adjuvant (FIA) was used, *only* immediate type of hypersensitivity reactions such as Arthus type or anaphylactic type of reaction could be obtained. Moreover, using FCA delayed type reactions could only be obtained when the injected antigen was previously emulsified with the adjuvant. If the antigen and the adjuvant were injected in different sites, no delayed type of reactivity was obtainable with soluble proteins. Several years ago, it was shown (*3*) in my laboratory that *C. parvum* could be substituted to *Mycobacteria* in FCA for inducing delayed type of reactivity with soluble proteins in the guinea pig.

More recently, in collaboration with Rahman (*4*) we succeeded in inducing delayed type of reactivity in the guinea pig in two different conditions: (1) intradermal injection of egg albumin mixed with *C. parvum* in absence of mineral oil; (2) separate injections of *C. parvum* and antigen.

In the first type of experiments, guinea pigs received *an intradermal* injection of either 10 µg of crystalline egg albumin alone (control group) or of the same dose of ovalbumin mixed in *saline* with 500 µg (dry weight) of heat-killed *C. parvum*. None of the animals in the control group developed delayed hypersensitivity to the antigen nor they produced detectable amounts of circulating antibody. In contrast, in the *C. parvum*-treated group *all* animals developed a strong "tuberculin type" reaction when challenged 4–6 weeks later by an intradermal injection of the same dose of ovalbumin.

In the second group, the control animals were injected in a foot pad with 10 µg of ovalbumin in saline. The animals of the treated group received concurrently an injection of 10 µg of ovalbumin in the back and 500 µg of *C. parvum* in the foot pads. None of the control animals reacted when challenged 4 weeks later with ovalbumin. Nearly 75% of the animals of the second group of animals responded with "tuberculin type" reaction to the antigen. In this group of animals low amount of circulating antibody could also be evidenced.

These results show clearly that delayed type of reactivity to ovalbumin can be readily induced in guinea pigs using *C. parvum* as adjuvant. The peculiar feature is that this phenomenon has been obtained without using paraffin oil emulsion. Moreover, delayed type of hypersensitivity to egg albumin was obtained by injecting *C. parvum* and the antigen in two different sites.

2. *Antibody synthesis*

It has been previously reported that *C. parvum* strongly enhances antibody synthesis to both thymus-dependent (*2, 5*) and thymus-independent antigens (*6*).

Furthermore, *C. parvum* determined in "B mice" (thymectomized, irradiated and bone-marrow repopulated) a 19S and 7S response, comparable to intact animals (*6*).

The data reported here (*7*) provide evidence that *C. parvum* exerts a remarkable intensification and prolongation of the immunological memory.

Groups of adult rabbits were immunized by intravenous injections of 2.5 mg of bovine serum albumin (BSA)/kg, which is known to be a rather weak antigen in this animal species. The animals were divided into two groups: the control group and the *C. parvum*-treated group. *C. parvum*-treated animals received a *single* intravenous injection of 2 mg/kg (dry weight) of *C. parvum* 4 days *before* the immunizing injection of the antigen. The animals of both groups were subsequently boostered at spaced intervals of time with the same dose of BSA and the serum antibody levels were measured with the classical precipitation method. The results are summarized in Fig. 2.

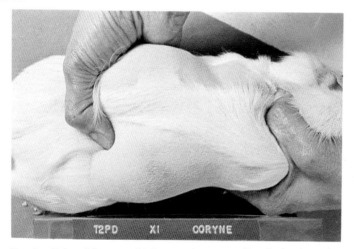

FIG. 1. Delayed hypersensitivity reactions to ovalbumin in the guinea pig after treatment with *C. parvum*. Guinea pigs were immunized intradermally either with 10 μg of ovalbumin alone or with 10 μg of ovalbumin mixed in saline with 500 μg of *C. parvum* on day 0. Skin tests were performed on day 49 by intradermal injection of 10 μg of ovalbumin. Controls, treated with 10 μg ovalbumin alone, showed only negative reactions. All animals immunized with the mixture ovalbumin and *C. parvum* developed strong "tuberculin type" (delayed) skin reactions.

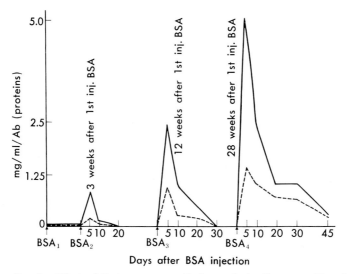

FIG. 2. Effect of *C. parvum* on antibody synthesis. *C. parvum* (2 mg/kg) was administered intravenously, once, 5 days before the intravenous immunizing dose of 2.5 mg/kg of BSA. The primary response was not greatly affected by *C. parvum*. However, the antibody synthesis rates were markedly increased in *C. parvum*-treated groups, following the anamnestic injections. The long-lasting effect of *C. parvum* is emphasized. —— *C. Parvum*-treated rabbits; - - - - control rabbits.

For the dose of BSA used, the primary antibody response was too low to be measured with the technique used. However, using passive haemagglutination technique, it was found that both groups of animals synthesized certain amounts of antibodies, the *C. parvum*-treated animals having produced somewhat higher levels. But striking differences appeared when the animals were boostered with subsequent anamnestic injection. Two main features should be emphasized: (a) from the first booster on and for the other subsequent booster, spaced by several weeks or even several months, both groups of animals have produced increasing amounts of antibody; (b) however, the amounts of antibody synthesized by *C. parvum*-treated animals were in *all* cases more than the double of those produced by the control animals.

Emphasis should be laid on the incredibly long-lasting immunological memorisation in the *C. parvum*-treated animals, since the anamnestic effects were almost of the same magnitude nearly a year after. Similar results have been obtained in guinea pigs using egg albumin as antigen. The cellular basis of this highly enhanced and long-lasting immunological memory is still conjectural.

3. Action on tumour invasion

Increasing evidence is accumulating from animal model, but also from studies in man to suggest that *C. parvum* is capable of tumour growth inhibition (8–16).

It is my intention to report here some of our most recent results concerning the effect of *C. parvum* on the growth and dissemination of certain isogeneic grafted malignant tumours. The material accumulated is too vast to be reported here exhaustively. I shall limit myself to a few examples which are particularly evocative.

YC8 tumour in Balb/c mice: A great part of our investigations were performed with an isogeneic lymphoma called YC8, induced by Moloney virus in Balb/c mice and maintained by serial passages in ascitic form in this strain. *C. parvum* was obtained from Institut Mérieux (69003 Lyon, France) in form of heat-killed suspension containing 2 mg/ml (dry weight) of bacterium added with 8‰ of formaldehyde.

The ascitic cells were obtained from Balb/c recipients which received 8 days before an intraperitoneal inoculum of 180,000 living tumour cells. The cells were obtained from ether asphyxiated donors by sterile puncture of the peritoneal cavity following an intraperitoneal injection of 2 ml of warm sterile Hank's solution added with 10 IU/ml of heparine. The tumour cells concentration was adjusted to have the inoculum dose contained in 0.2 ml.

C. parvum was administered at a uniform dose of 500 μg, either by intraperitoneal or intravenous route, in a volume of 0.25 ml. The time interval between the tumour inoculation and the injection of *C. parvum* varied in different groups of experiments and will be indicated accordingly.

Experimental group I: In this group of experiments the animals received a high dose, *i.e.*, 5×10^5 of tumour cells intraperitoneally while *C. parvum*, at a dose of 500 μg, was also administered intraperitoneally at different time intervals. The results are reported in Fig. 3. The results show clearly a significant prolongation of survival time in all groups treated with *C. parvum*. Important differences were observed depending on time intervals.

Experimental group II: In this experimental group, the tumour inoculum size varied, while the time of *C. parvum* administration was fixed on day 0. The results are reported in Fig. 4.

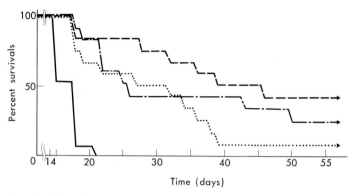

FIG. 3.   Mortality rates in control and *C. parvum*-treated animal groups receiving intraperitoneal inoculation of YC8 cells. Balb/c mice received an intraperitoneal uniform inoculum of 5×10^5 live YC8 cells on day 0. The animals were divided into four groups: (a) control group (——); (b) animals injected with 500 μg of *C. parvum* on day −6 (···); (c) animals injected with 500 μg of *C. parvum* on day 0 (—·—); (d) animals injected with 500 μg of *C. parvum* on day −2 (——). Median survival time (MST) : —— 16.60; ······ 30.58; ——— 45.58; —·— 37.08.

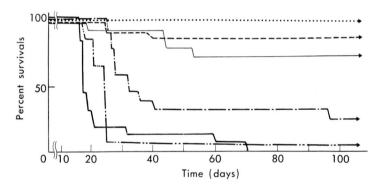

FIG. 4.   Mortality rates in control and *C. parvum*-treated groups of animals receiving YC8 tumour inocula by intraperitoneal route. In the control groups Balb/c mice received respectively by intraperitoneal route 10^3 (—·—), 10^4 (—··—), and 10^5 (——) of YC8 cells on day 0. The *C. parvum*-treated groups of the animals received respectively 10^3 (······), 10^4 (———), and 10^5 (——) tumoural cells 2 days preceding the intraperitoneal injection of 500 μg of *C. parvum*. There is a highly significant increase in the MST in all three groups treated with *C. parvum* and a high percentage (reaching 100% with the lowest tumoural inoculum) of definitive survivors. MTS: —·— 52.26; —··— 26.13; —— 25.73; ······ 65; ——— 61.46; —— 58.80.

In the control groups the mortality was of 100% in the subgroups receiving 10^5 and 10^4 tumour cells and of 70% in the subgroup receiving 10^3 cells.

In the treated groups, no mortality was noted within the 150 days of observation in the subgroups receiving 10^3 cells, and definitive survival rates were respectively of 80% and 70% in the subgroups receiving 10^4 and 10^5 of tumour cells.

These results emphasize a remarkable increase in host resistance to tumour invasion following administration of *C. parvum* 2 days before the tumour inoculation.

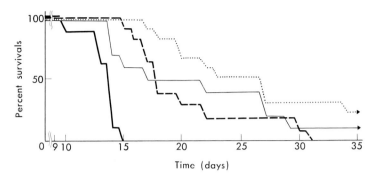

Fig. 5. Mortality rates in control and *C. parvum*-treated animals receiving the tumour inocula and *C. parvum* by intravenous route. The Balb/c mice were divided into four groups. Two of the subgroups served as control and received respectively on the day 0 an intravenous inoculum of 10^5 cells or 10^3 cells. The two treated groups received intravenously 500 μg of *C. parvum* on day -4 followed on the day 0 by an intravenous injection of 10^5 cells or 10^3 cells. Significant prolongation of the median survival time was observed with both the tumoural inocula. For the lower dose of tumoural cells 25% of definitive survivors were noted. ······ control 10^3 cells; ⎯⎯ control 10^5 cells; ⁃⁃⁃⁃ *C. parvum* treated 10^3 cells; ⎯⎯ *C. parvum* treated 10^5 cells. MST: ⎯⎯ 13.35; ⎯⎯ 24.50; ⁃⁃⁃⁃ 20; ······ 33.83.

Experimental group III: In this experimental group the animals received malignant inocula of respectively 10^5 and 10^3 cells intravenously on day 0 while *C. parvum* was administered equally by intravenous injection at a uniform dose of 500 μg on day -4. The results are reported in Fig. 5.

From the results reported in Fig. 5 it can be deduced that in the control groups the mortality was regularly of 100% with both doses of the malignant cells inoculated, the differences laying in the median survival time.

In the treated groups consistent prolongation of the survival time was observed in both subgroups. With the smaller inoculum about 25% of definitive survivors were observed.

Attempts to quantify the antitumoural action of C. parvum: Figure 6 represents a series

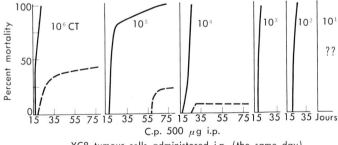

Fig. 6. An attempt to quantify the protective effect of *C. parvum* against YC8 lymphoma in Balb/c mice. An inoculum of 10^3 tumoural cells causes nearly 100% of mortality. In this experiment, treatment with *C. parvum* injected intraperitoneally on day 0 afforded full protection against 10^3, 10^4, and 10^5 cells and about 50% of protection against 10^6 cells. ⎯⎯ controls; ⁃⁃⁃⁃ *C. parvum*-treated on day 0.

of results in which we attempted to quantify the protective antitumoural action of
C. parvum (28). It was first established that an intraperitoneal inoculation of 10^2
YC8 cells causes in the control group nearly 100% of mortality in less than 2 months
in the Balb/c mice.

Groups of animals were therefore administered an intraperitoneal injection of
a uniform dose of 500 μg of C. parvum and challenged 2 days later with increasing doses of tumoural cells, i.e., 10^3, 10^4, 10^5, and 10^6, respectively.

As evidenced by the data summarized in Fig. 6 full protection has been afforded by C. parvum against 10, 100, and 1,000 lethal doses of cancerous cells and
about 50% against 10,000 lethal doses.

The interest of these data should be considered in view of some recent theories
on immunological surveillance, which claim that a normal organism can dispose,
by its own immune defenses, of a certain number of tumoural cells. Actually, this
number remains highly hypothetical in humans.

The results reported above imply that treatment with C. parvum affords a
considerable increase in the resistance of the host against several doses of thousands
of 100% lethal tumour cells. However, the magnitude of this resistance is influenced
by a certain number of factors.

Augmentation of host resistance was impressive when tumoural cells and C.
parvum were given both intraperitoneally. With lower tumoural burdens survival
rates approaching 100% versus 100% of mortality in the control groups were observed.

Treatment by intravenous route has yielded less consistently favorable results,
however a certain percentage of definitive survivors were noted in conditions in
which 100% mortality was observed in the control groups.

Time factors are also important. The best results were obtained when C.
parvum was given on day −2 or on day 0. Even better results were observed when
C. parvum was administered both on day −2 and repeated on +4 (not reported
here).

4.   Protection with C. parvum against metastatic dissemination

Milas and Mujagic (17) reported in 1972 that subcutaneous injection of C.
parvum into $C_{57}BL$ mice, before or after intravenous injection of syngeneic fibrosarcoma cells, reduced to a great extent the number of lung nodules 25 days
after the tumour cell injection. Bomford and Olivotto (18, 19) reported similar
results using another fibrosarcoma murine strain, the T3 cells, given intravenously.
Regression of hamster melanoma by intralesional injection of C. parvum has been
recently reported by Dimitrov et al. (14).

More recently Pot-Deprun and Chouroulinkov (20) carried out studies on the
effects of C. parvum on the evolution and metastatic dissemination of Lewis
pulmonary fibrosarcoma. This tumour, which appeared spontaneously in the $C_{57}BL$
mouse, is transplantable by subcutaneous inoculation. The growth of this tumour
is rapid and the animals develop rapidly in almost all cases pulmonary metastases
from the 3rd week on after the graft. The results are summarized in Fig. 7.

In all cases 10^6 tumoral cells were injected subcutaneously. The C. parvum-

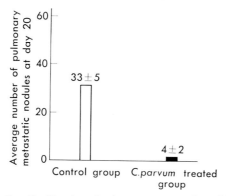

F<small>IG</small>. 7. Number of pulmonary metastatic nodules in mice grafted with Lewis fibrosarcoma in control group (□) and in *C. parvum* treated group (■).

treated animals received 500 µg of the bacterial suspension intraperitoneally on day −4.

In the control group the lethality was of 100% and the median survival time was of about 34 days. In the *C. parvum*-treated animals the median survival time was of 53 days.

The most remarkable feature is the action of *C. parvum* on the metastatic dissemination. In the control group the average number of pulmonary nodules on the 20th day was of 34; it was reduced to 4 in the *C. parvum* treated group (Fig. 7).

The results reported above are in agreement with those found by other authors and emphasize the remarkable protective action of *C. parvum* on metastatic tumoural dissemination.

5. Action of C. parvum on bone marrow colony-forming cells

There is indirect clinical evidence that tumour invasion may exert a depressive action on erythro- and myelogenesis. On the other hand, the myelotoxicity of many cytostatic drugs justified the study of the effect of *C. parvum* on bone marrow colony-forming cells. The technique of culture used was that described by Minz and Sachs (*21*).

The bone marrows were obtained from adult male $C_{57}BL$ mice by perfusion of the femurs. The cells were dispersed by pushing the cell suspension in a syringe through a tiny needle. The cells were plated in a medium made of 0.6 pecent of agar dissolved in blood serum supplemented with Eagle medium and recovered with soft agar (0.3%). The cultures were placed at 37°C in a gassed and humid incubator. The colonies were counted after 7 days of culture. Clusters of less than 30 cells were not comprised.

The *C. parvum*-treated animals received during 2 consecutive days an intraperitoneal injection of 500 µg of the bacterial suspension. The results are summarized in Fig. 8.

Bone marrow from control mice produced only 5 to 10 colonies. Bone marrow from *C. parvum*-treated animals produced 24 hr after the second injection about 50 colonies.

Following a transient regression on the 3rd day, a logarithmic increase in the

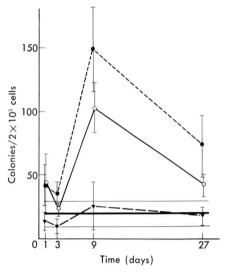

Fɪɢ. 8.   Action of *C. parvum* on bone marrow colony-forming cells. In the control group the number of colony-forming cells varied between 10 and 15 colonies. Treatment with *C. parvum* (500 μg intraperitoneally on two consecutive days) determined a rapid and sustained augmentation of the number of colony-forming cells. ● bone-marrow from *C. parvum* treated animals+normal serum ; ○ bone-marrow from *C. parvum* treated animals+serum from *C. parvum* treated mice ; ▼ bone-marrow from control mice+serum from *C. parvum* treated mice ; ■ bone-marrow on serum from control mice.

number of colonies was observed. After having reached the peak on the 5th day with 150 of $>2 \times 10^5$ cell colonies, the number was progressively declining, approaching the normal level 27 days later.

In conclusion:

1)   *C. parvum* increased considerably the bone marrow colony-forming cell production.

2)   The duration of the stimulating activity overpasses any other presently known similar effect.

3)   The stimulating factor resides in the cell and not in the serum since the addition of serum from *C. parvum*-treated animals to the culture medium resulted rather in a depression of bone marrow colony-forming cells.

DISCUSSION

The mechanisms by which *C. parvum* influences the various forms of immune reactions and consequently inhibits tumour growth and invasion remain still a matter of speculation. Evidence has been provided here that *C. parvum* promoted delayed type of hypersensitivity to soluble proteins, even in the absence of the emulsifying agents, which are essential in FCA. Similar effects have been obtained even when *C. parvum* and the soluble antigens were injected in two remote sites.

C. parvum enhances also antibody synthesis to a variety of proteins. In contrast to FCA the primary response is but little enhanced. The surprising feature is the long vigorous potentiation of the anamnestic responses and even more the incredibly long lasting immunological memory attaining the order of a year.

These two orders of phenomena emphasize the potency of the action of *C. parvum* on the cell population which are implicated in the immune reaction.

The inhibitory action of *C. parvum* on tumour growth and dissemination must be related to the strengthening of the host immune system.

How can they be explained on the basis of our present immunological concepts? It is admitted that delayed hypersensitivity is mediated by (T) cells. It is also accepted that memory cells are T cells, while antibody synthesis is the attribute of bone marrow derived (B) cells. On the other hand conclusive evidence has been provided that *C. parvum* is a potent stimulator of the macrophage functions resulting in new properties of the so-called "activated" macrophages. How can the tumour growth repression be explained on the basis of these presently prevalent concepts? Attempts to identify a particular cell type participating in *C. parvum*-induced immunological disruption and tumour regression have resulted in divergent observations. It has been reported by Howard *et al.* (6) that thymus-deprived animals were able to develop a normal response to thymus-dependent antigens (SRBC) when pretreated with *C. parvum*, including synthesis of both 19S and 7S antibody. Findings from several sources, including our own results, it was demonstrated that restraint of tumour growth, as a consequence of *C. parvum* administration, can proceed in animals whose T cells have been depleted (22) or who have been treated with antilymphocytic serum (23) tending to minimize the effector function of that cell type in the *C. parvum* suppression of tumour growth. The demonstration that such a phenomenon is independent of host capacity to produce humoral antibody lessens the likelihood of B cells participation (12, 24).

While those observations tend to diminish the importance of lymphocytes in *C. parvum*-mediated tumour repression, increasing attention has been focused on the role of macrophage (1, 25).

Our recent investigations proved that *C. parvum*-activated peritoneal macrophages display non-specific cytostatic and cytotoxic effects on tumoural cells (5, 26).

In summary, *C. parvum* produces some bewildering changes in the immune reactions and among them a remarkable inhibition of the growth and invasion of malignant tumours. The accumulated results point to the central implication of the activated macrophages in these events.

REFERENCES

1. Halpern, B., Prevot, A. R., Biozzi, G., Stiffel, C., Mouton, D., Morard, J. C., Bouthillier, Y., and Decreusefond, C. Stimulation de l'activité phagocytaire du système réticuloendothélial provoquée par *Corynebacterium parvum*. J. Reticulo-endothelial Soc., *1*: 77–96, 1964.

2. Volkman, A. and Gowans, J. L. The origin of macrophages from bone marrow. Brit. J. Pathol., 46, 62–70 (1965).

3. Neveu, T., Branellec, A., and Biozzi, G. Propriétés adjuvantes de *Corynebacterium*

parvum sur la production d'anticorps et sur l'induction de l'hypersensibilité retardée envers les propriétés conjuguées. Ann. Inst. Pasteur, *106*: 771–777, 1964.

4. Rahman, S. and Halpern, B. Unpublished results.

5. Halpern, B., Fray, A., Crepin, Y., Platica, O., Lorinet, A. M., Rabourdin, A., Sparros, L., and Isac, R. *Corynebacterium parvum*, a potent immunostimulant in experimental infections and in malignancies. *In;* G.E.W. Wolstenholme and J. Knight (eds.), Immunopotentiation (Ciba Foundation Symposium), vol. 18, pp. 217–236, Elsevier/Excerpta Medica/North Holland, Amsterdam/London/New York, 1973.

6. Howard, J .G., Scott, M. T., and Christie, G. H. Cellular mechanisms underlying the adjuvant activity of *Corynebacterium parvum*: Interaction of activated macrophages with T and B lymphocytes. *In;* G.E.W. Wolstenholme and J. Knight (eds.), Immunopotentiation (Ciba Foundation Symposium), vol. 18, pp. 101–120, Elsevier/Excerpta Medica/North Holland, Amsterdam/London/New York, 1973.

7. Halpern, B. and Parlebas, J. Unpublished results.

8. Halpern, B., Biozzi, G., Stiffel, C., and Mouton, D. Inhibition of tumour growth by administration of killed *Corynebacterium parvum*. Nature, *212*: 853–859, 1966.

9. Woodruff, M.F.A. and Boak, J. L. Inhibitory effect of injection of *Corynebacterium parvum* on the growth of tumour transplants in isogeneic hosts. Brit. J. Cancer, *20*: 345–355, 1966.

10. Currie, G. A. and Bagshawe, K. D. Active immunotherapy with *Corynebacterium parvum* and chemotherapy in murine fibrosarcomas. Brit. Med. J., *1*: 541–544, 1970.

11. Fisher, J. C., Grace, W. R., and Mannick, J. A. The effect of nonspecific immune stimulation with *Corynebacterium parvum* on patterns of tumor growth. Cancer, *26*: 1379–1382, 1970.

12. Halpern, B., Crepin, Y., and Rabourdin, A. An analysis of the increase in host resistance to isogeneic tumor invasion in mice by treatment with *Corynebacterium parvum*. *In;* B. Halpern (ed.), *Corynebacterium parvum*: Its Application in Experimental and Clinical Oncology, vol. 1, pp. 193–200, Plenum Press, New York, 1975.

13. Fisher, B., Wolmark, N., and Fisher, E. R. Results of investigations with *C. parvum* in an experimental animals system. *In;* B. Halpern (ed.), *Corynebacterium parvum*: Its Application in Experimental and Clinical Oncology, Vol. 1, pp. 220–245, Plenum Press, New York, 1975.

14. Dimitrov, N., Chouroulinkov, I., Israel, L., and O'Rangers, J. Regression of hamster melanoma by *Corynebacterium parvum*. *In;* B. Halpern (ed.), *Corynebacterium parvum*: Its Application in Experimental and Clinical Oncology, vol. 1, pp. 278–285, Plenum Press, New York, 1975.

15. Israel, L. and Halpern, B. Le *Corynebacterium parvum* dans les cancers avancés. Première évaluation de l'activité thérapeutique de cette immunostimuline. La Nelle Presse Méd., *1*: 19–23, 1972.

16. Israel, L. Preliminary results of nonspecific immunotherapy for lung cancer. Cancer Chemother. Rep., *4*: 283–286, 1973.

17. Milas, L. and Mujagic, H. Protection by *Corynebacterium parvum* against tumor cells injected intravenously. Rev. Eur. Clin. Biol., *17*: 498–502, 1972.

18. Bomford, R. and Olivotto, M. The mechanism of inhibition by *Corynebacterium parvum* of the growth of lung nodules from intravenously injected tumour cells. Int. J. Cancer, *14*: 226–235, 1974.

19. Bomford, R. and Olivotto, M. Inhibition by *C. parvum* of nodule formation by intraveously injected fibrosarcoma cells. *In;* B. Halpern (ed.), *Corynebacterium parvum*:

Its Application in Experimental and Clinical Oncology, vol. 1, pp. 270–276, Plenum Press, New York, 1975.

20. Pot-Deprun, J. and Chouroulinkov, I. Effect de l'immunostimulation par *Corynebacterium parvum* sur l'évolution de la tumeur de Lewis chez la souris $C_{57}Bl_6$. C. R. Acad. Sci. (Paris), *280*: 685–688, 1975.

21. Minz, V. and Sachs, L. Differences in inducing activity for human bone marrow colonies in normal serum and serum from patients with leukemias. Blood, *42*: 331–339, 1973.

22. Woodruff, M.F.A., Dunbar, N., and Ghaffar, A. The growth of tumours in T cell deprived mice and their response to treatment with *Corynebacterium parvum*. Proc. Roy. Soc. Lond. (Biol.), *184*: 97–102, 1973.

23. Castro, J. E., Medawar, P. B., and Hamilton, D. N. Orchidectomy as a method of immunopotentiation in mice. *In;* G.E.W. Wolstenholme and J. Knight (eds.), Immunopotentiation (Ciba Foundation Symposium), vol. 18, pp. 237–258, Elsevier/Excerpta Medica/North Holland, Amsterdam/London/New York, 1973.

24. Biozzi, G., Stiffel, C., Mouton, D., Bouthillier, Y., and Decreusefond, C. Importance of specific and nonspecific immunity in anti-tumor defence. Ann. Inst. Pasteur (Paris), *122*: 685–694, 1972.

25. Evans, R. and Alexander, P. Mechanism of immunologically specific killing of tumour cells by macrophages. Nature, *236*: 168–170, 1972.

26. Fray, A., Sparros, L., Lorinet, A. M., and Halpern, B. Nonspecific cytotoxic activity of peritoneal exudate cells against tumoral cells in *C. parvum* treated animals. *In;* B. Halpern (ed.), *Corynebacterium parvum*: Its Application in Experimental and Clinical Oncology, vol. 1, pp. 181–186, Plenum Press, New York, 1975.

27. Puvion, F., Fray, A., and Halpern, B. A comparative study with the scanning electron microscope of the interaction between stimulated or unstimulated mouse peritoneal macrophages and tumour cells. *In;* B. Halpern (ed.), *Corynebacterium parvum*: Its Application in Experimental and Clinical Oncology, vol. 1, pp. 137–146, Plenum Press, New York, 1975.

28. Fray, A., Crepin, Y., Platica, O., Sparros, L., Lorinet, A. M., and Rabourdin, A. Action inhibitrice de *Corynebacterium parvum* sur le développement des tumeurs malignes syngéniques et son mécanismes. C. R. Acad. Sci. (Paris), *276*: 1911–1915, 1973.

Discussion of Paper of Dr. Halpern

DR. ALEXANDER: There are two processes by which macrophages can be rendered non-specifically cytotoxic, (1) adding antigen to a pre-sensitized system or, (2) by pharmacologic means, such as with endotoxin, peptoglycan, or double-stranded RNA. Do you believe such macrophages arise following treatment with *C. parvum* because all animals carry a certain degree of immunity to this microorganism, so its administration is equivalent to challenging a BCG-sensitized animal with PPD, or is there perhaps something in the cell wall of *C. parvum* which, analogous to endo-toxin, activates the macrophages directly?

DR. HALPERN: We have been able to identify agglutinins to *C. parvum* antibodies in mice which have never received *C. parvum*. Probably all laboratory mice have been to some degree infected with this saprophyte and carry "spontaneous" anti-bodies.

Peritoneal macrophages induced by various chemicals, such as thioglycolate, glycogene, and peptone, display morphological changes which are grossly similar to those observed with *C. parvum*. However, there is a fundamental difference in their immunological properties. The macrophages induced by chemicals did not show evidence of cytotoxic action against the YC8 lymphoma cells while those induced by *C. parvum* were highly cytotoxic.

DR. KENNEDY: In your experiments in which you examined the effect of injection of *C. parvum* on the colony-forming cells of the recipient, did you determine whether the increase in number of colonies following administration of the microorganisms involved mostly monocytes colonies or mostly granulocyte colonies? If monocyte colonies were preferentially increased, an increase in host macrophage numbers might be expected. Also, was there an increase in the number of cells per colony?

DR. HALPERN: In non-treated animals one can easily count individual colonies and microscopically distinguish between monocyte and granulocyte precursor populations. Following *C. parvum* administration, however, individual colonies were no longer distinct but rather fused into large masses containing both granulocytic and monocytic colonies. Our results are so far preliminary, and we thus do not know if *C. parvum* is promoting one precursor line over the other. Dr. Dimitrov and I published a paper (Dimitrov *et al.*, Proc. Soc. Expl. Biol. Med., *148:* 440, 1975) on these preliminary results obtained 48 hr after *C. parvum* injection. We have evidence presently that this effect is rather long lasting, persisting more than 2 months.

DR. JERNE: Has the active component of the *C. parvum* cell wall been isolated and characterized?

DR. HALPERN: Several groups are working on this project, but unfortunately most of used extractive reagents destroy its activity. Dr. Jolles has found that all the activity is present in the cell wall, and none in the bacterial body. This activity must be due to a chemical, as, unlike BCG which is usually only active in live form, heat-killed *C. parvum* does not lose its anti-tumour effect.

We have not yet isolated a substance equal in activity to the whole bacterium.

HOST DEFENSE AGAINST CANCER AND ITS POTENTIATION, D. MIZUNO ET AL. (EDS.), UNIV. OF TOKYO PRESS, TOKYO / UNIV. PARK PRESS, BALTIMORE, PP. 421-433, 1975

Immunopotentiation with Mycobacterial Cell Wall Skeletons and Its Application to Tumor Immunotherapy

Yuichi YAMAMURA, Ichiro AZUMA, Tadayoshi TANIYAMA, and Fumio HIRAO

The Third Department of Internal Medicine, Osaka University Medical School, Osaka, Japan

Abstract: Adjuvanticity and anti-tumor activity of the cell wall skeletons (CWS) prepared from mycobacteria, nocardia, and corynebacteria were examined. The CWS prepared from *Mycobacterium bovis* BCG (BCG-CWS) stimulated helper function of carrier-specific thymus-derived lymphocytes (T cells) and enhanced cell-mediated cytotoxicity. It was also shown that BCG-CWS acted on T cells and bone-marrow derived cells (B cells) as mitogen. Tumor growth was suppressed in mice which were inoculated intradermally with a mixture of oil-attached CWS and living tumor cells. It is shown that systemic and specific tumor immunity to mastocytoma P815-X2 was induced by the inoculation of a mixture of oil-attached BCG-CWS and mitomycin C-treated or X-irradiated mastocytoma P815-X2 cells in syngeneic mice. The intravenous injection of oil-attached BCG-CWS prevents the incidence of lung cancer in rabbits by the instillation of 3-methylcholanthrene and 4-nitroquinoline 1-oxide.

A successful case of melanoma, which was firstly treated with BCG-CWS, was reported.

It is well known that Freund's complete adjuvant (FCA), which contains heat-killed mycobacterial cells in mineral oil, is one of the most potent adjuvant currently used (*1, 2*). So-called "wax D" fraction has been shown to be adjuvant-active principle of mycobacteria. Recently, it has been shown that methanol extracted residue (MER), peptidoglycolipids, whole cell wall, water-soluble materials (adjuvants) from delipidated cell residue or cell wall, cord factor, RNA fraction and tuberculin protein are reported to be adjuvant-active principle of mycobacterial cells.

Previously (*3–5*), it has been shown that "mycolic acid-arabinogalactan-mucopeptide" complex (Fig. 1) is the principle structure of the cell wall skeleton (CWS) of mycobacteria, nocardia, and corynebacteria, and also suggested that this principle structure, especially mucopeptide moiety, is responsible for the adjuvanticity of the CWS (*6*). Recently, it has been demonstrated that CWS prepared from *Mycobacterium bovis* BCG (BCG-CWS) suppressed the tumor growth of sarcoma 180, mastocytoma P815-X2, EL4 leukemia, melanoma B16, and line 10 hepatoma in allogeneic or syngeneic mice or guinea pigs (*7–9*).

In this paper, the authors will review the adjuvanticity, especially on thymus-derived lymphocytes (T cells), mitogenicity and antitumor activity of the CWS prepared from mycobacteria, nocardia, and corynebacteria. A patient of melanoma, who was treated successfully by oil-attached BCG-CWS, was reported. Remarkable side effects were not observed.

Preparation of CWS

The cell walls were prepared from the cells of *M. bovis* BCG, *Mycobacterium tuberculosis* H37Rv and H37Ra strains, *Mycobacterium kansasii*, *Mycobacterium smegmatis*, *Nocardia asteroides* 131, *Nocardia rubra*, *Corynebacterium diphtheriae* PW8, and *Corynebacterium fermentans* by the method described previously (*10*). The cells were disrupted with Sorvall cell fractionator (Model RF-1) at 35,000 psi at 5 to 10°C. The disrupted product was centrifuged to remove unbroken cells and cell debris, after which the cell wall fraction was collected by centrifugation at 20,000 g, 60 min. The whole cell wall fraction was treated several times with trypsin, chymotrypsin, and pronase followed by repeated washing with buffer, saline, water, and acetone. The proteinase-treated cell walls were extracted consecutively with diethyl ether-ethanol (1:1), chloroform and chloroform-methanol (2:1). The cell wall residue thus obtained was designated as "cell wall skeleton (CWS)." The CWS fraction was obtained in yields of 5 to 7% of intact cells of mycobacteria, nocardia, and corynebacteria. The CWS of *M. bovis* BCG is shown to be composed of mycolic acid (34.2%), arabinose and galactose as neutral sugars (32.6%) in a molar-ratio of 2.8:1, and amino acids and amino sugars (20.1%) consisting mainly of alanine, glutamic acid, α,ε-diaminopimelic acid, muramic acid, and glucosamine (*10*). Similarly, the authors have reported that the principle chemical structure of the CWS of nocardia and corynebacteria is also shown to be "mycolic acid (nocardomycolic acid or corynomycolic acid)-arabinogalactan-mucopeptide" complex as was expressed in the CWS prepared from the cells of mycobacteria (Fig. 1). The detailed chemical properties of each components of the CWS of mycobacteria, nocardia, and corynebacteria have been described in detail previously (*10, 11*).

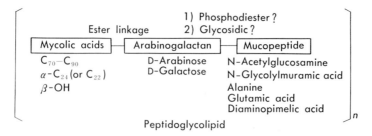

FIG. 1. Chemical structure of CWS prepared from *M. bovis* BCG.

Adjuvanticity of CWS of Mycobacteria, Nocardia, and Corynebacteria

1. Adjuvanticity of CWS on primary response to sheep erythrocytes (SRBC) in vitro

It has been shown that BCG-CWS augmented the primary immune response to SRBC *in vitro* (*12*) by using Marbrook's method (*13*). The adjuvant effect was observed on the formation of 19S-antibody *in vitro* culture method. Primary anti-hapten response of mouse spleen cells to dinitrophenylated keyholelympet hemocyanin (DNP-KLH) was also found when BCG-CWS was added to culture medium (*12*). As shown in Table 1, the CWS prepared from the cells of myco-bacteria, nocardia, and corynebacteria showed potent adjuvant effect on the primary immune response to SRBC *in vitro*. It has also been shown that these CWS of mycobacteria, nocardia, and corynebacteria augmented the circulating antibody formation and development of cell-mediated immunity to bovine serum albumin, SRBC, and sulfanylazo-bovine serum albumin in mice and guinea pigs *in vivo* (*11*).

TABLE 1. Adjuvanticity of CWS Prepared from Mycobacteria, Nocardia, and Corynebacteria

CWS (100 μg) of	PFC/culture		Adjuvanticity
	Exp. 116	Exp. 162	
M. bovis BCG	360± 17	1,890± 337	⊹
M. tuberculosis H37Rv	339± 9		⊹
M. tuberculosis H37Ra	287± 40		++
M. kansasii	675± 64		⊹
M. smegmatis		10,560± 960	⊹
N. asteroides 131	1,194±284		⊹
N. rubra		5,542±1,437	⊹
C. diphtheriae PW8	2,301± 86		⊹
—	60± 52	945± 236	

The normal spleen cells (2×10^7/tube) were cultured with SRBC (4×10^6/tube) and CWS (100 μg/tube). PFC responses were assayed on day 4 of culture. Each value represents the arithmetic mean of dupli-cate cultures ±1 standard error (SE) of the mean. Adjuvant effect of BCG-CWS is represented by ⊹.

2. Stimulation of helper activity of carrier-primed cells with BCG-CWS

In the previous paper (*12*), the authors have shown that BCG-CWS stimulated helper activity of carrier-specific T cells *in vitro* where a double chamber system separated by a cell impermeable nucleopore membrane was used.

In this experiment, two groups of C57BL/6J mice were immunized with 100 μg of KLH (carrier-primed mice) in the presence or absence of BCG-CWS, or 100 μg of dinitrophenylated bovine γ-globulin (DNP-BGG) (hapten-primed mice). At 37 days after immunization, spleen cells primed with DNP-BGG were mixed with KLH-primed spleen cells and DNP-KLH (10 μg) *in vitro* and transferred into 650 R X-irradiated recipient mice of C57BL/6J. Anti-hapten plaque-forming cells (PFC) were assayed at 7 days after cell transfer. As shown in Table 2, anti-hapten antibody response was stimulated by the helper cells which were obtained from the donor mice treated with BCG-CWS. These results suggest that BCG-CWS stimulates carrier-primed helper T-cells in an adoptive transfer system.

TABLE 2. Stimulation of Helper Activity of Carrier-primed Cells with CWS Prepared from *M. bovis* BCG

Exp.	Carrier (KLH)-primed cells		Hapten (DNP-BGG)-primed cells (No. of cells)	Anti-hapten antibody (TNP-PFC/spleen)
	Adjuvant	No. of cells		
1	BCG-CWS (100 μg)	3×10^7	3×10^7	$11,050 \pm 5,188$[a] $(n=3)$
	—	3×10^7	3×10^7	$2,678 \pm$ 720 $(n=3)$
2	BCG-CWS (100 μg)	5×10^7	5×10^7	$23,900 \pm 2,347$ $(n=5)$
	—	5×10^7	5×10^7	$4,844 \pm 2,182$ $(n=5)$

KLH-primed spleen cells, DNP-BGG-primed cells, and DNP-KLH (10 μg) were mixed *in vitro* and transferred into 650 R X-irradiated recipient mice. Anti-hapten PFC were assayed 7 days after cell transfer.
[a] Mean $\pm$ SE.

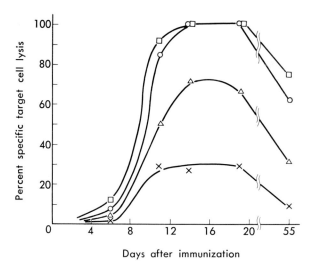

Days after immunization

Fig. 2.   Appearance of cytotoxic effector cells in spleen of mice. C57BL/6J mice were immunized i.p. with mastocytoma P815-X2 cells (1×10^4) with ($\bigcirc$) or without ($\times$) oil-attached BCG-CWS (100 μg), or oil droplets ($\triangle$), or mastocytoma P815-X2 cells (3×10^7) alone ($\square$). Several days later, cell-mediated cytotoxicity of spleen cells of mice was determined by incubation of spleen cells (1×10^7) and ^{51}Cr-labelled mastocytoma P815-X2 cells (1×10^5) at ratio of 100 : 1 for 20 hr at 37°C.

3.   *Effect of BCG-CWS on cell-mediated cytotoxicity*

The mice of C57BL/6J (H-2^b) were immunized with mastocytoma P815-X2 (H-2^d) cells with or without BCG-CWS attached to oil droplets or suspended in phosphated-saline, and cell-mediated cytotoxicity was determined by the method of Brunner *et al.* (*14*) using ^{51}Cr-labelled mastocytoma P815-X2 cells (target cells) and spleen cells (effector cells) obtained from C57BL/6J mice immunized with mastocytoma P815-X2 cells. As shown in Fig. 2, oil-attached BCG-CWS enhanced significantly cell-mediated cytotoxicity of mice spleen cells obtained from the groups immunized with mastocytoma P815-X2 cells in dose of 10^4, and cytotoxic activity of this group is almost similar to that of spleen cells of mice immunized

TABLE 3.   Effect of Oil-attached CWS of Mycobacteria, Nocardia, and Corynebacteria on Cell-mediated Cytotoxicity

Group	C57BL/6J mice were immunized with:	% of specific target cell lysis
	Mastocytoma P815-X2 (1×10^4)+oil-attached CWS (100 μg) of	
1	M. bovis BCG	65.9
2	N. rubra	94.0
3	C. diphtheriae PW8	66.2
4	+oil droplets	48.0
5	+medium	15.3

Mice of C57BL/6J were immunized intraperitoneally (i.p.) with a mixture of mastocytoma P815-X2 cells (1×10^4) and oil-attached CWS (100 μg), oil droplets, or medium. Eleven days later, cell-mediated cytotoxicity of spleen cells of immunized mice was determined by incubation of spleen cells (effector cells) and ^{51}Cr-labelled mastocytoma P815-X2 at ratio of 100:1 for 20 hr.

with 3×10^7 of mastocytoma P815-X2 cells. The cytotoxic activities of spleen cells of various treated mice were still high on day 55 after tumor immunization and then decreased gradually. It was observed that BCG-CWS which was suspended in phosphate buffered-saline (PBS) is also active for the stimulation of cell-mediated cytotoxicity, however, adjuvanticity of BCG-CWS suspended in PBS is lower than that of oil-attached BCG-CWS. As shown in Table 3, oil-attached CWS of N. rubra, C. diphtheriae PW8 also potently stimulated cell-mediated cytotoxicity of spleen cells in mice.

In order to determine the specificity of cytotoxic lymphocytes generated in mice, ^{51}Cr-labelled mastocytoma P815-X2 cells (H-2^d) and EL-4 leukemia cells (H-2^b) were used as target cells. The C57BL/6J mice spleen cells activated against H-2^d lysed mastocytoma P815-X2 cells only, but failed to lyse EL4 leukemia target cells. These result indicates that specificity of cytotoxic response of C57BL/6J spleen cells exhibited immunological specificity. It was shown that oil-attached BCG-CWS did not influence the effector phase of cytotoxic response in vitro, and might influence the induction stage of cytotoxic lymphocytes. It was also confirmed by treatment with AKR anti-θ C$_3$H serum that T cells are responsible for cytotoxicity.

It was shown that oil-attached BCG-CWS augmented the induction of cell-mediated cytotoxicity rather than humoral antibody when mastocytoma P815-X2 cells or trinitrophenylated (TNP)-mastocytoma P815-X2 cells were used as antigens in C57BL/6J mice. Mice were once immunized with mastocytoma P815-X2 cells (10^4) with or without 100 μg of oil-attached BCG-CWS. Eleven days later, cytotoxic activity of spleen cells was determined by chromium release assay and anti-mastocytoma P815-X2 antibody in mice sera was titrated by Wigzell's method (15). Cytotoxic activity of spleen cells from mice treated with mastocytoma P815-X2 cells (10^4) and 100 μg of oil-attached BCG-CWS reached a maximum level, whereas cytotoxic activities with the mastocytoma P815-X2 cells (10^4) in oil droplets and medium were 84% and 13% of the maximum respectively. On the other hand, anti-mastocytoma P815-X2 antibodies produced in mice treated with mastocytoma P815-X2 cells and 100 μg of oil-attached BCG-CWS was almost similar to those of oil droplets and medium.

TABLE 4. Effect of Oil-attached BCG-CWS on Humoral and Cellular Responses to Viable TNP-mastocytoma P815-X2 Cells in Mice

Group	C57BL/6J mice were immunized with[a] :	Specific target cell lysis[b] (%)	Anti-TNP PFC/ spleen
1	TNP-mastocytoma + oil-attached P815-X2 (10⁴) BCG-CWS (100 μg)	90.2	1,495± 97[c]
2	" +oil droplets	60.0	1,320±209
3	" +medium	42.5	1,485± 79
4	TNP-mastocytoma + oil-attached P815-X2 (3×10⁷) BCG-CWS (100 μg)	100.0	4,750±329
5	" +oil droplets	100.0	4,520±202
6	" +medium	95.3	4,300±161

[a] C57BL/6J mice were immunized i.p. with TNP-mastocytoma P815-X2 cells with or without oil-attached BCG-CWS, oil droplets, or medium. Eleven days later, cytotoxic activity and anti-hapten responses of spleen cells obtained from immunized mice were determined. [b] ^{51}Cr-release assay was performed at 100 : 1 of effector cells to target cells. [c] Mean ± SE.

Above results were further confirmed by the following experiment. We determined humoral and cellular responses to viable TNP-mastocytoma P815-X2 cells in mice. The viability of mastocytoma P815-X2 cells was not significantly decreased by trinitrophenylation using sodium 2,4,6-trinitrobenzenesulfonate under alkaline condition. As shown in Table 4, cell-mediated cytotoxicity was induced in mice with viable TNP-mastocytoma P815-X2 cells as well as viable mastocytoma P815-X2 cells. The enhancing activity of oil-attached BCG-CWS on cell-mediated cytotoxicity using viable TNP-mastocytoma P815-X2 cells was observed..

On the other hand, anti-hapten responses to viable TNP-mastocytoma P815-X2 cells in mice treated with oil-attached BCG-CWS did not increase significantly on the 11th day after tumor injection. These results suggest that oil-attached BCG-CWS is a potent adjuvant for potentiating cell-mediated immunity rather than humoral response to mastocytoma P815-X2 cells in mice. Recently, Mitchell et al. (16) have shown that living BCG injected intravenously enhanced nonspecifically cell-mediated cytotoxicity in which T cells were effector cells. The treatment of mice with oil-attached BCG-CWS alone stimulates somewhat nonspecifically cell-mediated cytotoxicity to mastocytoma P815-X2.

Mitogenicity of BCG-CWS

It was found that BCG-CWS which was suspended in PBS or attached to oil droplets acts on lymphocytea as mitogen. Spleen cells of C57BL/6J mice were cultured with BCG-CWS and ^{3}H-thymidine, and the incorporation of ^{3}H-thymidine was determined. As shown in Table 5, BCG-CWS at the concentration of 10–100 μg is mitogenic on normal spleen cells of C57BL/6J mice. It was also shown that BCG-CWS acted as mitogen on the cortisone-treated thymocytes of C57BL/6J mice and the spleen cells of nude mice (BALB/c-nu/nu). These results suggest that BCG-CWS is a T- and B-cell mitogen.

TABLE 5. Mitogenic Activity of BCG-CWS

Incubated with[a]	cpm (ratios)
Normal spleen cells (2×10^6)	
+medium (control)	$10,377 \pm 1,264$ (1.0)
+PBS-BCG-CWS[b] (10 μg)	$19,803 \pm$ 786 (1.90)
+PBS-BCG-CWS[b] (100 μg)	$30,133 \pm$ 631 (2.90)
+oil droplets	$16,749 \pm 2,357$ (1.61)
+oil-attached BCG-CWS (10 μg)	$25,171 \pm 1,494$ (2.42)
+oil-attached BCG-CWS (100 μg)	$27,883 \pm 3,273$ (2.68)

[a] Spleen cells (2×10^6) of C57BL/6J mice were cultured with BCG-CWS for 48 hr. ^{3}H-Thymidine (1 μCi) was added 24 hr before the end of culture and measured incorporation of ^{3}H-thymidine. [b] BCG-CWS suspended in phosphate-buffered saline.

Anti-tumor Activity of CWS

1. Suppression of tumor growth in syngeneic mice

The CWS prepared from mycobacteria, nocardia, and corynebacteria were treated with mineral oil (Drakeol 6VR) and suspended as oil-in-water in 0.85% NaCl containing 0.2% Tween 80 as described previously (*8*). The suspension of tumor cells, mastocytoma P815-X2, EL4 leukemia, or melanoma B16, was mixed with oil-attached CWS and a 0.05 ml amount of mixture was inoculated intradermally in the flank of each mouse. As shown in Table 6, oil-attached CWS of various mycobacteria, *M. kansasii*, *M. tuberculosis* strains H37Rv and H37Ra, and *M. smegmatis*, were as effective as that of *M. bovis* BCG in the dose of 100 μg for the suppression of the growth of mastocytoma P815-X2, EL4 leukemia, and melanoma B16 in syngeneic mice. Oil-attached CWS prepared from *N. asteroides* 131, *N. rubra*, *C. diphtheriae* PW8, and *C. fermentans* also suppressed the growth of mastocytoma P815-X2 and EL4 leukemia in syngeneic mice (Table 7). In these syngeneic tumor systems in mice, living cell suspension of *M. bovis* BCG (2 mg/mouse) mixed

TABLE 6. Suppression of Tumor Growth with Oil-attached CWS Prepared from Mycobacteria

CWS of	Dose (μg)	No. of mice tested	Mastocytoma P815-X2[a]	EL4 leukemia[b]	Melanoma B16[c]
M. bovis BCG (lot No. 181)	100	10	10/10[d]	2/6	9/10
(lot No. 182)	100	10	6/6	2/6	
M. kansasii	100	10	8/8	0/1	9/10
M. tuberculosis H37Rv	100	10	5/6	2/8	3/8
M. tuberculosis H37Ra	100	10	6/7	1/8	9/10
M. smegmatis	100	10	6/6	7/9	
Control (oil droplets)	100	10	0/0	0/0	0/0

[a] A mixture of mastocytoma P815-X2 (2×10^4) and oil-attached mycobacterial CWS was inoculated intradermally (i.d.) in mice of (C57BL/6J$\times$DBA/2)F$_1$, and measured at 43 days after inoculation. [b] A mixture of EL4 leukemia (5×10^4) and oil-attached mycobacterial CWS was inoculated (i.d.) in mice of C57BL/6J and measured at 23 days after inoculation. [c] A mixture of melanoma B16 (1×10^5) and oil-attached mycobacterial CWS was inoculated (i.d.) in mice of C57BL/6J and measured at 35 days after inoculation. [d] No. of tumor-free mice/No. of mice survived.

TABLE 7. Suppression of Tumor Growth with Oil-attached CWS Prepared from Nocardia and Coryne-bacteria

CWS of	Dose (μg)	No. of mice tested	Mastocytoma P815-X2[a]	EL4 leukemia[b]
M. bovis BCG (lot No. 181)	100	10	5/5[c]	4/8
N. asteroides 131	100	10	2/2	1/4
N. rubra	100	10	10/10	4/9
C. diphtheriae PW8	100	10	4/5	2/6
C. fermentans	100	10	2/4	
Control (oil droplets)		10	0/0	0/0

[a], [b] See Table 6. [c] No. of tumor-free mice/No. of mice survived.

with tumor cells have shown to be less active for the suppression of tumor growth, and in some cases enhanced the growth of tumor.

When the tumor growth was suppressed in mice by the intradermal inoculation of a mixture of oil-attached CWS and tumor cells, mice showed systemic and specific resistance to subsequent challenge of tumor cells. The mice of (C57BL/6J×DBA/2)F$_1$ were inoculated intradermally with a mixture of mastocytoma P815-X2 (2×10^4) and oil-attached BCG-CWS (100 μg), and tumor growth was suppressed in 6 out of 10 mice. These 6 mice in which tumor growth was suppressed were reinoculated intradermally in the right flank with mastocytoma P815-X2 cells (1×10^5). The growth of mastocytoma P815-X2 reinoculated was suppressed completely. On the other hand, EL4 leukemia (1×10^5) transplanted intradermally in the mice in which the growth of mastocytoma P815-X2 was suppressed grew progressively and killed all the mice at 3 weeks after transplantation of EL4 leukemia. Above results suggest that systemic and specific tumor immunity was induced in mice by the intradermal inoculation of a mixture of oil-attached BCG-CWS and tumor cells.

TABLE 8. Induction of Tumor Immunity by the Inoculation of Mitomycin C-treated or Irradiated Mastocytoma P815-X2 Cells in (C57BL/6J×DBA/2)F$_1$ Mice[a]

Tumor cells	Tumor cells were inoculated with:	No. of mice tested	No. of tumor-free mice/ No. of mice survived
Mitomycin C-treated[b] masto-cytoma P815-X2 (1×10^6)	Oil-attached BCG-CWS (100 μg)	10	8/10
	Oil droplets	10	2/3
Irradiated[c] mastocytoma P815-X2 (1×10^6)	Oil-attached BCG-CWS (100 μg)	10	5/5
	Medium (MEM) (oil-attached BCG-CWS separately)	10	0/3
	Oil droplets	10	1/3
	Medium (MEM)	10	0/2

[a] A mixture of mitomycin C-treated or irradiated tumor cells and oil-attached BCG-CWS, oil droplets, or medium (MEM: minimum essential medium) in 0.05 ml was inoculated i.d. in mice of (C57BL/6J× DBA/2)F$_1$. Two weeks later, mastocytoma P815-X2 cells (2×10^4) were transplanted i.d. and mice were examined at 28 days after challenge of tumor cells. [b] Tumor cells (1×10^6) were treated with mitomycin C (40 μg/ml) for 30 min. [c] Tumor cells (1×10^6) were irradiated in a dose of 5,000 rads.

2. Induction of tumor immunity in mice with mitomycin C-treated or X-irradiated tumor cells and oil-attached BCG-CWS in mice

Systemic tumor immunity was induced in mice by the inoculation of mixture of mitomycin C-treated or irradiated mastocytoma P815-X2 and oil-attached BCG-CWS. As shown in Table 8, a mixture of mitomycin C-treated or irradiated mastocytoma P815-X2 cells (1×10^6) and oil-attached BCG-CWS (100 μg) was inoculated intradermally in (C57BL/6J $\times$ DBA/2)F$_1$ mice. Two weeks later, mastocytoma P815-X2 cells were inoculated intradermally and the growth of challenged tumor at inoculated site was examined. The mice which were inoculated with mitomycin C-treated mastocytoma P815-X2 cells and oil-attached BCG-CWS showed the development of potent systemic resistance to subsequent challenge of mastocytoma P815-X2 cells. It is shown that the inoculation of oil-attached BCG-CWS separately from irradiated tumor cells could not induce systemic resistance to subsequent challenge of tumor cells.

3. Prevention of experimental lung cancer in rabbit with oil-attached BCG-CWS

Previously, the authors have reported that experimental lung cancer was induced in rabbit by the instillation of chemical carcinogens (3-methylcholanthrene and 4-nitroquinoline 1-oxide) into the lower bronchus with the use of specially made bronchoscope (17). In this experiment, the authors have examined the activity of oil-attached BCG-CWS for the prevention of lung cancer in rabbit. As shown in Table 9, in the rabbits which had received a single intravenous injection of 5 mg of oil-attached BCG-CWS at the start of experiment (group C), the incidence of lung cancer was almost the same as that in the rabbits of control group (group A). On the other hand, there is no incidence of lung cancer in the rabbits which received intravenously 5 mg of oil-attached BCG-CWS at the start of experiment, and 2 mg of BCG-CWS every 30 to 40 days and survived 200 to 300 days after the first instillation of carcinogens (group E). In the control group (group D), there are 28% of incidence of lung cancer. Experiment in group B was designed to examine the effect of thymus on the carcinogenesis in rabbits. The rabbits which were thymectomized (group B) developed the lung cancer by the instillation of carcinogens in the incidence of 93% levels in comparison with that of 45% in control group (group A). It is not clear the reason why the intravenous injection of oil-

TABLE 9. Effect of Oil-attached BCG-CWS on the Incidence of Lung Cancer in Rabbit by Instillation of Carcinogens[a]

Group	Rabbits used	Intravenous injection of oil-attached BCG-CWS	Survival periods (days)	Incidence of lung cancer
A	Normal	No treatment	300<	15/33 (45%)
B	Thymectomized	No treatment	300<	13/14 (93%)
C	Normal	5 mg (1×)	300<	5/10 (50%)
D	Normal	No treatment	200–300	7/25 (28%)
E	Normal	5 mg (1×), 2 mg every 30 to 40 days	200–300	0/17 (0%)

[a] Rabbits were instilled intrabronchially with a mixture of 3-methylcholanthrene (40 mg) and 4-nitroquinoline 1-oxide (0.4 mg) in rabbit plasma every 30 to 40 days using special bronchoscope.

attached BCG-CWS prevents the incidence to lung cancer in rabbits, however, above results may suggest that the continuous stimulation of T cells by the intravenous injection of oil-attached BCG-CWS exhibits the suppression effect on the incidence of lung cancer in rabbits.

4. Clinical application of oil-attached BCG-CWS on immunotherapy of malignant melanoma

Oil-attached BCG-CWS was applied for the immunotherapy on the patient who was a 70-year-old farmer with malignant melanoma on the pad of the right big toe (primary tumor) and two enlarged lymph nodes in the right inguinal region (metastatic lesion). The primary lesion received 5 injections of the oil-attached BCG-CWS, 100–300 μg for each time, every 10 to 14 days, during 3 months. At the first injection, 200 μg of oil-attached BCG-CWS was also administrated into a metastatic inguinal lymph node. At the second time, 100 μg of oil-attached BCG-CWS together with irradiated autologous and allogeneic melanoma cells (0.83×10^6) were administrated intracutaneously in the right upper arm. The growth of the primary lesion was progressive until the start of the injection of oil-attached BCG-CWS, however, after the third injection the primary tumor showed degenerative change, and finally it reduced from 15 mm $\times$ 12 mm to 6 mm $\times$ 6 mm in size and became atrophic. The metastatic inguinal tumor and other metastatic lesions on the right lower leg which had not received oil-attached BCG-CWS injection showed either inhibition or slight regression after the treatment.

Leucocytosis due to lymphocytosis was found in peripheral blood after injections of oil-attached BCG-CWS into the primary or metastatic lesions. The lymphocytosis lasted for 3 to 4 days after the injection. The reactivity of DNCB increased after the injection of oil-attached BCG-CWS. The cytotoxic activity of the peripheral blood lymphocytes of patient to allogeneic melanoma cells was stimulated and killed the target cells much more than normal lymphocytes did.

As complication by the treatment with oil-attached BCG-CWS, high fever (up to 38°–39°C) was seen after the first injection of oil-attached BCG-CWS into right inguinal lymph node, and only slight fever (about 37°C) was noted after each injection. Other complications including chills, headache, nausea, vomiting, and pain at the injected area occurred occasionally 4–7 hr after injection and persisted for one day. These symptoms were, however, generally mild and responded promptly with symptomatic therapy.

REFERENCES

1. Freund, J. The mode of action of immunologic adjuvants. Adv. Tuberculol., *7*: 130–148, 1956.
2. Munoz, J. Adjuvant effects of mycobacteria and endotoxin in antibody response. Adv. Immunol., *4*: 397–440, 1964.
3. Azuma, I., Yamamura, Y., and Fukushi, K. Fractionation of mycobacterial cell wall. Isolation of arabinose mycolate and arabinogalactan from cell wall fraction of *Mycobacterium tuberculosis* strain Aoyama B. J. Bacteriol., *96*: 1885–1887, 1968.
4. Kanetsuna, F. Chemical analysis of mycobacterial cell walls. Biochim. Biophys. Acta, *158*: 130–148, 1968.

5. Lederer, E. The mycobacterial cell wall. Pure Appl. Chem., *25*: 135–165, 1971.
6. Azuma, I., Kishimoto, S., Yamamura, Y., and Petit, J. F. Adjuvanticity of mycobacterial cell walls. Japan. J. Microbiol., *15*: 193–197, 1971.
7. Yamamura, Y., Azuma, I., Taniyama, T., Ribi, E., and Zbar, B. Suppression of tumor growth and regression of established tumor with oil-attached mycobacterial fractions. Gann, *65*: 179–181, 1974.
8. Meyer, T. J., Ribi, E., Azuma, I., and Zbar, B. Biologically active components from mycobacterial cell walls. II. Suppression and regression of strain-2 guinea pig hepatoma. J. Natl. Cancer Inst., *52*: 103–111, 1974.
9. Zbar, B., Ribi, E., Meyer, T. J., Azuma, I., and Rapp, H. J. Immunotherapy of cancer: Regression of established intradermal tumors after intralesional injection of mycobacterial cell walls attached to oil droplets. J. Natl. Cancer Inst., *52*: 1571–1577, 1974.
10. Azuma, I., Ribi, E., Meyer, T. J., and Zbar, B. Biologically active components from mycobacterial cell walls. I. Isolation and composition of cell wall skeleton and components P_3. J. Natl. Cancer Inst., *52*: 95–101, 1974.
11. Azuma, I., Kanetsuna, F., Taniyama, T., Yamamura, Y., Hori, M., and Tanaka, Y. Adjuvant activity of mycobacterial fractions. I. Purification and *in vivo* adjuvant activity of cell wall skeletons of *Mycobacterium bovis* BCG, *Nocardia asteroides* 131 and *Corynebacterium diphtheriae* PW8. Biken J., *18*: 1–13, 1975.
12. Taniyama, T., Watanabe, T., Azuma, I., and Yamamura, Y. Adjuvant activity of mycobacterial fractions. II. *In vitro* adjuvant activity of cell walls of mycobacteria, nocardia and corynebacteria. Japan. J. Microbiol., *18*: 415–426, 1974.
13. Marbrook, J. Primary immune response in cultures of spleen cells. Lancet, *ii*: 1279–1281, 1967.
14. Brunner, K. T., Mauel, J., Rudolf, H., and Chapuis, B. Studies of allograft immunity in mice. I. Induction, development and *in vitro* assay of cellular immunity. Immunology, *18*: 501–515, 1970.
15. Wigzell, H. Quantitative titration of mouse H-2 antibodies using ^{51}Cr-labelled target cells. Transplantation, *3*: 423–431, 1965.
16. Mitchell, M. S., Kirkpatrick, D., Mokyr, M. B., and Gery, I. On the mode of action of BCG. Nature New Biol., *243*: 216–218, 1973.
17. Hirao, F., Fujisawa, T., Tsubura, E., and Yamamura, Y. Experimental cancer of the lung in rabbits induced by chemical carcinogens. Cancer Res., *32*: 1209–1217, 1972.

Discussion of Paper of Drs. Yamamura et al.

DR. HALPERN: The cell wall extract you employed is a complex macromolecule. Was it prepared by a method analogous to that developed by Medewar?

DR. YAMAMURA: Our CWS was obtained from BCG cell walls by treatment with proteolytic enzymes followed by organic solvent extraction. We have now isolated another water-soluble derivative having adjuvant properties, which is composed principally of polysaccharide and mucopeptide and does not include mycolic acid, as does CWS.

DR. HALPERN: A group at the Pasteur Institute has isolated a very small molecule, of three constituents, from the cell wall of BCG, which still retains many of the properties of the intact preparation. Such simple units may eventually be characterized and synthesized.

DR. YAMAMURA: We are also examining small molecular weight components isolated from both BCG and other mycobacteria, but these do not reveal as remarkable adjuvant and anti-tumor effects as the intact preparations.

DR. HALPERN: In the clinical cases you described, how was the CWS administered?

DR. YAMAMURA: Intratumorally and also intradermally, either alone or combined with autologous or cultured allogeneic malignant melanoma cells.

DR. HALPERN: Did you ever recognize tumor enhancement with CWS treatment?

DR. YAMAMURA: No.

DR. NISHIOKA: In man, you did not observe an alteration in the T to B cell ratio in the peripheral blood. Was this also true in your animal models?

DR. YAMAMURA: We have not determined this ratio in our experimental animals.

DR. HOBBS: In addition to the lymphocytosis and increase in specific cytotoxicity to malignant melanoma cells which you observed, did you also note a general augmentation of a non-specific cytotoxicity?

Dr. Yamamura: Yes.

HOST DEFENSE AGAINST CANCER AND ITS POTENTIATION, D. MIZUNO ET AL. (EDS.),
UNIV. OF TOKYO PRESS, TOKYO / UNIV. PARK PRESS, BALTIMORE, PP. 435-443, 1975

Selection of Anti-hormonal Therapy of Some Cancers

J. R. Hobbs, A. Barrett, I. De Souza, L. Morgan, P. Raggatt, and
H. Salih

Tumour Biology Group, Westminster Hospital and Medical School, London, U.K.

Abstract: Histochemical assessments of enzyme induction in 24-hr cultures of
cancers by added oestrogen or androgen or prolactin or growth hormone or
placental lactogen, *etc.*, provide an *in vitro* test for hormonodependence or its
antagonism. Application to 400 human breast cancers has already revealed 7
different patterns of response, hitherto undetectable by previous urinary assays or
receptor assays. The *in vitro* results successfully predicted *in vivo* responses in 83% of
the first 89 patients receiving only anti-hormonal treatments. The test can be
applied to other tumours, especially carcinoma of the prostate or ovary or uterus.
It has also become clear that to be successful appropriate tumours, hypophysectomy
must abolish both growth hormone and prolactin, and where only the latter
remains, oral bromocriptine (CB 154) can complete the treatment.

Recent measurements (*1*) suggest that on average the first metastases to later
be shown as established are seeded from primary breast cancers of a size from 100–
1,000 cells (undetectable by any current or foreseeable method). Indeed in only 8
of 776 patients was there evidence of the smallest found metastasis having been
seeded from a primary of above 10^9 cells (the size of a small pea). If this is correct
it would explain the difficulties, ever since good data were available, in showing
any major improvement in the initial treatment of breast cancer. The implications
are that all current attempts to diagnose and treat at an earlier stage will still be
too late for the vast majority of patients: those tumours that metastasise will largely
have already done so. In this light the Tumour Biology Group of Westminster
Hospital are continuing to put their effort into the better management of the 80%
of patients who will be coming back with metastases during our working lives.

Four lines of therapy are currently under investiagtion: radiotherapy, cytotoxic
drugs, immunotherapy, and hormonal measures. Already the tests we have developed are indicating that if radiotherapy or cytotoxic drugs are used before hormonal
measures, then during relapses the breast cancers show a much lower incidence

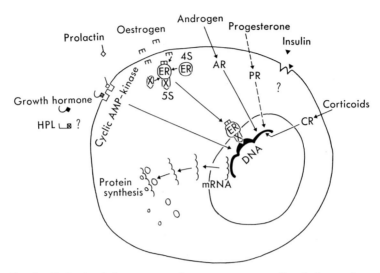

Fig. 1. Endocrine influences upon human mammary cells. It is now known cytoplasmic 4s oestrogen receptors upon binding oestrogen fix an X protein which can then, as a 5s complex, bind to nuclear DNA (5). The other steroid hormones probably work similarly. The polypeptide hormones have membrane receptors and we believe that for prolactin can be shared by GH or HPL; exactly how their influence reaches the nucleus is not known but it is blocked by mitomycin (so presumably requires translation of mRNA).

of hormone dependence. The conclusion is that hormonal measures should be the first to be tried, especially if hormone dependence can be shown to be present. Conversely if hormone independence could be reliably indicated, unnecessary hypophysectomy *etc.* could be avoided.

In the tests we use (2–4) a fresh biopsy of breast cancer tissue is taken and from the results of frozen section is selected (by our histopathologists) where possible to be of low fat content and with largely viable cells. One slice is frozen in liquid nitrogen as the reference to what the tumour was like in the patient, and adjacent slices submitted to tissue culture. One control slice is grown in the culture medium only, free of any added proteins or relevant hormones. Others are grown in media to which a single concentration of either oestrogen, androgen, prolactin, growth hormone (GH), human placental lactogen (HPL) *etc.*, has been added. After 24 hr all the slices are frozen, and, for each, adjacent sections are stained by haematoxylin and eosin or developed histochemically to indicate their total dehydrogenase activity. It is then possible to see if the presence of a hormone has enhanced tumour activity above that of the fresh-frozen (as it was in the patient) or medium only controls. If it has, this is defined as *in vitro dependence* on that hormone. Where this is not seen, the tumour is defined as showing *in vitro independence*.

In a nutshell, the added hormones (with little interference from proteins or antibodies) are allowed to bind to any receptors in the cultured slices. Within 8–12 hr hormones bound from the culture medium will have overruled any previously there in the patient, as their $T_{1/2}$ are known to be only 5–8 hr. They act through to the nucleus to increase messenger RNA synthesis to result in increased

TABLE 1. *In Vitro* Results for 400 Women with Breast Cancer

47% Independent	
53% Dependent	
Prolactin/GH	16%
Prolactin/GH or oestrogen	11
Prolactin/GH or androgen	11
Prolactin/GH or androgen or oestrogen	1
Androgen only	6
Oestrogen only	8
All prolactin	39
All oestrogen	20
All androgen	18

In pregnancy—1 patient, prolactin/GH or HPL

In men—2 patients, prolactin/GH or androgen

synthesis of enzymes *etc.* (Fig. 1). By assaying enzyme activity a small increase in enzyme protein can be magnified in visible terms.

Table 1 shows that about half the breast cancers show *in vitro dependence* of 7 classes. Where more than one hormone is involved, any one will promote the tumour *in vitro*, and there is as yet little evidence of synergism. The implication is that if only one is abolished *in vivo* (*e.g.*, prolactin by α-bromergocryptine) another (*e.g.*, GH) can continue to promote the tumour. This incidence is the same whether the primary tumour or its metastasis are biopsied. In 14 patients who did not have hormonal treatments (or the menopause) between the testing of the primary tumour and a second biopsy at the time of returning with metastases (6/12–2 1/2 years) there was no change in the *in vitro* findings. However, in 2 patients where oestrogen-dependence was initially shown and a regression induced on androgens, subsequent relapse has revealed a tumour now dependent on androgens. Anti-androgen therapy then induced a second regression. More often, however, relapses after hormonal measures are showing *in vitro* independence, *e.g.*, 6 patients initially had tumours showing dependence or oestrogens which responded to removal of oestrogens, but when later their tumours finally relapsed they had acquired *in vitro* independence.

In relation to menopausal status, there is a significant excess (57%) of GH + prolactin dependence before the menopause, being only 29% five years thereafter. There is also a significant excess of androgen dependence (26%) 5 years after the menopause, being only 7% before the menopause. Oestrogen dependence while somewhat higher before the menopause (32%) continues to 14% at 5 years thereafter.

Some advantages of these tests are (i) tumour, only 24 hr in culture, is similar to how it was in the patient, (ii) interference from plasma factors, binding-proteins, antibodies *etc.* is reduced to a minimum, (iii) histochemistry confines assessment to viable tumour cells and results are not diluted by irrelevant tissues (dead cells) as with homogenisation, (iv) the effects of many hormones can be tested (ACTH, FSH, LH, TSH, and HCG have so far been ineffective; oestriol can act like 17-β-oestradiol; dihydrotestosterone can act like testosterone whereas dehydroepiandrosterone cannot), (v) the effects of inhibitors can also be tested as can inhibition by an added hormone (*e.g.*, prolactin occasionally causes this; oestrogen often, but not always, inhibits a testosterone-dependent tumour, and *vice versa*), (vi) the final assay depends on receptors that have worked (not just those that may be present in a homogenate but do not work), and (vii) the results can be available within 26 hr of biopsy.

So much for the *in vitro* findings.   What is their relevance to *in vivo* behaviour? Preliminary results have been assessed in all those patients who received hormonal measures only, without any other treatment, hitherto leaving the clinician a free choice. Regressions were scored according to the criteria of the British Breast Cancer Group, permitting a regression maintained for 3 months to count. Where they occurred, in all cases they were observed within 6 weeks (so it does not seem necessary to wait longer than this if such treatment fails).

TABLE 2.   Results Where Correct Treatment Was Given *In Vivo* according to the *In Vitro* Prediction

In vitro dependence	Number patients	Objective response
Oestrogen only	10	9
Androgen only	7	6

For oestrogen-only dependence, hormonal measures were oophorectomy and/or Tamoxifen. For androgen-only dependence, hormonal measures were Linoral or total adrenalectomy. Table 2 shows the results of such treatments.

Because of the initial free choice some patients received treatments not based on the *in vitro* predictions. Two oestrogen-dependent tumours received oestrogens and visibly effloresced: similarly two androgen-dependent tumours worsened on androgens.

Initially we tried the effect of oral CB154 (Sandoz, α-bromergocryptine) on patients with tumours which had shown *in vitro* dependence on prolactin. Some had trouble tolerating the drug, but since then it has been found that starting on a low dose (0.5 mg t.i.d.) and working up to a full dose 2 mg on rising, 2 mg at 14.00 hr and 3 mg in bed (to last through the night) gets better control of prolactin levels which can be reduced to the limit of our radioimmunoassay (<2 mg/ml). In 10 patients so maintained no benefit was seen in 9, confirming findings of the the European Organization for Research on Treatment of Cancer (E.O.R.T.C.) Breast Cancer Group. Later when we found GH (and probably HPL) seems to share the same receptor as prolactin, we believe abolition of prolactin alone is inadequate for our patients. Table 3 shows the clinical results of hypophysectomy in some of our patients.

It has become clear this operation can often fail to abolish prolactin (20/24 patients so far), presumably by allowing residual anterior pituitary cells to escape from the influence of prolactin inhibitory factor (PIF). It is therefore important to monitor the levels after operation (*6*) when GH can also be detected in some 30%. Where however hypophysectomy had abolished GH but not prolactin we are now using oral CB154 to complete the abolition of prolactin. In 5 such patients, suc-

TABLE 3. Results of Hypophysectomy

Patient number	Post-op. prolactin (ng/ml)	Result	*In vitro* predictions correct
A. For tumours showing *in vitro* independence			
35	Not done	P	Yes
68	<2	P	Yes
82	5	P	Yes
334	7	P	Yes
430	3	P	Yes
B. For tumours showing *in vitro* dependence on prolactin (above 6 ng/ml)			
66	<2	R	Yes
76	5	P	No
105	8	R	Yes
191	9	P	No
216	3	R	Yes
265	6	R	Yes
C. For tumours showing *in vitro* dependence on prolactin at 6 ng/ml			
48	<2	R	Yes
133	4	P	Probably
183	2	R	Yes
196	<2	R	Yes
213	5	P	Probably
308	6	S	Yes
383	7	S	Yes
411	5	S	Probably
424	12	S	Yes

R : regression by criteria of British Breast Cancer Group. P : progression of disease. S : no progression ± relief of pain.

cessful responses (3R+2S as in Table 3) have resulted, so we will continue to try this therapy for prolactin/GH-dependent tumours. Of the 4 failures which progressed in Table 3, B, C, three had died before we realised this and did not receive CB154. The fourth has had a regression on CB154. In the future it may be possible to have a long-acting growth hormone inhibitor (STIH) and this with CB154 might achieve a medical hypophysectomy. For 18 tumours showing *in vitro* independence, anti-hormonal treatments failed in 16.

Table 4 summarises the above results together with all those for which we now have adequate clinical follow-up data, and in which only anti-hormonal treatments were given up to the assessment.

TABLE 4. Predictive Value of *In Vitro* Assays

	No.	%
Patients assessed after only anti-hormonal treatments	89	100
Predictions Wrong	15	17
Correct	74	83

TABLE 5. *In Vitro* Results for Other Tumours

Carcinoma of prostate	
Prolactin (GH)- or testosterone-dependent	3
Independent	1
Adenocarcinoma of ovary	
Prolactin (GH)-dependent	1
Neuroblastoma	
Prolactin (GH)-dependent	5
Prolactin (GH)- or oestrogen-dependent	1
Malignant melanoma	
Oestrogen-dependent	2
Independent	19
Myeloma	
Independent	2
Hypernephroma	
Independent	1

These results are encouraging us to apply the test in prospective trials, incorporating objective criteria such as urinary hydroxyproline excretion, bone scintiscans, and serum levels of human casein.

Other implications which follow are, (i) blind trials of oestrogens (or other hormones) will worsen some tumours while antagonising others; it is time for trials with preselection or better knowledge of the patients, (ii) measurements of urinary androgens cannot find most of the 7 classes of dependent patients listed in Table 1, (iii) finding of oestrogen receptors (60%) does not necessarily mean they work (our results 20%, and see also Ref. 7) and again it logically only includes 3 of the 7 classes, (iv) all the above dependences seem to occur at normal plasma levels of the relevant hormones, (v) the tests can be applied to other tumours (Table 5).

To conclude, at Westminster, the teamwork is trying to abolish the lottery facing patients with metastatic breast cancer.

ACKNOWLEDGMENTS

We are most grateful to Mr. H. Flax and our clinical colleagues for the clinical follow-up of the patients, and to our histopathologists, especially Professor D. H. Mackenzie and Dr. W. Brander for their cooperation. We also thank the Dame Barbara Hepworth, Lawson and Fane Trusts, and Sandoz Ltd. for their financial support.

REFERENCES

1. Bauer, W. C. and Legal, Y. An estimation of the size of breast carcinoma at time of first lymph node metastasis. Lab. Invest., *28*: 377–378, 1973.
2. Salih, H., Flax, H., and Hobbs, J. R. *In-vitro* oestrogen sensitivity of breast-cancer tissue as a possible screening method for hormonal treatment. Lancet, *I*: 1198–1202, 1972.
3. Salih, H., Flax, H., Brander, W., and Hobbs, J. R. Prolactin dependence in human breast cancers. Lancet, *II*: 1103–1105, 1972.
4. Flax, H., Salih, H., Newton, K., and Hobbs, J. R. Are some women's breast cancers androgen dependent? Lancet, *I*: 1204–1207, 1973.

5. Yamamoto, K. R. Characterization of the 4s and 5s forms of the estradiol receptor protein and their interaction with deoxyribonucleic acid. J. Biol. Chem., *249*: 7068–7075, 1974.
6. Hobbs, J. R., Salih, H., Flax, H., and Brander, W. Prolactin dependence in human breast cancer. Proc. Roy. Soc. Med., *66*: 866, 1973.
7. Braunsberg, H., James, V.H.T., Irvine, W. T., Jamieson, C. W., James, F., and Sellwood, R. A. Prognostic significance of oestrogen uptake by human-breast cancer tissue. Lancet, *I*: 163–165, 1973.

Discussion of Paper of Drs. Hobbs et al.

DR. HALPERN: Do you kill hormone-dependent tumour cells when you add the appropriate antagonistic hormone *in vitro*?

DR. HOBBS: No, for although we do observe inhibition in our culture system, it is difficult to interpret as many of the cultures, if the period of incubation is slightly extended, will reveal cell death anyway. In a preliminary series, we have noted 90% favorable clinical responses by administering androgens to patients whose oestrogen-dependent tumours are inhibited by androgen *in vitro*. Similar treatment of individuals whose oestrogen-dependent neoplasms grow independently of androgens yields no response, and a bilateral ovariectomy must then be performed.

DR. WELSCH: How accurate is your histochemical quantification of dehydrogenase activity?

DR. HOBBS: We have compared results with 200 tumours analyzed over two years by a histoquantimet machine and visual observation of histochemically localized enzyme activity, and noted only two discrepancies. We now rely solely on the latter procedure. Whatever we're reading is reproducible, as we obtained almost identical results with 20 tumours read initially and then re-examined several months later. The concentrations of oestrogen and androgen we employ *in vitro* are unphysiologic, but again they seem to offer valid results.

DR. WELSCH: One apparently requires such levels to form any type of response.

DR. HOBBS: That's true for the steroid hormones, but not for prolactin, growth hormone, and placental lactogen, which are used in physiologic amounts. However, these have membrane receptors, which may be more easily accessible than the steroid hormone receptors.

DR. WELSCH: Were most of the specimens you examined primary biopsies or metastatic foci?

DR. HOBBS: We've studied about an equal number of primary and secondary lesions. In patients who relapse after a regression induced or prolonged by hormonal therapy, many are found to have become hormone-independent, or dependent on the treatment being administered.

DR. WELSCH: How many neuroblastomas and ovarian carcinomas were shown to be prolactin sensitive?

DR. HOBBS: Eight of eight neuroblastomas and one of two ovarian carcinomas were dependent on both growth hormone and prolactin.

DR. ALEXANDER: You stated that one ought to consider hormonal therapy early in the management of human breast cancer. Does this imply its primary or prophylactic use in stages I and II?

DR. HOBBS: I don't have any conclusive evidence on which to suggest the usefulness of primary or prophylactic hormonal therapy in the early stages of mammary carcinoma. If the patient presents with metastases I would consider anti-hormonal therapy as a first attempt if one can successfully determine the appropriate regime by tests such as ours.

DR. CASTRO: What are the clinical signs of tumour promotion produced by treatment in hormone-dependent tumours?

DR. HOBBS: We measure such objective criteria as tumour size with calipers, urinary hydroxyproline excretion, bone scans, and serum casein levels by radio-immunoassay. We observed two patients with androgen-dependent breast cancers who were given androgens, and their hydroxyproline outputs increased 3-fold in 2 days, which I feel is clear evidence of promotion of those tumours by the hormone. Our surgeons thus no longer routinely administer androgens to these patients, for, if one uses hormonal therapy blindly, tumour enhancement may occur. Also, simple determination of oestrogen receptors or urinary steroid levels is not equivalent to the variety of different possibilities our sequence of *in vitro* hormonal dependency tests detect.

Closing Remarks

Prof. Yuichi Yamamura

The three days Symposium on "Host Defense against Cancer and Its Potentiation" has come to an end and it seems that now I am to close the Symposium with some remarks.

In closing the Fifth International Symposium of the Princess Takamatsu Cancer Research Fund, first of all, allow me to express our sincere appreciation to the gracious patronage of her Imperial Highness, Princess Takamatsu and to the generous support of the Princess Takamatsu Cancer Research Fund.

Also, may I extend my cordial gratitude to all active participants who presented many interesting papers and exciting discussions during this Symposium.

We know that there are various kinds of defense mechanisms of the host against cancer, however, among them the immunological defense mechanism was suggested to be the most distinctive and attractive one. As pointed out in Dr. Jerne's lecture, vast and rapid progress of immunology in the last decade enabled us to know in detail about the mechanism of immune response and immune regulation. Formerly unrecognizable tumor specific antigens and antibodies against tumor came to be detected by recently developed immunological techniques. Various methods how to potentiate or enhance the immunological response against tumor cells, which seem to be effective in the suppression of tumor growth, were presented by many researchers.

It is quite clear that the general area of immunotherapy of cancer is one of bright promise, although many important problems remained unsolved.

The breath of this Symposium was so great that it is not possible to summarize all the scientific papers and comments. Therefore, I shall try to make some generalizations that may express the idea of the Symposium and make personal observations concerning the directions in which I saw things moving.

The papers presented in this Symposium may be divided into several topics. The first topic was on the immune surveillance system in cancer. Many recent studies have revealed that cell-mediated immunity plays an important role in immune surveillance in cancer. In this connection, selective immunopotentiation and selective immunosuppression, particularly T-cell oriented, were discussed. The *in vitro* method of lymphocyte-mediated cytotoxicity and a newly devised method of detecting and characterizing small numbers of sensitized cytotoxic T lymphocytes presented by Dr. Brunner will give us an excellent tool for studying cell-mediated immunity against cancer. The important role of macrophage, such as immunologically specific cytotoxic macrophage, was stressed and emphasized by Dr. Halpern, Dr. Alexander and Dr. Dukor ; these papers were very stimulative for understanding the cellular mechanism of immune response against cancer.

The second topic was various approaches to tumor immunotherapy. Amplification of the immune response has been attempted by immunization with allogeneic tumor cells or xenogeneic tumor cells with syngeneic or autochthonous tumor cells with immunopotentiating agents added. Experimental and clinical studies on tumor immunotherapy were extensively studied by using microorganisms, fungi, plants or some biological and chemical materials.

BCG, *Corynebacterium parvum*, lentinan, cholera neuraminidase, Coley's toxin, PS-K, low molecular derivatives of antibiotics such as pyranylsecalonic acid and others were also reported.

I don't want to list and compare all the materials, which are being used in tumor immunotherapy. The problems to be solved are 1) what material will be used effectively and successfully in cancer patients without serious side effects ; 2) what is the common mechanism of immunopotentiation which leads to the success of immunotherapy of cancer. I think we are still at the beginning of immunotherapy. But a fantastic experimental model using an autochthonous tumor graft was presented by Drs. Nakahara and Tokuzen, which will give many suggestions to the researchers, who have used allogeneic or syngeneic tumors as models of cancer immunotherapy.

Decreased immune response and its mechanism in tumor-bearing animals constituted the third topic. T-cell functions were shown to be impaired and immunosuppressive substances were isolated from tumor culture cells or ascites fluid as reported by Dr. Kitagawa and Dr. Kennedy. These immunosuppressive substances were reevaluated from the point of view on "toxohormone," which was discovered and named many years ago by Drs. Nakahara and Fukuoka. Lymphocyte trapping was also impaired or inhibited by tumors as suggested by Dr. Frost.

Such research is expected to relate in the future to the method on how to eliminate these immunosuppressive effects of the tumor, resulting in the enhancement of the defense mechanism of tumor-bearing animals.

The last topic was the host factors influencing tumor growth or tumor genesis. The effects of adrenocortical and thyroid hormones, prolactin, brown adipose, serum properdin level, chalones, and other factors were discussed. Clinical use of *in vitro* assay of various hormones on breast cancer and its usefulness in the treatment reported by Dr. Hobbs was an excellent example of an application of laboratory research on host factors to a clinical approach.

The ultimate goal in cancer research is either to find out a means of preventing or curing cancer. The way to reach the goal must be very distant and difficult, but our job for the coming years, whether it be in immunotherapy or in other kinds of therapy, is to achieve this goal.

I believe that host defense mechanism against cancer and its potentiation play an important role in guiding us to that goal.

Thank you very much,
good by